MEDICINE AND BIOLOGY RESEARCH DEVELOPMENTS

# BENEFICIAL EFFECTS OF PROPOLIS ON HUMAN HEALTH AND CHRONIC DISEASES

## VOLUME 1

# MEDICINE AND BIOLOGY RESEARCH DEVELOPMENTS

*TSISANA SHARTAVA – SERIES EDITOR –*
TBILISI, GEORGIA

**Parasitology Research Trends**
*Olivier De Bruyn and Stephane Peeters (Editors)*
2010. ISBN: 978-1-60741-436-0

**General Anesthesia Research Developments**
*Milo Hertzog and Zelig Kuhn (Editors)*
2010. ISBN: 978-1-60876-395-5

**Venoms: Sources, Toxicity and Therapeutic Uses**
*Jonas Gjersoe and Simen Hundstad (Editors)*
2010. ISBN: 978-1-60876-448-8

**Type III Secretion Chaperones: A Molecular Toolkit for all Occasions**
*Matthew S. Francis*
2010. ISBN: 978-1-60876-667-3

**A Guide to Hemorrhoidal Disease**
*Pravin Jaiprakash Gupta*
2010. ISBN: 978-1-60876-431-0

**Recent Advances in BIS Guided TCI Anesthesia**
*David A. Ferreira and Luís Antunes, Pedro Amorim and Catarina Nunes*
2010. ISBN: 978-1-61668-627-7

**Biomaterials Developments and Applications**
*Henri Bourg and Amaury Lisle (Editors)*
2011. ISBN: 978-1-60876-476-1

**TRP Channels in Health and Disease: Implications for Diagnosis and Therapy**
*Arpad Szallasi (Editor)*
2011. ISBN: 978-1-61668-337-5

**Biological Aspects of Human Health and Well-Being**
*Tsisana Shartava (Editor)*
2011. ISBN: 978-1-61209-134-1

**Tracing the Drainage Divide: The Future Challenge for Predictive Medicine**
*Enzo Grossi*
2011. ISBN: 978-1-61209-232-4

**Nanotechnology and Advances in Medicine**
*Maysaa El Sayed Zaki (Editor)*
2011. ISBN: 978-1-61209-640-7

**Beneficial Effects of Propolis on Human Health and Chronic Diseases. Volume 1**
*Tahira Farooqui and Akhlaq A.Farooqui (Editors)*
2012. ISBN: 978-1-62081-440-6

**Beneficial Effects of Propolis on Human Health and Chronic Diseases. Volume 2**
*Tahira Farooqui and Akhlaq A.Farooqui (Editors)*
2012. ISBN: 978-1-62081-483-3

MEDICINE AND BIOLOGY RESEARCH DEVELOPMENTS

# BENEFICIAL EFFECTS OF PROPOLIS ON HUMAN HEALTH AND CHRONIC DISEASES

## VOLUME 1

TAHIRA FAROOQUI
AND
AKHLAQ A. FAROOQUI
EDITORS

nova
publishers
*New York*

**Library of Congress Cataloging-in-Publication Data**

ISBN: 978-1-62081-440-6

ISSN: 2167-3071

*Published by Nova Science Publishers, Inc. † New York*

"Do not go where the path may lead;
go instead where there is no path and leave a trail"

*Ralph Waldo Emerson quotes*
*(American Poet, Lecturer and Essayist, 1803-1882)*

# CONTENTS

# FOREWORD

*George A. Burdock*[*]
American Board of Toxicology, NC, US
American College of Nutrition, FL, US

I am flattered the editors requested I write a forward for each of the two volumes on propolis. It would be disingenuous of me to state that when I wrote a review[1] of the (then) current literature on the safety of propolis in 1998, I expected the paper to receive so many citations. As of this writing (February, 2012), it is the second most cited paper in *Food and Chemical Toxicology*, having been referenced nearly 500 times. At the time of my original research of the literature, the amount of published information was rather limited, but this status could also have been an artifact of fewer and smaller electronic databases available for searching the scientific literature. However, I was able to obtain copies of some of the seminal papers, including the works of Bankova, Ghisalberti, Marcucci and others which enabled me to "stand on the shoulders of giants."[2]

Propolis can be roughly translated as "defense of the city" and in this role, propolis is astoundingly multifunctional. Propolis is used as a sealing compound to protect the hives from climatic intrusions (drafts and water) because of its physical nature of as a sticky polymer that, when dry, leaves a smooth, non-porous surface. Propolis can act as a barrier to vegetation, including vines or branches from growing into the hive, through some as yet undescribed herbicidal effect. Propolis can also halt the establishment and propagation of a very broad spectrum of microbial pathogens or opportunists (including bacteria, fungi and viruses). As a general purpose sealant, propolis also provides a physical barrier to small intruders such as insects and a means to seal up the remains of larger intruders such as mice or lizards, promoting the mummification of the corpse and avoiding formation of the products and consequences of decomposition.

Incredibly, all the functionalities provided in the previous paragraph (and more to be cited in the following chapters) are produced from a variety of botanical sources including

---

* gburdock@burdockgroup.com.

1 Burdock, G.A. (1998). Review of the biologic properties and toxicity of bee propolis (propolis). *Food and Chemical Toxicology* 36:347-363.

2 Attributed to Bernard of Chartres, but popularized by Sir Isaac Newton (http://en.wikipedia.org/wiki /Standing_on_the_shoulders_of_giants site visited 12Feb2012).

many species of trees, fruits and other vegetation – the only commonality between the various environments where propolis has been sampled, seems to be the very lack of commonality of vegetal sources. For example, the reader will see in the following chapters, that although propolis may be made from *Populus* spp. and was originally thought to be the sole source for propolis production, and although the two (i.e., propolis and *Populus*) may share a number of common constituents, *Populus* is proving not to be the sole feedstock for propolis production. Indeed, propolis feedstock may have many sources, even in places where no members of the genus *Populus* may grow. In the chapter by Isla and co-authors on Argentine-sourced propolis, the authors note that other species used by bees include pine, birch, elm, beech and horse chestnut; further, the authors describe behavior of bees in Uganda which selectively forage on *Alnus* species, to the point where the trees can be exfoliated. Other authors describe additional sources of propolis to include flowers, fruit and potentially any vegetation having resinous exudates. Sources also vary according to the season, as the result of local weather conditions and probably countless other factors; although despite these variables, the need for propolis does not diminish. The point being, that the bees have proven to be very resourceful in obtaining the right mix of feedstock for a remarkably multifunctional ingredient.

In as much as the following chapters will note that the feedstock for propolis can vary with area, season and climatic conditions, the ability of the bees to process the propolis is limited. As noted in the chapter by Kumazawa (and other chapters), the process by which bees gather the needed feedstock resin has been described and includes scraping the source with their mandibles, tucking it into the corbiculae on their hind legs and a subsequent unloading process by nest mates upon arrival at the hive. How much undocumented processing takes place during this gathering, transportation and delivery process, in addition to post-arrival processing, might be important in the production of some key propolis constituents. We know, for example, apian flavonoid glucosidases are involved and (from Farooqui and Farooqui in Volume II), the enzymes of propolis include glucose-6-phosphatase, ATPase, succinic dehydrogenase and glycoside hydrolase are present in propolis and are obviously contributed by the bee. However, what we do not know at this point is which of these enzymes, mechanical process or even simple oxidation, are key variables in the production and activity of propolis. We know that different batches of propolis will have certain different characterizing constituents or ratios of constituents, but are these differences a product of the variability of the feedstock or of the need for batches of propolis with different activities? It is hard to believe that propolis is a "one size fits all" substance and there is no difference in the processing that takes place by the bee. Secondary to the preceding is, of course, the question of how much control do the bees have over the constituents and functionality of propolis? Is there a signaling mechanism turning genes on and off according to certain prevailing conditions in the hive?

Several authors have reported the constituents of propolis. El-Hady describes the composition of Egyptian propolis and explains that the color of propolis depends on its origin and may vary from dark-brown to reddish brown with a greenish one and the odor, which can vary from sample to sample, with some even having no odor at all. The chapters by El-Hady, Popova, Bellik and Boukraa and others, describe specific properties of propolis in terms of its activity against bacteria, including but not limited to *Streptococcus mutans* and *S. veridans; Staphlococcus epidermidis* and *S. aureus; Lactobacillus; Bacillus cereus; Klebsiella pneumonia* and others and; the variable susceptibility of various strains to various types of propolis. Propolis is active against *Candida albicans, C. tropicalis* and *C. glabrata* and;

viruses including influenza, hepatitis B, *Herpes simplex* type 1, *Herpes simplex* type 2, vesicular stomatitis virus, adenovirus type 2, polio virus type 2, herpes zoster virus and others. Although not all propolis samples were equally effective in halting activity or replication of these organisms or viruses, there seemed to be a wide range of organisms against which propolis is efficacious. Many of these activities *in vitro* have given rise to applications in supplements and personal products, many of which are described in Volume II.

Again, I would like to thank the editors for giving me the opportunity to write a Foreword for this book and I hope the reader enjoys the following chapters as much as I have.

# PREFACE

Propolis, a resinous substance collected by honeybees from various plant sources. The color, consistency, and chemical composition of propolis vary according to the geographical region, botanical origin, and the season in which it is collected by honeybees. In addition, biological activities of propolis also vary from one geographical region to other due to differences in its composition. Propolis not only contains several flavonoids (galangin, quercetin, kaempferol, pinocembrin, and pinobanksin), but also possess cinnamic acid and its derivatives (chlorogenic acid, ferrulic acid, caffeic acid phenethyl ester), along with various steroids, amino acids and volatile aldehydes and ketones. Among propolis constituents flavonoids mediate antioxidant effects, where as caffeic acid phenethyl ester (CAPE) inhibits NF-kB activation and produces anti-inflammatory effects. CAPE also mediates antiviral and immunomodulatory properties. It also inhibits the growth of different types of transformed cells. Presence of flavonoids and phenolic acids provides propolis with antibacterial, antifungal, antiviral, antiparasitic, antineoplastic, hepatoprotective, immunomodulating, antioxidative, and anti-inflammatory properties. Since propolis has so many above mentioned properties, it is likely that in future it can be used for the development of new drugs in fields of immunology, carcinogenesis, infectious diseases, neurological disorders, allergy, and ulcers. Information on the effect of propolis on above conditions is scattered throughout the literature in the form of original papers, and reviews. We have decided to provide readers with a comprehensive and cutting edge description on metabolism and molecular mechanism associated with the beneficial effects of propolis on human health in a manner that is useful not only to students and teachers but also to researchers and physicians.

Our attempts to assemble literature on propolis have resulted in two books entitled "Beneficial effects of propolis on human health and chronic diseases", Volume I and "Beneficial effects of propolis on human health and chronic diseases", Volume II. Volume I of this book contains a comprehensive description of chemical composition and biological activities of propolis, whereas Volume II deals with the potential therapeutic aspects of propolis for treating chronic diseases such as neurodegenerative diseases, heart disease, and cancer.

Volume I contains 13 chapters. Chapters 1 and 2 deal with the chemical properties of different propolis types in relation to their biological activity and updates the chemical composition of propolis. Chapters 3 and 4 describe cutting edge information on the seasonal variation in the composition and the antimicrobial and antioxidant activities of propolis as well as shed light on its flavonoids responsible for the anti- inflammatory and anti-allergic activities. Chapter 5 focuses on the immunomodulatory action of propolis, discusses the problem of propolis standardization, concentration, intake period, its pro- or anti-inflammatory activity, and its association with vaccines. Chapters 6-9 deal with specific biological activities of Egyptian, Japanese, Argentine, and Mediterranean propolis. Chapter 10 describes the antimicrobial properties of propolis. Chapter 11 demonstrates the protective effect of propolis in conjunction with N-2-hydroxy ethyl ethylene diamine triacetic acid (HEDTA) against beryllium-induced hepatorenal dysfunction. Chapter 12 unravels the health benefits of polyphenols in propolis. Finally, chapter 13 provides readers and researchers a sequence of protocols, discussing and comparing qualitative and quantitative methods used as a means of standardization for propolis and honey, which can be ideal for the screening of new biodynamic molecules.

This edited book would not have been possible without the help and patience of our publisher, Nadya S. Gotsiridze-Columbus, President at Nova Science Publishers, Inc. We would also like to thank her for cooperation, understanding, and help. We are also thankful to staff of Nova Science Publishers, Inc., for the professional handling of the manuscript. We hope that our attempts to assemble information from International group of authors from 8 countries to describe propolis composition would result into more advances on standardization of propolis composition.

In: Beneficial Effects of Propolis on Human Health ... ISBN: 978-1- 62081-440-6
Editors: Tahira Farooqui and Akhlaq A. Farooqui 

*Chapter 1*

# Chemical Profiles of Different Propolis Types in Relation to their Biological Activity

***Vassya Bankova* and Boryana Trusheva***
Institute of Organic Chemistry with Centre of Phytochemistry,
Bulgarian Academy of Sciences, Sofia, Bulgaria

## Abstract

In the last decade, the paradigm shift in propolis research was completed: the awareness that propolis is a product of variable chemical composition and that there are many propolis types became common knowledge. For this reason and unlike previous review articles, the present review on propolis is organized in agreement with this concept. Recent findings in propolis research are summarized and discussed, concerning chemical profiles, new constituents, biological activity and active principles of different propolis types, as determined by their plant source(s). European poplar propolis, Brazilian green (*Baccharis*) propolis, Brazilian and Cuban red propolis (*Dalbergia*) and other recently discovered propolis types are considered.

## 1. Introduction

Propolis (bee glue) is a bee product with double application in the beehive. Bees make use of the sticky texture of this resinous material by applying it for blocking holes and cracks, repairing combs, strengthening the thin borders of the comb, etc. On the other hand, they make use also of its biological properties: propolis contains the putrefaction of "embalmed" intruders, killed in the hive and too large to be carried out, and it is responsible for the lower incidence of bacteria and moulds within the hive than in the atmosphere outside [1]. The

* Correspondence concerning this article should be addressed to: Vassya Bankova, Institute of Organic chemistry with Centre of Phytochemistry, Bulgarian Academy of Sciences, Acad. B, Bonchev str. Bl.9, 1113 Sofia, Bulgaria. bankova@orgchm.bas.bg; Telephone: ++3592-9606-149; Fax: ++3592 8700 225.

property to fight and prevent infections is one of the most essential characteristics of propolis, which has been recognized and used by humans since ancient times. Nowadays, propolis is still among the most popular home made remedies in some regions of the world, and it is a valued ingredient of numerous health foods and drinks, food supplements, cosmetics and over-the-counter preparations [2,3]. For this reason, and inspired by the general interest in natural products, modern science took notice of propolis. The attention of researchers to this bee product has been constantly growing for the last 50 years. Over the period 2000 – 2010 the research articles on propolis increased from about 70 to over 200 per year (Scopus database). After the year 2000, many new propolis constituents have been isolated and structurally elucidated, and a lot of new data has been published concerning its beneficial biological properties. In the course of this research, numerous samples from different geographic origins have been studied and it has become obvious that the chemical composition of propolis is extremely variable. As propolis is a plant derived product, its chemistry depends on the source plant, respectively on the specificity of the local flora at the site of collection and the choice of plant resin for propolis production made by bees. It turned out that in a particular phytogeographic region honeybees demonstrate unambiguous and constant preference to particular plant source(s) and as a results, different propolis chemical types exist [4,5]. Basic information on the most widespread propolis types is represented in Table 1.

**Table 1. Chemical profiles of the most widespread propolis types**

| Propolis type | Geographical distribution | Major plant source | Chemical profile (characteristic constituents) | References |
|---|---|---|---|---|
| Poplar type | Europe, Western Asia, China, South Africa, North America, New Zealand | Bud exudates of poplar trees, mainly Populus nigra | Pinocemnrin, galangin chrysin, pinobanksin 3-O-acetate, pentelyl caffeates, phenethyl caffeate (CAPE), caffeic acid, ferulic and isoferulic acid | [6-12] |
| Brazilian green | Brazil (Sao Paulo, Rio de Janeiro, Minas Gerais) | Leaf exudates of *Baccharis dracunculifolia* | Artepillin C, baccharin, drupanin, aromadendrine, caffeoylquinic acids | [13,14] |
| South American red | Brazil (North-East part), Cuba, Mexico | Exudates of *Dalbergia ecastophyllum*, other *Dalbergia* species | Medicarpin, vestitol, 3-O-methyl vestitol | [15-17] |
| Mediterranean | Southern Greece and Greek islands, Crete, Sicily, Malta, Adriatic Coast of Croatia | *Cupressus sempervirens* resin | isocupressic acid, pimaric acid, imbricataloic acid, totarol, ferruginol | [18-20] |
| Pacific | Okinawa, Taiwan, Indoinesia | Fruit exudates of *Macaranga tanarius* | Propolin C, propolin D, propolin F | [21,22] |

The observed biological activities of bee glue are due to the plant-derived secondary metabolites but surprisingly, different chemical composition doesn't always result in drastic differences in pharmacological effects. However, there is some specificity, and for this reason pharmacological studies must always be accompanied by chemical characterization of the propolis used in the experiments, or at least by determining the chemical type of this propolis. This was the paradigm shift in propolis research that was completed in the last decade: the awareness that propolis is a product of variable chemical composition and that there are many propolis types became common knowledge. Nevertheless, a significant number of pharmacological studies on propolis are yet published without any chemical analysis of the bee glue, and this makes them practically useless. This fact is most unfortunate because among them, there are investigations of high quality, regarding the pharmacological part, and also ones that report valuable activities.

In this chapter, we focus on the scientifically sound information about distinct propolis types, published in the years after 2000, grouped in accordance of the source plant and the respective chemical profiles, characteristic for the particular propolis type. The composition-activity relationship for these propolis types is discussed.

## 2. Poplar Type Propolis

Propolis has been a traditional European remedy since the times of Ancient Greece and Rome. For this reason the first studies on propolis chemistry and biological activity were performed in European laboratories and with European bee glue. In the 1970's and 1980's it became clear that in Europe the plant source of propolis are the bud exudates of poplar trees, mainly *Populus nigra* L. [7,23,24]. Hence, this propolis type contains the typical poplar bud constituents: flavonoid aglycones (flavanones, flavones and flavonols), phenolic acids (caffeic, ferulic, isoferulic, *p*-coumaric) and their esters. Most abundant are the flavonoids pinocembrin (Fig. 1), galangin and chrysin, and the esters phenethyl caffeate (CAPE) (Fig. 1), pentenyl caffeates, benzyl ferulate, etc. Over 150 individual constituents have been found in poplar type propolis so far [25].

There is an impressive number of articles dedicated to the pharmacological activities of poplar type propolis. The information (published after 2000) about pharmacological activities of this propolis type and the responsible constituents is summarized in Table 2.

Of course, among the most studied ones is the most popular property of propolis: action against bacteria and fungi, and, to a lesser extent, against viruses. A long list of bacterial species and strains has been tested for their susceptibility towards poplar propolis extracts, including important human pathogens. Most often, ethanol propolis extracts have been used for the experiments. Numerous publications report that poplar bee glue is more active against Gram-positive bacteria than to Gram-negative ones [103-110]. Of practical importance are the observations that poplar propolis inhibits methicillin resistant *Staphylococcus aureus* (MRSA) [30], *Campylobacter jejuni* [111], *Helicobacter pylori* [112-114], *Listeria monocytogenes* [110]. The activity against oral pathogens, such as *Streptococcus mutans*, *Lactobacillus fermentum*, etc., is also of clinical interest and has been studied by many authors [26,106,115-118]. In general, the antibacterial activity of poplar propolis is attributed to its phenolic constituents [119,120], among them caffeic acid phenethyl ester (CAPE) [29,121], pinocembrin [30,122] and pinobanksin-3-O-acetate [26].

**Table 2. Biological activities of poplar type propolis and responsible constituents**

| Type of activity | Responsible molecules | References |
|---|---|---|
| Antibacterial | Galangin, pinocembrin, pinobanksin-3-O-acetate, CAPE, quercetin | [26-30] |
| Antifungal | Galangin, pinocembrin, pinobanksin | [31,32] |
| Antiviral | Galangin, chrysin | [33-36] |
| Antioxidant | CAPE, tectochrysin, caffeic acid, ferulic acid, galangin | [37-43] |
| Antitumor, cytotoxic | CAPE, quercetin, chrysin, naringenin, caffeic acid, galangin; benzylcaffeate, cinnamyl caffeate; 2-acetyl-1,3-dicoumaroyl glycerol; 2-acetyl-1-coumaroyl-feruloyl glycerol | [44-62] |
| Antiinflammatory | Chrysin, kaempferol, CAPE, galangin, quercetin | [29,63-66] |
| Radioprotective | Quercetin, chrysin, naringenin, caffeic acid | [67-73] |
| Immunomodulatory | CAPE, quercetin, caffeic acid | [74-77] |
| UV-protecting | Not identified | [78] |
| Mitigaion of amnesia | Not identified | [79] |
| Clinical reports on use of topical preparation containing poplar propolis | Not identified | [80-86] |
| Prevention of hepatorenal injury | Not identified | [87] |
| Allergenic | Benzyl caffeate, 3-methyl-2-butenyl caffeate, CAPE | [88-100] |
| Inhibition of xanthine oxidase | CAPE, chrysin, galangin | [101] |
| Action against *Varroa destructor* (bee parasite) | Not identified | [102] |

Poplar propolis extracts have been found capable of inhibiting the development of fungal human pathogens such as *Candida albicans* [123-125], but also of phytopathogenic fungi [31,32,126]. Filamentous fungi were generally less sensitive to poplar propolis than yeasts [105]. The active components were proved to be chrysin, pinocembrin and galangin [31,32].

Poplar type propolis demonstrated significant activity also against Herpes simplex virus type 1 and type 2 [33,35,36]. Alcohol extract was active against HSV-1 and HSV-2, of the tested individual compounds only galangin and chrysin exhibited antiviral activity. In both cases the extracts exhibited high anti-herpetic activity when viruses were pretreated with them prior to infection.

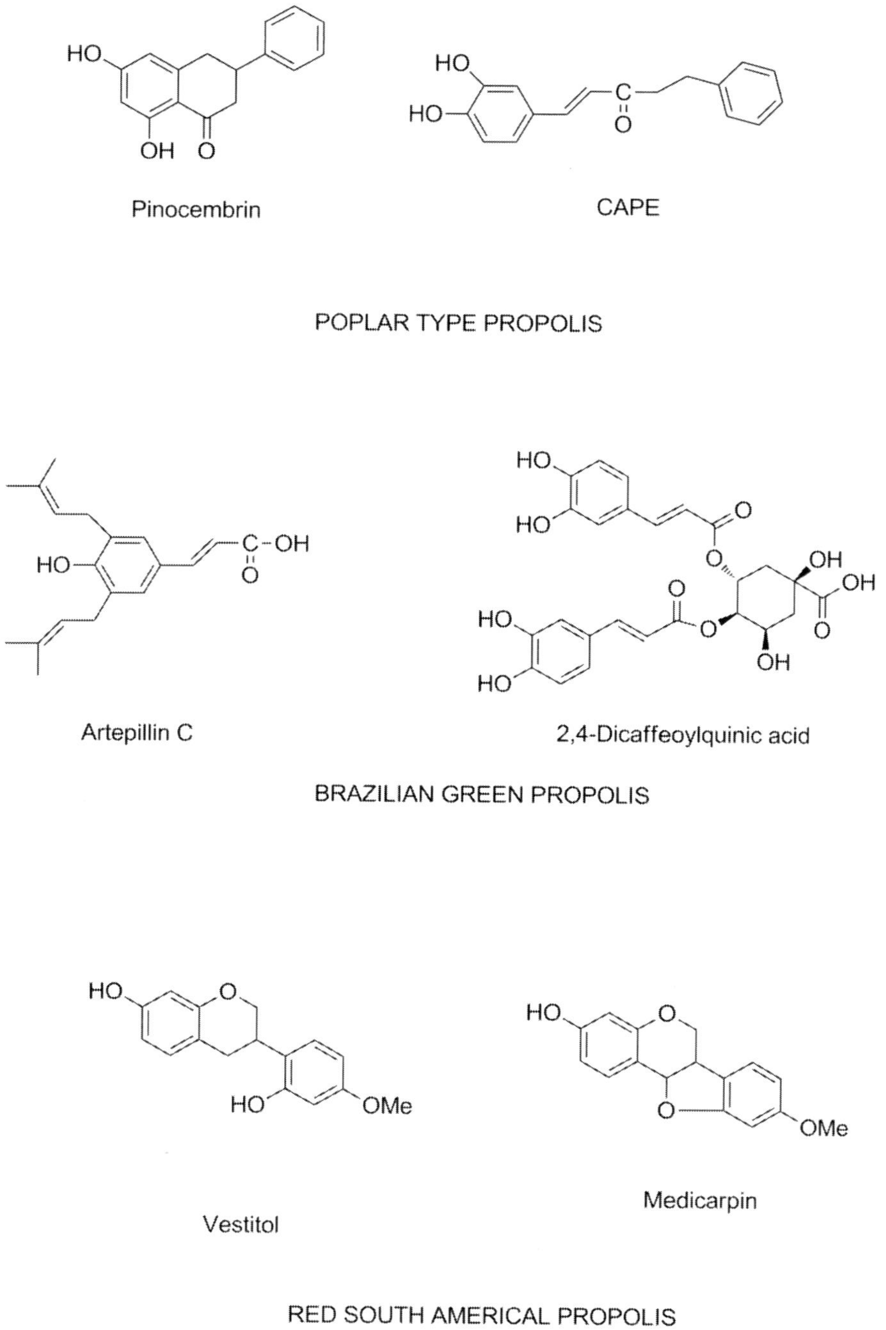


Figure 1. Important biologically active compounds in most widespread propolis types.

It is important to note that all investigations on the antibacterial action of individual substances, isolated from propolis, showed that not a single propolis component has an activity much higher than that of the total extract [121,127]. It seems that propolis has general antiinfective pharmacological value as a natural mixture and not as a source of new powerful antimicrobial, antifungal and antiviral individual compounds.

Antioxidant properties of propolis have attracted the attention of researchers and the general public especially during the last decade. Many studies confirm the radical scavenging potential of poplar propolis, using the 1,1-diphenyl-2-picrylhydrazyl radical (DPPH) and the 2,2'-azinobis(3-ethylbenzothiazoline-6-sulfonic acid) radical cation decolorization (ABTS) assays [39-42,128-135]. Evaluation of beta-carotene bleaching [39,128], of the ferric reduction antioxidant power (FRAP-assay) [135,136] and of the change of thiobarbituric acid reactive species (TBARS) [137] were also applied to poplar propolis, proving its antioxidant potential. Some further specialized tests have also confirmed this potential: microsomal lipid peroxidation test [138], test based on the modulation of ascorbate peroxidase activity of hemoglobin [139]. *In vivo* experiments proved that poplar propolis as food supplement modulated antioxidant enzymes and significantly decreased lipid peroxidation processes in mice [136]. Similar effects were observed also in an experiment with healthy humans [140]. The responsible constituents are again the poplar phenolics and flavonoids [131,135,137]. As individual antioxidant principles, CAPE [39,40,128], caffeic and ferulic acid [39,128] and galangin [42] were identified.

Since the beginning of the new Millennium, there has been a great number of publications considering the antitumor action of poplar propolis and its constituents. For example, poplar propolis and some isolated polyphenolic compounds (caffeic acid, CAPE and quercetin) decreased the number of tumor nodules in the lung; however, the antimetastatic effectiveness of poplar propolis was higher than that presented by its constituents [75]. The same authors found that poplar propolis, caffeic acid and CAPE modulate immune responses and increase host resistance to tumor cells [54,141]. Poplar propolis, caffeic acid and CAPE could be useful tools in the control of tumor growth according to Orsolic et al. [52], who reported that poplar propolis antitumor action could be the consequence of synergistic activities of its polyphenolic compounds.

The most important antitumor constituent of poplar propolis is the caffeic acid phenethyl ester (CAPE). This relatively simple compound is also the most studied propolis constituent of all, regardless the propolis type. Its popularity with researchers increased significantly after 1988, when it was identified as the main cytotoxic compound in propolis with preferential cytotoxicity on tumour cells [142]. Ever after, different aspects of the biological and pharmacological activities of CAPE have been studied, including the mechanism of its action. Many new aspects of its biological properties have been revealed, including anti-inflammatory, anti-HIV, antibacterial, antioxidant. CAPE has been shown to inhibit the ornithine decarboxylase, protein tyrosine kinase and lipoxygenase activities. It has also been reported that CAPE suppresses lipid peroxidation and inhibits the activation of nuclear transcription factor NF-kB, etc. [143,144]. The story of CAPE demonstrates the potential of propolis for identification of natural products with valuable activities [144].

Propolis in general is regarded as non-toxic but it is known to cause allergic reactions, mainly contact dermatitis. Practically all reports concerning propolis allergy involve poplar type propolis [90,95-97,99]. The main contact allergens in poplar propolis were identified as benzyl caffeate and 3-methyl-2-butenyl caffeate [90]. It is not clear whether other propolis types might cause allergic reactions as well.

Speaking of poplar propolis, it is important to mention a variety of poplar propolis which is encountered in locations of high altitude (over 1200 – 1500 m) and in the Northern regions of Europe. Its major plant source is the common aspen *Populus tremula* and it contains higher amounts of phenolic acids and less flavonoids, compared to the one coming from *P. nigra.*

This propolis type contains also phenolic glycerides (dicoumaroyl acetyl glycerol, diferuloyl acetyl glycerol, feruloyl coumaroyl acetyl glycerol, caffeoyl coumaroyl acetyl glycerol) [46,145]. The latter compounds contribute to the biological activity of the corresponding propolis, they have been proved to possess antiproliferative activity against different cell lines, antiradical and hepatoprotective action [44,46].

Available information about the abovementioned and about further biological activities of poplar type propolis and the responsible molecules is represented in Table 2.

Obviously, poplar propolis possesses valuable activities that have been well documented. In many cases, the active principles have also been identified. This knowledge gives the reason for a standardization of poplar propolis, based on the concentration of active principles. However, it has been demonstrated in many cases that the activity of propolis of any type is the result of simultaneous and synergistic action of several active molecules. For this reason it seems that, for the purposes of standardization and quality control, measuring the concentration of only one (or a couple of) individual constituent(s) could be inappropriate. A combination of three spectrophotometric methods has been proposed to quantify total phenolics, total flavones/flavonols and total flavanones/dihydroflavonols in poplar propolis [146]. This procedure is simple, easy to perform, gives results with good repeatability and accuracy, and provides reliable characterization of the chemical profile of poplar type propolis for the purposes of its use in different preparations and health foods.

## 3. Green Brazilian Propolis

In the last two decades, Brazilian propolis has become a subject of increasing commercial and scientific interest, because Brazil exports large amounts of propolis at the international market. Brazil is a large country comprising diverse phyto-geographical regions and therefore 12 distinct chemical types of Brazilian propolis have been described according to their botanical origin [5]. Without any doubt, green Brazilian propolis (GBP) is the most commercialized and most widely used Brazilian propolis type, greatly popular also in Japan. This propolis type is collected by bees from the shoot apices of *Baccharis dracunculifolia* (alecrim), an asteracean plant commonly found in the states Minas Gerais, Parana, Sao Paulo and Rio de Janeiro [14,147]. Its chemical composition differs significantly from the one of poplar type propolis. Most characteristic chemical constituents of green Brazilian propolis are prenylated phenylpropanoids, mostly prenylated coumaric acid derivatives (artepillin C, baccharin, drupanin), some flavonoid aglycones (although different from the ones in poplar propolis and in much lower concentration), diterpenic acids and caffeoylquinic acids [148].

Despite the impressive chemical difference, green Brazilian propolis has demonstrated biological activity which is similar to a great extent to that of poplar propolis. Expectedly, GBP is active against different bacteria, fungi and viruses. Among the susceptible microorganisms are the bacteria *Staphylococcus aureus* [149-153], *Streptococcus pneumoniae* [150], *Sterptococcus pyogenes* [152], *Klebsiela pneumoniae* [150], *Listeria monocytogenes* [153], the pathogenic fungi *Candida albicans* [150,154], *Trichophyton* species [155], *Paracoccidioides brasiliensis* [150], *Criptococcus neophormans* [156], the moulds *Cladosporium cladosporioides* and *C. sphaeroides* [157]. The activity *in vitro* against *Helicobacter pylori* is comparable to the one of poplar propolis [158] but the results of a pilot clinical study were inconclusive [159]. A series of studies deal with the activity of GBP against oral pathogens, causing caries and periodontitis [160-163] and with the use of GBP preparations in treatment of root canals, periodontitis and stomatitis [164-167]. Significant inhibition of the important bee pathogen *Paenibacillus larvae* has also been documented [168].

Active antimicrobial substances of GBP were found to be mainly phenolic compounds, details are displayed in Table 3.

**Table 3. Biological activities of green Brazilian propolis and responsible constituents**

| Type of activity | Responsible molecules | References |
|---|---|---|
| Antibacterial | artepillin C, drupanin, 3-hydroxy-2,2-dimethyl-8-prenylchromane-6-propenoic acid, (*E*)-3-[2,3-Dihydro-2-(1-methylethenyl)-7-prenyl-5-benzofuranyl]- 2-propenoic acid, 15-acetoxyisocupressic acid, caffeoylquinic acids | [149-153,158-163,168-172] |
| Antifungal | Artepillin C, drupanin | [150,154-157,164,173-175] |
| Antiviral | 3,4-dicaffeoylquinic acid, 3,5-dicaffeoylquinic acid, 3,4,5-tricaffeoylquinic acid | [34,176-179] |
| Antiparasitic | Not identified | [180-183] |
| Antitumor, cytotoxic | 3,4-dicaffeoylquinic acid, 3,5-dicaffeoylquinic acid, 3,4,5-tricaffeoylquinic acid, 3-[2-dimethyl-8(3-m3thyl-2-butehyl)benzopyran]-6-propenoic acid, baccharin, drupanin, aromadendrin-4-methyl ether | [184-208] |
| Antioxidant | Artepillin C, baccharin; chlorogenic acid, 3,4-dicaffeoylquinic acid, 3,5-dicaffeoylquinic acid, kaempferid | [44,170,209-222] |
| Antiinflammatory | Artepillin C; baccharin, kaempferid | [223-228] |
| Wound-healing | Not identified | [229-231] |
| UV-protecting | phenolics | [232,233] |
| Immunomodulatory | phenolics | [234-239] |
| Antihypertensive | 3,4-dicaffeoylquinic acid 3,5-dicaffeoylquinic acid 3,4,5-tricaffeoylquinic acid, dihydroquercetin, isosakuranetin | [240-242] |
| Antihypercholesterolemic and antihyperlipidemic | Not identified | [243-246] |
| Suppressive effect on toxicity of different toxic agents | Baccharin | [247-252] |
| Neuroprotective | Not identified | [253-255] |
| Antiulcer | Caffeic, ferulic, *p*-coumaric, cinnamic acids | [256-259] |
| Inhibition of xanthine oxidase | Artepillin C, *p*-coumaric acid | [101] |
| Anti-emetic | (E)- and (Z)-3-(2,2-dimethyl-2*H*-1-benzopyran-6-yl)-2-propenoic acid, dihydrocinnamic acid; dihydrohautriwaic aicd | [260] |
| Relaxant action of guinea-pig trachea *in vitro* | Not identified | [261] |

The antiviral action of GBP has been studied in the last decade much more that the one of poplar propolis. GBP demonstrated efficacy against herpes simplex virus type 1 [178] but also against influenza virus (H1N1) ([176,179], poliovirus type 1 [177], and anti-HIV-1 activity in CD4(+) lymphocyte and microglial cell cultures [34]. Caffeoylquinic acids have been identified as major antiinfluenza agents in GBP [179].

GBP has also potential to be used against two parasitic diseases which are of importance in tropical countries. Activity against *Leishmania braziliensis* [180,181] and activity *in vitro* and *in vivo* against *Tripanozoma cruzi* (causing Shaga's disease) have been reported [182,183].

GBP contains significant amounts of phenolic substances, so it is not surprising that it possesses antioxidant activity. Radical scavenging activity against DPPH radicals has been repeatedly demonstrated [215-218,221,222]. Da Silva et al. (2006) found correlation between the antiradical activity and the total phenolic and flavonoid levels in GBP [170]. Other authors demonstrated the anti-lipid peroxidation potential of GBP [209,214]. In addition, GBP was able to inhibit the oxidative stress in neutrophiles [211,219]. Its potential to act as UV-photoprotector was found promising [232,233].

The antioxidant activity is believed to be related to the anti-inflammatory properties in general [262] and GBP was found to exert anti-inflammatory action in several models [224,228,230]. Individual compounds with antiinflammatory properties are artepillin C, baccharin and kaempferid [225,227]. The anti-inflammatory and antibacterial properties contribute to the positive effect of GBP on tissue repair of cutaneous wounds in rats [229,231].

Research on the antitumor and cytotoxic activity of GBP has received much attention since the year 2000 (See Table 3). Cytotoxicity of GBP against different tumor cell lines has been demonstrated [184,194,197,202]. Apoptosis induced by GBP and its constituents artepillin C and caffeoylquinic acids was observed by several research groups [186,189,190,206-208]. GBP and artepillin C can play a cancer-preventing role against chemically induced carcinogenesis in rats and mice [185,187,192,196,205].

Many of the pharmacological properties of GBP have been connected, at least partly, to the *p*-coumaric acid derivative artepillin C. Analogously to CAPE in poplar propolis, this compound has been the subject of numerous pharmacological studies and has demonstrated diverse and valuable activities. A comprehensive review on its synthesis, biological activities and pharmacokinetics has been published recently [263].

Unlike poplar propolis, there is no publication claiming allergy toward GBP. There is only one communication reporting on acute renal failure in a patient with cholangiocarcinoma due to ingestion of GBP [264]. The allergenic properties of GBP haven't been studied so far. In a study aimed to search for side effects of GBP after long-term administration (30 days), no significant changes in the serum biochemical parameters of rats were observed [265].

Further data concerning the abovementioned and further biological activities of green Brazilian (alecrim) propolis, and the corresponding active constituents, are represented in Table 3.

Concerning standardization and quality control of GBP, a combination of spectrophotometric methods has been proposed [266,267] to quantify total phenolics and total flavonoids. This approach is similar but not identical to the one used for poplar type propolis. It is important to note that the content of flavonoids in GBP is much lower than the one in poplar propolis. Another important point is the need to use different standards for calibration for the measurements in case of GBP and in case of poplar propolis, because of the difference in their chemical composition.

## 3. Red South American Propolis

The first communications about red propolis and its biological activities came from Cuba and appeared in the 1990's. [268]. The major constituents in Cuban red propolis were identified as isoflavonoids [269-271]. With the beginning of the 21 century, red propolis has been detected also in the North-Eastern parts of Brazil, in the states of Alagoas, Bahia and Paraiba [272,273]. Red Brazilian propolis attracted the attention of propolis researchers and it turned out that isoflavonoids and pterocarpans were its major constituents [272]. Their plant source was identified as the red resinous exudates of *Dalbergia ecasophyllum* [15,274,275]. A comparative study of Brazilian and Cuban red propolis showed their similar chemical profiles and confirmed that they both originated from *Dalbergia* spp. [17]. However, Brazilian samples contained also prenylated benzophenones, typical for *Clusia* species, and this makes them specific [17,272]. Recently, a red-type propolis from the Southern region of Mexico was studied and found to contain *Dalbergia* isoflavonoids and pterocarpans, too [16]. Obviously, there is a red propolis type (RP), typical for South America. The published research papers concerning this propolis type are increasing from year to year, and the communicated results on its biological activity are encouraging, so we believe it deserves a more detailed overview.

Brazilian RP and some of its constituents (see Table 4) possess antimicrobial activity against *S. aureus* ([272,276-280], *Streptococcus mutans* [280,286], *Candida albicans* [272], *Trichophyton rubrum, T. tonsurans* and *T. mentagrophytes* [155]. Potent cytotoxic activity of Brazilian RP and isolated compounds against different cancer cell lines has been reported [276,281,283]. Atheroproprotecive properties of Brazilian RP are described, and attributed to its phenolic constituents [287]; it also improved dermal wound healing in a rodent model [284]. Red propolis contains isoflavonoids and its radical scavenging activity against DPPH radicals [272,276,288], as well as its high antioxidant activity by β-carotene/linoleic acid test [288] are not surprising. But maybe the most attractive and promising property of Brazilian red propolis is its ability to promote adypocite differentiation through PPARy activation, which suggests that it has the potential, when used as food additive, to prevent obesity and obesity associated disorders [285].

The data concerning biological activities and active constituents of red South American propolis are summarized in Table 4.

## 4. Other Propolis Types from Tropical and Subtropical Regions

The remarkable chemical variability of propolis is, of course, due to its' plant origin and to the fact that at different geographic locations the source plants might vary with respect to the local flora at the site of collection. The chemical composition of propolis is directly dependant on the availability of resinous plant materials in different geographic regions. This is especially true for tropical and subtropical regions, with their huge biodiversity. However, there is another important but often neglected factor: the choices bees make. In any environment, bees tend to choose as propolis sources plants with pronounced antimicrobial, antioxidant and cytotoxic properties, because propolis is very important as chemical defense of the hive [144]. Moreover, in environments with similar flora, as a rule, they choose the same source material, which leads to the existence of specific propolis types.

In the last decade, several new propolis types "emerged" in the scientific literature and in this chapter we are going to discuss briefly the most important ones of them.

The oldest known tropical propolis type, different from Green Brazilian and Red South-American ones, is the *Clusia*-type propolis. It was first noticed by the group of Tomas-Barberan in 1993, when they studies Venezuelan bee glue: they found in it (by LC-MS) polyprenylated benzophenones, and the propolis chemical profile coincided with the profile of the resins exuded by the flowers of *Clusia major* (autograph tree) [289]. The prenylated benzophenones exuded from the flowers of *Clusia* species were isolated later from propolis from Venezuela [290], Cuba [291,292] and Brazil [293,294]. The biological activities of the *Clusia*-type propolis are due to the properties of the prenylated benzophenones. Nevertheless, they are typical for propolis in general: antibacterial, antioxidant, cytotoxic (see Table 5). Propolis rich in prenylated benzophenones was active against *Staphylocosccus aureus* [290,293], *Streptococcus mutans* [293-295], *S. sorbinus*, *S. oralis, S. mitis, S. salivarius* and *Actinomycetes aeslundii* [293,294]. In addition, it suppressed the formation of mutans streptococci biofilms [295,296]. Of interest is the antiretroviral activity against HIV-1, displayed by two prenylated benzophenones isolated from Caribbean propolis [298]. Antioxidant potential of *Clusia*-type propolis has also been reported [291,333], as well as cytotoxic activity against human tumor cell lines [299-301].

**Table 4. Biological activities of South American red propolis and responsible constituents**

| Type of activity | Responsible molecules | References |
|---|---|---|
| Antibacterial | Isosativan, medicarpin, vestitol, neovestitol,isoliquiritgenin | [272,276-280] |
| Antifungal | Isosativan, medicarpin | [155,272] |
| Antitumor, cytotoxic | 3,8-dihydroxi-9-methoxypterocarpan, 7-hydroxy-6-methoxyflavanon, mucronulatol | [276,281-283] |
| Antioxidant | Vestitol, neovestitol, Isosativan, medicarpin | [272,280] |
| Against *Leishmania* | Not identified | [180] |
| Wound healing | Not identified | [284] |
| Anti-obesity | Not identified | [285] |

Bees in the Pacific islands in the Far East have been reported to collect a specific propolis type of bright green colour. From this propolis type from Okinawa [334] and Taiwan [312], prenylated flavanones (propolins) with radical scavenging activity were isolated. Further studies on chemical profiles and bee behaviour revealed the corresponding plant source: the resinous material on the surface of the fruits of *Macaranga tanarius* [22]. This propolis type and its major constituents the propolins, possess antibacterial activity [307,308], including activity against methicillin-resistant *Staphylococcus aureus* (MRSA) [311]. Its antiradical and antioxidant properties [309,313] are similar to the ones demonstrated by other propolis types. Pacific propolis and propolins have attracted the attention of researchers mainly with their cytotoxic and anticancer effect [21,61,314,315,335]. Details about the active constituents are displayed in Table 5. Recently, propolins have been identified in propolis from the Solomon Islands [311] and Indonesia [332], confirming the appropriateness of the term "Pacific propolis". Interestingly, prenylated *Macaranga* flavonoids were found also in some African propolis samples [310,331].

**Table 5. New propolis types, some of them possibly with limited distribution**

| Propolis type | Geographical distribution | Plant source(s) | Biological activity | Responsible molecules | References |
|---|---|---|---|---|---|
| ***Clusia type*** | **South America (Cuba, Brazil, Venezuela)** | **Frower resin of *Clusia species*** | | | |
| | | | Antibacterial | Prenylated benzophenones: hyperibone A; 7-*epi*-nemorosone, 7-*epi*-clusianone, xanthochymol, gambogenone | [293-297] |
| | | | Antiretroviral | 7-*epi*-nemorosone, plukenetione A | [298] |
| | | | Antitumor, cytotoxic | Nemorosone, plukenetione A | [291,299-301] |
| **Mediterrane-an type** | **Southern Greece, Krete, Sicily, Malta** | ***Cupressus sempervirens* resin** | | | |
| | | | Antibacterial | Totarol, totarolone, 14,15-dinor-13-oxo-8(17)-labden-19-oic acid, epi-manool, unicedric acid | [19,302-305] |
| | | | Antioxidant | | [303] |
| | | | Antiproliferati ve | Diterpenes | [306] |
| **Pacific type** | **Okinawa, Taiwan, Indonesia** | **Fruit resin of *Macaranga tanarius*** | | | |
| | | | Antibacterial | Nymphaeol B, isonymphaeol B; propolisns C, G, D and H | [307-311] |
| | | | Antioxidant | Propolins | [22,309,312, 313] |
| | | | Anticancer | Nymphaeols A, B and C, propolin A, propolin B, propolin H, propolin G | [21,61,312,3 14,315] |
| | | **Other propolis t ypes** | | | |
| Argentinean Andean | San Juan Province, Argentina | *Larrea nitida* resinous exudates | Antifungal | 3´methyl-nordihydroguaiaretic acid,,nordihydroguaiaretic acid; (4-[4-(4-hydroxy-phenyl)-2,3-dimethyl-butyl]-benzene-1,2-diol | [316] |

| Propolis type | Geographical distribution | Plant source(s) | Biological activity | Responsible molecules | References |
|---|---|---|---|---|---|
| *Zuccagnia* type | Tucuman Province, Argentina | *Zuccagnia punctata* | Cytotoxic, Antifungal | 2',4'-dihydroxy-3'-methoxychalcone, 2',4'-dihydroxychalcone, pinocembrin, galangin, 7-hydroxy-8-methoxyflavanone | [317,318] |
| Unknown Argentinean | Catamarca Province, Argentina | Unknown | Antibacterial, antioxidant | 2',4'-dihydroxy-3'-methoxychalcone, 2',4'-dihydroxychalcone, 2',4',4-trihydroxy-6'- methoxychalcone, 5-hydroxy-4',7-dimethoxyflavone, 4',5-dihydroxy-3,7,8-trimethoxyflavone and 7-hydroxy- 5,8-dimethoxyflavone | [319] |
| Nepalese | Nepal | *Dalbergia sissoo* | Inhibitory activity on nitric oxide production | Neoflavonoids | [320] |
| Unknown | Mexico | Unknown | cytotoxic | (2*R*,3*S*)-8-[4-phenylprop-2-en-1-one]-4',7-dihydroxy-3',5-dimethoxyflavan-3-ol | [321] |
| *Rhus* type | Okayama, Japan | *Rhus javanica* var. *chinensis* sap | antioxidant | Unidentifed flavonoids | [322] |
| Unknown | Piaui State, Brazil | *Anacardium occidentale ??* | Antimicrobial | Cardanols, cardols, anacardic acid | [323] |
| Unknown | Brazil | Unknown | Ani-HIV | Moronic acid | [324] |
| Unknown | Myanmar | Unknown | Cytotxic | 3α,27-dihydroxycycloart-24E-en-26-oic acid, (22*Z*,24*E*)-3-oxocycloart-22,24-dien-26-oic acid, (24*E*)-3-oxo-27,28-dihydroxycycloart-24-en-26-oic acid | [325,326] |
| Unknown | Algeria | Unknown | Stromelysin-1 inhibition | (+)-chickoric acid and its methyl ester, caffeic acid | [327] |
| Unknown | Henan Province, China | Unknown | Cytotoxic | 8-C-Cinnamoyl flavan-3-ols | [328] |
| Unknown | Jeju Island, Korea | Unknown | Inhibition of soybean lipoxygenase | 4'-Methoxy-bavachromanol | [329] |
| Unknown | Nigeria | Unknown | Antibacterial | Unknown | [330] |
| Africna Macaranga | Kenya | *Macaranga schweinfurthii* ?? | Antibacterial, antioxidant | Macarangin, schweinfurthins A and B | [331] |
| Unknown | Kenya | Unknown | Antibacterial | Tetrahydrojusticidin B, phyllamyricinC | [331] |
| Mixed type | Malta | *Cupressus sempervirens* + *Ferula communis* | Antifungal | Dierpenic acids, ferutin, teferin, jaeschkeanadiol, 2-acetoxy-6-p-hydroxybenzoyl jaeschkeanadiol | [305] |
| Mixed type | Indonesia | *Mangifera indica* + *Macaranga tanarius* | Antioxidant | Alkylresorcinols | [332] |

Recent studies have revealed a new type of European propolis: Mediterranean propolis, distinguished by a high concentration of diterpenoids. This propolis type was found in the South of Greece, in Sicily and in some Croatian Adriatic islands and Malta [18,20,304,305]. Its chemical profile is characterized by the presence of substantial amounts of diterpene acids:

isocupressic, communic, pimaric and imbricatoloic acid, together with totarol and 13-epitorulosal. It also possesses antibacterial [18,19,303-305] and antiproliferative activity [306]. A separate chapter in this book is dealing with this propolis type, so it will not be discussed further in this chapter.

There are numerous research papers reporting on the biological activity and chemical composition of propolis types, different from the already discussed. Maybe some of these propolis types will become as popular and important in propolis research as the red-type propolis or the Pacific type propolis. The available data of these propolis types are collected and represented in Table 5.

## Conclusion

There is no doubt that in further specific ecosystems, for example such in Sub-Saharan Africa, Australia, etc.; propolis plant sources and respectively the chemical composition of propolis will continue to surprise scientists. The search for new active propolis constituents in samples from unexplored regions is a promising direction for further propolis research, especially in the search for new antimicrobial, antioxidant and anticancer agents. The results summarized in this chapter demonstrate once again that propolis remains a fascinating subject for further studies and we can expect further exciting findings, further surprises that bees have prepared for us.

## References

[1] Ghisalberti E. L. Propolis: a review. *Bee World*. 1979;60:59-84.

[2] Burdock G. A. Review of the biological properties and toxicity of bee propolis (propolis). *Food Chemistry and Toxicology*. 1998;36:347-363.

[3] Pietta P. G., Gardana C., Pietta A. M. Analytical methods for quality control of propolis. *Fitoterapia*. 2002;73 Suppl 1:S7-20.

[4] Bankova V. Chemical diversity of propolis and the problem of standardization. *Journal of Ethnopharmacology*. 2005;100:114-117.

[5] Park Y. K., Alencar S. M., Aguiar C. L. Botanical origin and chemical composition of Brazilian propolis. *Journal of Agricultural and Food Chemistry*. 2002;50:2502-2506.

[6] Bankova V. S., Popov S. S., Marekov N. L. A study on flavonoids of propolis. *Journal of Natural Products*. 1983;46:471-474.

[7] Nagy E., Papay V., Litkei G., Dinya Z. Investigation of the chemical constituents, particularly the flavonoid components of propolis and *Populi gemma* by the GC/MS method. In: Farkas L, Gabor M, Kallay F, eds. Flavonoids and bioflavonoids. Amsterdam: *Elsevier*. 1985:233-240.

[8] Greenaway W., Scaysbrook T., Whatley F..R. Composition of propolis of Oxfordshire, UK and its relation to poplar bud exudate. *Zeitschrift fur Naturforschung*. 1988;43c:301-304.

[9] Bankova V., Dyulgerov A., Popov S., Evstatieva L., Kuleva L., Pureb O., Zamjansan Z. Propolis produced in Bulgaria and Mongolia: phenolic compounds and plant origin. *Apidologie*. 1992;23:79-85.

[10] Markham K. R., Mitchell K. A., Wilkins A. L., Daldy J. A., Lu Y. HPLC and GC-MS identification of the major organic constituents in New Zealand propolis. *Phytochemistry*. 1996;42:205-211.

[11] Sawaya A. C. H. F., Tomazela D. M., Cunha I. B. S., Bankova V. S., Marcucci M. C., Custodio A. R., Eberlin M. N. Electrospray ionization mass spectrometry fingerprinting of propolis. *Analyst*. 2004;129:739-744.

[12] Cao W., Fu J., Suo Z., Chen W., Zheng J. A comparative study on chemical compositions of Chinese propolis and poplar resin. *Food and Fermentation Industries*. 2007;33:162-166.

[13] Bankova V., Boudourova- Krasteva G., Sforcin J. M., Frete X., Kujumgiev A., Maimoni-Rodella R., Popov S. Phytochemical evidence for the plant origin of Brazilian propolis from Sao Paulo state. *Zeitschrift fur Naturforschung C*. 1999;54:401-405.

[14] Teixeira E. W., Negri G., Meira R. M. S. A., Message D., Salatino A. Plant origin of green propolis: bee behavior, plant anatomy and chemistry. *Evidence-Based Complementary and Alternative Medicine*. 2005;2:85-92.

[15] Daugsch A., Moraes C. S., Fort P., Park Y. K. Brazilian red propolis—chemical composition and botanical origin. *Evidence-Based Complementary and Alternative Medicine*. 2008;5:435–441.

[16] Lotti C., Fernandez M. C., Piccinelli A. L., Cuesta-Rubio O., Hernandez I. M., Rastrelli L. Chemical constituents. *Journal of Agricultural and Food Chemistry*. 2010;58:2209-2213.

[17] Piccinelli A. L., Lotti C., Campone L., Cuesta-Rubio O., Fernandez M. C., Rastrelli L. Cuban and Brazilian red propolis: botanical origin and comparative analysis by high-performance liquid chromatography-photodiode array detection/electrospray ionization tandem mass spectrometry. *Journal of Agricultural and Food Chemistry*. 2011;59:6484-6491.

[18] Trusheva B., Popova M., Bankova V., Tsvetkova I., Naydenski C., Sabatini A. G. A new type of European propolis, containing bioactive labdanes. *Rivista Italiana EPPOS*. 2003;13:3-8.

[19] Melliou E, Chinou I. Chemical analysis and antimicrobial activity of Greek propolis. *Planta Medica*. 2004;70:1-5.

[20] Popova M. P., Graikou K., Chinou I., Bankova V. S. GC-MS profiling of diterpene compounds in Mediterranean propolis from Greece. *Journal of Agricultural and Food Chemistry*. 2010;58:3167-3176.

[21] Chen C. N., Wu C. L., Lin J. K. Apoptosis of human melanoma cells induced by the novel compounds propolin A and propolin B from Taiwenese propolis. *Cancer Letters*. 2007;245:218-231.

[22] Kumazawa S., Nakamura J, Murase M, Miyagawa M., Ahn M. R., Fukumoto S. Plant origin of Okinawan propolis: honeybee behavior observation and phytochemical analysis. *Naturwissenschaften*. 2008;95:781-786.

[23] Lavie P. The relationship between propolis, poplar buds (*Populus* spp.) and castor. In: Lavie P, ed. *Proceedings of the XXV$^{th}$ International Beekeeping Congress, Grenoble 1975*. Bucharest: Apimondia Publishing House. 1976:227–231.

[24] Greenaway W., Scaysbrook T., Whatley F. R., The analysis of bud exudate of *Populus x euramericana* and of propolis by gas chromatography-mass spectrometry. *Proceedings of the Royal Society B*. 1987;232:249-272.
[25] Greenaway W., May J., Scaysbrook T., Whatley F. R. Identification by gas-chromatography mass-spectrometry of 150 compounds in propolis. *Zeitschrift fur Naturforschung C*. 1991;46:111-121.
[26] Koo H., Rosalen P. L., Cury J. A., Park Y. K., Bowen W. H. Effects of compounds found in propolis on *Streptococcus mutans* growth and on glucosyltransferase activity. *Antimicrobial Agents and Chemotherapy*. 2002;46:1302-1309.
[27] Pepeljnjak S., Kosalec I. Galangin expresses bactericidal activity against multiple-resistant bacteria: MRSA, *Enterococcus* spp. and *Pseudomonas aeruginosa*. *FEMS*. 2004;240:111-116.
[28] Cushnie T. P., Lamb A. J. Detection of galangin-induced cytoplasmic membrane damage in *Staphylococcus aureus* by measuring potassium loss. *Journal of Ethnopharmacology*. 2005;101:243-248.
[29] Du Toit K., Buthelezi S., Bodenstein J. Anti-inflammatory and antibacterial profiles of selected compounds found in South African propolis. *South African Journal of Science*. 2009;105:470-472.
[30] Darwish R. M., Abu Fares R. J., Abu Zarga M. H., Nazer I. K. Antibacterial effect of Jordanian propolis and isolated flavonoids against human pathogenic bacteria. *African Journal of Biotechnology*. 2010;9:5966-5974.
[31] Quiroga E. N., Sampietro D. A., Soberon J. R., Sgariglia M. A., Vattuone M. A. Propolis from the northwest of Argentina as a source of antifungal principles. *Journal of Applied Microbiology*. 2006;101:103-110.
[32] Yang S. Z., Peng L. T., Su X. J., Chen F., Cheng Y. J., Fan G., Pan S. Y. Bioassay-guided isolation and identification of antifungal components from propolis against *Penicillium italicum*. *Food Chemistry*. 2011;127:210-215.
[33] Huleihel M., Isanu V. Anti-herpes simplex virus effect of an aqueous extract of propolis. *The Israel Medical Association Journal*. 2002;4 Suppl:923-927.
[34] Gekker G., Hu S., Spivak M., Lokensgard J. R., Peterson P. K. Anti-HIV-1 activity of propolis in $CD4^+$ lymphocyte and microglial cell cultures. *Journal of Ethnopharmacology*. 2005;102:158–163.
[35] Nolkemper S., Reichling J., Sensch K. H., Schnitzler P. Mechanism of herpes simplex virus type 2 suppression by propolis extracts. *Phytomedicine*. 2010;17:132-138.
[36] Schnitzler P., Neuner A., Nolkemper S., Zundel C., Nowack H., Sensch K. H., Reichling J. Antiviral activity and mode of action of propolis extracts and selected compounds. *Phytotherapy Research*. 2010;24 Suppl 1:S20-S28.
[37] Lee S., Kim K. S., Park Y., Shin K. H., Kim B. K. In vivo anti-oxidant activities of tectochrysin. *Archives of Pharmacal Research*. 2003;26:43-46.
[38] Okutan H., Ozcelik N., Ramazan Yilmaz H., Uz E. Effects of caffeic acid phenethyl ester on lipid peroxidation and antioxidant enzymes in diabetic rat heart. *Clinical Biochemistry*. 2005;38:191-196.
[39] Ahn M. R., Kumazawa S., Usui Y., Nakamura J., Matsuka M., Zhu F., Nakayama T. Antioxidant activity and constituents of propolis collected in various areas of China. *Food Chemistry*. 2007;101:1383-1392.

[40] Velazquez C., Navarro M., Acosta A., Angulo A., Dominguez Z., Robles R., Robles-Zepeda R., Lugo E., Goycoolea F. M., Velazquez E. F., Astiazaran H., Velazquez J. H. C. Antibacterial and free-radical scavenging activities of Sonoran propolis. *Journal of Applied Microbiology*. 2007;103:1747-1756.

[41] Kumazawa S., Ahn M. R., Fujimoto T., Kato M. Radical-scavenging activity and phenolic constituents of propolis from different regions of Argentina. *Natural Product Research*. 2010;24:804-812.

[42] Laskar R. A., Sk I., Roy N., Begum N. A. Antioxidant activity of Indian propolis and its chemical constituents. *Food Chemistry*. 2010;122:233-237.

[43] Gocer H., Gulcin I. Caffeic acid phenethyl ester (CAPE): correlation of structure and antioxidant properties. *International Journal of Food Sciences and Nutrition*. 2011; doi:10.3109/09637486.2011.585963.

[44] Banskota A. H., Tezuka Y., Adnyana I. K., Midorikawa K., Matsushige K., Message D., Huertas A. A. G., Kadota S. Cytotoxic, hepatoprotective and free radical scavenging effects of propolis from Brazil, Peru, the Netherlands and China. *Journal of Ethnopharmacology*. 2000;72:239-246.

[45] Heo M. Y., Sohn S. J., Au W. W. Anti-genotoxicity of galangin as a cancer chemopreventive agent candidate. *Mutation Research*. 2001;488:135-150.

[46] Banskota A. H., Nagaoka T., Sumioka L. Y., Tezuka Y., Awale S., Midorikawa K., Matsushige K., Kadota S. Antiproliferative activity of the Netherlands propolis and its active principles in cancer cell lines. *Journal of Ethnopharmacology*. 2002;80:67-73.

[47] Usia T., Banskota A. H., Tezuka Y., Midorikawa K., Matsushige K., Kadota S. Constituents of Chinese propolis and their antiproliferative activities. *Journal of Natural Products*. 2002;65:673-676.

[48] Liao H. F., Chen Y. Y., Liu J. J., Hsu M. L., Shieh H. J., Liao H. J., Shieh C. J., Shiao M. S., Chen Y. J. Inhibitory effect of caffeic acid phenethyl ester on angiogenesis, tumor invasion, and metastasis. *Journal of Agricultural and Food Chemistry*. 2003;51:7907–7912.

[49] Lee K. W., Chun K. S., Lee J. S., Kang K. S., Surh Y. J., Lee H. J. Inhibition of Cyclooxygenase-2 expression and restoration of gap junction intercellular communication in H-ras-transformed rat liver epithelial cells by caffeic acid phenethyl ester. *Annals of the New York Academy of Sciences*. 2004;1030:501-507.

[50] Woo K. J., Jeong Y. J., Park J. W., Kwon T. K. Chrysin-induced apoptosis is mediated through caspase activation and Akt inactivation in U937 leukemia cells. *Biochemical and Biophysical Research Communications*. 2004;325:1215-1222.

[51] Orsolic N., Terzic S., Mihaljevic Z., Sver L., Basic I. Effects of local administration of propolis and its polyphenolic compounds on tumor formation and growth. *Biological and Pharmaceutical Bulletin*. 2005;28:1928-1933.

[52] Orsolic N., Sver L., Terzic S., Basic I. Peroral application of water-soluble derivative of propolis (WSDP) and its related polyphenolic compounds and their influence on immunological and antitumour activity. *Veterinary Research Communications*. 2005;29:575-593.

[53] Orsolic N., Terzic S., Sver L.., Basic T. Honey-bee products in prevention and/or therapy of murine transplantable tumours. *Journal of the Science of Food and Agriculture*. 2005;85:363-370.

[54] Orsolic N., Saranovic A. B., Basic I. Direct and indirect mechanism(s) of antitumour activity of propolis and its polyphenolic compounds. *Planta Medica*. 2006;72:20-27.

[55] Benkovic V., Knezevic A. H., Brozovic G., Knezevic F., Dikic D., Bevanda M., Basic I., Orsolic N. Enhanced antitumor activity of irinotecan combined with propolis and its polyphenolic compounds on Ehrlich ascites tumor in mice. *Biomedicine and Pharmacotherapy*. 2007;61:292-297.

[56] Orsolic N., Basic I. Suppression of tumor growth by water-soluble derivative of propolis and related polyphenolic compounds. *Periodicum Biologorum*. 2007;109:181-187.

[57] Draganova-Filipova M. N., Georgieva M. G., Peycheva E. N., Miloshev G. A., Sarafian V. S., Peychev L. P. Effects of propolis and CAPE on proliferation and apoptosis of McCoy-Plovdiv cell line. *Folia Medica*. 2008;50:53-59.

[58] Demestre M., Messerli S. M., Celli N., Shahhossini M., Kluwe L., Mautner V., Maruta H. CAPE (Caffeic acid phenethyl ester)-based propolis extract (Bio 30) suppresses the growth of human neurofibromatosis (NF) tumor xenografts in mice. *Phytotherapy Research*. 2009;23:226-230.

[59] Orsolic N., Stajcar D., Basic I. Propolis and its flavonoid compounds cause cytotoxicity on human urinary bladder transitional cell carcinoma in primary culture. *Periodicum Biologorum*. 2009;111:113-121.

[60] Szliszka E., Czuba Z. P., Domino M., Mazur B., Zydowicz G., Krol W. Ethanolic extract of propolis (EEP) enhances the apoptosis- inducing potential of TRAIL in cancer cells. *Molecules*. 2009;14:738-754.

[61] Chen C. N., Hsiao C. J., Lee S. S., Guh J. H., Chiang P. C., Huang C. C., Huang W. J. Chemical modification and anticancer effect of prenylated flavanones from Taiwanese propolis. *Natural Product Research*. 2011. doi:10.1080/14786419.2010.535146.

[62] Shvarzbeyn J., Huleihel M. Effect of propolis and caffeic acid phenethyl ester (CAPE) on NFκB activation by HTLV-1 Tax. *Antiviral Research*. 2011;90:108-115.

[63] Rossi A., Longo R., Russo A., Borrelli F., Sautebin L. The role of the phenethyl ester of caffeic acid (CAPE) in the inhibition of rat lung cyclooxygenase activity by propolis. *Fitoterapia*. 2002;73 Suppl 1:S30-S37.

[64] Beyer G., Melzig M. F. Effects of propolis on hypoxanthine-xanthine oxidase-induced toxicity in cultivated human cells and on neutrophil elastase activity. *Biological and Pharmaceutical Bulletin*. 2005;28:1183-1186.

[65] Woo K. J., Jeong Y. J., Inoue H., Park J. W., Kwon T. K. Chrysin suppresses lipopolysaccharide- induced cyclooxygenase-2 expression through the inhibition of nuclear factor for IL-6 (NF-IL6) DNA-binding activity. *FEBS Letters*. 2005;579:705-711.

[66] Xuan H., Zhu R., Li Y., Hu F. Inhibitory effect of chinese propolis on phosphatidylcholine-specific phospholipase C activity in vascular endothelial cells. *Evidence- Based Complementary and Alternative Medicine*. 2011;2011:985278.

[67] Orsolic N., Tadic Z., Benkovic V., Horvat A., Lojkic M., Basic I. Radioprotective effect of a water-soluble derivative of propolis in mice. *Mellifera*. 2004;4:45-52.

[68] Orsolic N., Basic I. Antitumor, hematostimulative and radioprotective action of water-soluble derivative of propolis (WSDP). *Biomedicine and Pharmacotherapy*. 2005;59:561-570.

[69] Orsolic N., Benkovic V., Horvat- Knezevic A., Kopjar N., Kosalec I., Bakmaz M., Mihaljevic Z., Bendelja K., Basic I. Assessment by survival analysis of the radioprotective properties of propolis and its polyphenolic compounds. *Biological and Pharmaceutical Bulletin*. 2007;30:946—951.

[70] Benkovic V., Orsolic N., Horvat-Knezevic A., Ramic S., Dikic D., Basic I., Kopjar N. Evaluation of the radioprotective effects of propolis and flavonoids in gamma-irradiated mice: the alkaline comet assay study. *Biological and Pharmaceutical Bulletin*. 2008;31:167-172.

[71] Benkovic V., Horvat-Knezevic A., Dikic D., Lisicic D., Orsolic N., Basic I., Kosalec I., Kopjar N. Radioprotective effects of propolis and quercetin in γ-irradiated mice evaluated by the alkaline comet assay. *Phytomedicine*. 2008;15:851-858.

[72] Benkovic V., Knezevic A. H., Dikic D., Lisicic D., Orsolic N., Basic I., Kopjar N. Radioprotective effects of quercetin and ethanolic extract of propolis in gamma-irradiated mice. *Archives of Industrial Hygiene and Toxicology*. 2009;60:129-138.

[73] Benkovic V., Knezevic A. H., Orsolic N., Basic I., Ramic S., Viculin T., Knezevic F., Kopjar N. Evaluation of radioprotective effects of propolis and its flavonoid constituents: in vitro study on human white blood cells. *Phytotherapy Research*. 2009;23:1159-1168.

[74] Ansorge S., Reinhold D., Lendeckel U. Propolis and some of its constituents down-regulate DNA synthesis and inflammatory cytokine production but induce TGF-β1 production of human immune cells. *Zeitschrift für Naturforschung*. 2003;58c:580-589.

[75] Orsolic N., Knezevic A. H., Sver L., Terzic S., Basic I I. Immunomodulatory and antimetastatic action of propolis and related polyphenolic compounds. *Journal of Ethnopharmacology*. 2004;94:307-315.

[76] Park J. H., Lee J. K., Kim H. S., Chung S. T., Eom J. H., Kim K. A., Chung S. J., Paik S. Y., Oh H. Y. Immunomodulatory effect of caffeic acid phenethyl ester in Balb/c mice. *International Immunopharmacology*. 2004;4:429-436.

[77] Draganova-Filipova M., Nikolova M., Mihova A., Peychev L., Sarafian V. A pilot study on the immunomodulatory effect of Bulgarian propolis. *Biotechnology and Biotechnological Equipment*. 2010;24:119-124.

[78] Gregoris E., Fabris S., Bertelle M., Grassato L., Stevanato R. Propolis as potential cosmeceutical sunscreen agent for its combined photoprotective and antioxidant properties. *International Journal of Pharmaceutics*. 2011;405:97-101.

[79] Chen J., Long Y., Han M., Wang T., Chen Q., Wang R. Water-soluble derivative of propolis mitigates scopolamine-induced learning and memory impairment in mice. *Pharmacology Biochemistry and Behavior*. 2008;90:441-446.

[80] Hartwich A., Legutko J., Wszołek J. Propolis: its properties and administration to patients treated for some surgical diseases. *Przeglad Lekarski*. 2000;57:191-194.

[81] Holcova S., Schmidt M. Showering gel and shampoo with a special concentrate from propolis for the treatment of seborrhoic eczema, psoriasis and atopic eczema- An observational study. *Haut*. 2005;16:311-315.

[82] Holcova S., Hladicova M. Effect and local tolerability of a shampoo containing the propolis special extract GH 2002 in dermatitis seborrhoica with distinct dandruff formation. *Kosmetische Medizin*. 2007;28:76-80.

[83] Sosa S., Bornancin A., Tubaro A., Loggia R. D. Topical antiinflammatory activity of an innovative aqueous formulation of Actichelated® propolis vs two commercial propolis formulations. *Phytotherapy Research*. 2007;21:823–826.

[84] Lozina L. A., Peichoto M. E., Boehringer S. I., Koscinczuk P., Granero G. E., Acosta O. C. Efficacy of Argentine propolis formulation for topical treatment of canine otitis externa. *Arquivo Brasileiro de Medicina Veterinaria e Zootecnia*. 2010;62:1359-1366.

[85] Marchisio P., Esposito S., Bianchini S., Desantis C., Galeone C., Nazzari E., Pignataro L., Principi N. Effectiveness of a propolis and zinc solution in preventing acute otitis media in children with a history of recurrent acute otitis media. *International Journal of Immunopathology and Pharmacology*. 2010;23:567-575.

[86] Akyol S., Armutcu F., Yigitoglu M. R. The medical usage of caffeic acid phenethyl ester (CAPE), an active compound of propolis, in neurological disorders and emergencies. *Spatula DD*. 2011;1:37-42.

[87] Zhu W., Li Y. H., Chen M. L., Hu F. L. Protective effects of Chinese and Brazilian propolis treatment against hepatorenal lesion in diabetic rats. *Human and Experimental Toxicology*. 2011;30:1246-1255.

[88] Kiec-Swierczynska M., Krecisz B., Swierczynska-Machura D. Most frequent causes of allergic contact dermatitis in farmers: based on material collected in the Nofer Institute of Occupational Medicine, Lodz. *Medycyna Pracy*. 2003;54:237-243.

[89] Giusti F., Miglietta R., Pepe P., Seidenari S. Sensitization to propolis in 1255 children undergoing patch testing. *Contact Dermatitis*. 2004;51:255-258.

[90] Hausen B. M. Evaluation of the main contact allergens in propolis (1995 to 2005). *Dermatitis*. 2005;16:127-129.

[91] Maria Y. Rhinitis and asthma triggered by nasal inhalation of a spray containing propolis in a beekeeper. *Revue Francaise d'Allergologie et d'Immunologie Clinique*. 2005;45:426-427.

[92] Seidenari S., Giusti F., Pepe P., Mantovani L. Contact sensitization in 1094 children undergoing patch testing over a 7-year period. *Pediatric Dermatology*. 2005;22:1-5.

[93] Walgrave S. E., Warshaw E. M., Glesne L. A. Allergic contact dermatitis from propolis. *Dermatitis*. 2005;16:209-215.

[94] Brailo V., Boras V. V., Alajbeg I., Juras V. Delayed contact sensitivity on the lips and oral mucosa due to propolis-case report. *Medicina Oral, Patología Oral y Cirugía Bucal*. 2006;11:E303-304.

[95] Munstedt K., Hellner M., Hackethal A., Winter D., von Georgi R. Contact allergy to propolis in beekeepers. *Allergologia et Immunopathologia*. 2007;35:95-100.

[96] Menniti-Ippolito F., Mazzanti G., Vitalone A., Firenzuoli F., Santuccio C. Surveillance of suspected adverse reactions to natural health products: the case of propolis. *Drug Safety*. 2008;31:419-423.

[97] Rajpara S., Wilkinson M. S., King C. M., Gawkrodger D. J., English J. S., Statham B. N., Green C., Sansom J. E., Chowdhury M. M., Horne H. L., Ormerod A. D. The importance of propolis in patch testing-a multicentre survey. *Contact Dermatitis*. 2009;61:287-290.

[98] Wagner E., Becker D., Dickel H., Geier J., John S. M., Lessmann H., Mahler V., Rogosky E., Skudlik C., Weisshaar E., Diepgen T. L. Impact of an occupational contact allergy to propolis in cases of occupational skin disease. *Dermatologie in Beruf und Umwelt*. 2009;57:77–80.

[99] Necas M., Dastychova E. Contact sensitization in patients with lower extremity dermatitis in the South Moravian region, Czech Republic. *Phlebology*. 2010;25:132-137.

[100] Holcova S., Hladikova M. Efficacy and tolerability of propolis special extract GH 2002 as a lip balm against *Herpes labialis*: a randomized, double-blind three-arm dose finding study Treatment of *Herpes labialis* by propolis lip balm. *Health*. 2011;3:49-56.

[101] Yoshizumi K., Nishioka N., Tsuji T. The xanthine oxidase inhibitory activity and hypouricemia effect of the propolis in rats. *Yakugaku Zasshi*. 2005;125:315-321.

[102] Garedew A., Lamprecht I., Schmolz E., Schricker B. The varroacidal action of propolis: a laboratory assay. *Apidologie*. 2002;33:41–50.

[103] El-Fadaly H., El-Badrawy E. E. Y. Flavonoids of propolis and their antibacterial activities. *Pakistan Journal of Biological Sciences*. 2001;4:204-207.

[104] Stepanovic S., Antic N., Dakic I., Svabic-Vlahovic M. In vitro antimicrobial activity of propolis and synergism between propolis and antimicrobial drugs. *Microbiological Research*. 2003;158:353-357.

[105] Garedew A., Schmolz E., Lamprecht I. Microbiological and calorimetric investigations on the antimicrobial actions of different propolis extracts: an *in vitro* approach. *Thermochimica Acta*. 2004;422:115-124.

[106] Boyanova L., Kolarov R., Gergova G., Mitov I. In vitro activity of Bulgarian propolis against 94 clinical isolates of anaerobic bacteria. *Anaerobe*. 2006;12:173-177.

[107] Scazzocchio F., D'Auria F. D., Alessandrini D., Pantanella F. Multifactorial aspects of antimicrobial activity of propolis. *Microbiological Research*. 2006;161:327-333.

[108] Silici S., Unlu M., Vardar-Unlu G. Antibacterial activity and phytochemical evidence for the plant origin of Turkish propolis from different regions. *World Journal of Microbiology and Biotechnology*. 2007;23:1797-1803.

[109] Yaghoubi M. J., Ghorbani G., Zad S. S., Satari R. Antimicrobial activity of Iranian propolis and its chemical composition. *DARU Journal of Pharmaceutical Sciences*. 2007;15:45-48.

[110] Marghitas L. A., Mihai C. M., Chirila F., Dezmirean D. S., Fit N. The study of the antimicrobial activity of Transylvanian (Romanian) propolis. *Notulae Botanicae Horti Agrobotanici Cluj-Napoca*. 2010;38:40-44.

[111] Campana R., Patrone V., Franzini I. T., Diamantini G., Vittoria E., Baffone W. Antimicrobial activity of two propolis samples against human *Campylobacter jejuni*. *Journal of Medicinal Food*. 2009;12:1050-1056.

[112] Boyanova L., Derejian S., Koumanova R., Katsarov N., Gergova G., Mitov I., Nikolov R., Krastev Z. Inhibition of *Helicobacter pylori* growth *in vitro* by Bulgarian propolis: preliminary report. *Journal of Medical Microbiology*. 2003;52:417–419.

[113] Boyanova L., Gergova G., Nikolov R., Derejian S., Lazarova E., Katsarov N., Mitov I., Krastev Z. Activity of Bulgarian propolis against 94 *Helicobacter pylori* strains *in vitro* by agar-well diffusion, agar dilution and disc diffusion methods. *Journal of Medical Microbiology*. 2005;54:481-483.

[114] Nostro A., Cellini L., Di Bartolomeo S., Di Campli E., Grande R., Cannatelli M. A., Marzio L., Alonzo V. Antibacterial effect of plant extracts against *Helicobacter pylori*. *Phytotherapy Research*. 2005;19:198-202.

[115] Uzel A., Sorkun K., Oncag O., Cogulu D., Gencay O., Salih B. Chemical compositions and antimicrobial activities of four different Anatolian propolis samples. *Microbiological Research*. 2005;160:189-195.

[116] Koru O., Toksoy F., Acikel C. H., Tunca Y. M., Baysallar M., Guclu A. U., Akca E., Tuylu A. O., Sorkun K., Tanyuksel M., Salih B. *In vitro* antimicrobial activity of propolis samples from different geographical origins against certain oral pathogens. *Anaerobe*. 2007;13:140-145.

[117] Liberio S. A., Pereira A. L. A., Araujo M. J. A. M., Dutra R. P., Nascimento F. R. F., Monteiro-Neto V., Ribeiro M. N. S., Goncalves A. G., Guerra R. N. M. The potential use of propolis as a cariostatic agent and its actions on mutans group streptococci. *Journal of Ethnopharmacology*. 2009;125:1-9.

[118] Saavedra N., Barrientos L., Herrera C. L., Alvear M., Montenegro G., Salazar L. A. Effect of Chilean propolis on cariogenic bacteria *Lactobacillus fermentum*. *Ciencia e Investigacion Agraria*. 2011;38:117-125.

[119] Kosalec I., Pepeljnjak S., Bakmaz M., Vladimir-Knezevic S. Flavonoid analysis and antimicrobial activity of commercially available propolis products. *Acta Pharmaceutica*. 2005;55:423-430.

[120] Popova M., Silici S., Kaftanoglu O., Bankova V. Antibacterial activity of Turkish propolis and its qualitative and quantitative chemical composition. *Phytomedicine*. 2005;12:221-228.

[121] Kujumgiev A., Bankova V., Ignatova A., Popov S. Antibacterial activity of propolis, some of its components and their analogues. *Pharmazie*. 1993;48:785-786.

[122] Chaillou L. L., Nazareno M. A. Bioactivity of propolis from Santiago del Estero, Argentina, related to their chemical composition. *LWT- Food Science and Technology*. 2009;42:1422-1427.

[123] Kacaniova M., Melich M., Knazovicka V., Felsociova S., Sudzinova J. The antimicrobial activity of honey and propolis against yeasts *Candida* species. *Lucrari Stiintifice Zootehnie si Biotehnologii*. 2009;42:167-173.

[124] Herrera C. L., Alvear M., Barrientos L., Montenegro G., Salazar L. A. The antifungal effect of six commercial extracts of Chilean propolis on *Candida* spp. *Ciencia e Investigacion Agraria*. 2010;37:75-84.

[125] Buchta V., Cerny J., Opletalova V. In vitro antifungal activity of propolis samples of Czech and Slovak origin. *Central Europe*. 2011;6:160-166.

[126] Yang S., Peng L., Cheng Y., Chen F., Pan S. Control of Citrus green and blue molds by Chinese propolis. *Food Science and Biotechnology*. 2010;19:1303-1308.

[127] Bonvehi J. S., Coll F. V. Phenolic composition of propolis from China and from South America. Zeitschrift für Naturforschung. 1994;49c:712–718.

[128] Ahn M. R., Kumazawa S., Hamasaka T., Bang K. S., Nakayama T. Antioxidant activity and constituents of propolis collected in various areas of Korea. *Journal of Agricultural and Food Chemistry*. 2004;52:7286–7292.

[129] Jasprica I., Bojic M., Mornar A., Besic E., Bucan K., Medic-Saric M. Evaluation of antioxidative activity of Croatian propolis samples using DPPH$^{\cdot}$ and ABTS$^{\cdot+}$ stable free radical assays. *Molecules*. 2007;12:1006-1021.

[130] Rzepecka-Stojko A., Kurek-Gorecka A., Maciejewska-Paszek I., Stec M., Pawlowska-Goral K., Gastolek-Soltysik K. The determination of flavonoid content of ethanol

extracts of propolis and the antioxidant capacity of flavonoids. *Farmaceutyczny Przeglad Naukowy*. 2009;11:33-36.

[131] Gregoris E., Stevanato R. Correlations between polyphenolic composition and antioxidant activity of Venetian propolis. *Food and Chemical Toxicology*. 2010;48:76-82.

[132] Savickas A., Ramanauskiene K., Pukalskas A., Kasparaviciene G., Briedis V., Inkeniene A., Zilius M., Kasparavicius S. The influence of solvent on the quantity and antioxidant activity of ethanolic extracts of Lithuanian propolis. *Chemija*. 2010;21:118-122.

[133] Mot A. C., Silaghi-Dumitrescu R., Sarbu C. Rapid and effective evaluation of the antioxidant capacity of propolis extracts using DPPH bleaching kinetic profiles, FT-IR and UV—vis spectroscopic data. *Journal of Food Composition and Analysis*. 2011;24:516-522.

[134] Sulaiman G. M., Al Sammarrae K. W., Ad'hiah A. H., Zucchetti M., Frapolli R., Bello E., Erba E., D'Incalci M., Bagnati R. Chemical characterization of Iraqi propolis samples and assessing their antioxidant potentials. *Food and Chemical Toxicology*. 2011;49:2415-2421.

[135] Yang H, Dong Y, Du H, Shi H, Peng Y, Li X. Antioxidant compounds from propolis collected in Anhui, China. *Molecules*. 2011;16:3444-3455.

[136] Sobocanec S., Sverko V., Balog T., Saric A., Rusak G., Likic S., Kusic B., Katalinic V., Radic S., Marotti T. Oxidant/antioxidant properties of Croatian native propolis. *Journal of Agricultural and Food Chemistry*. 2006;54:8018–8026.

[137] Katalinic V., Radic S., Ropac D., Mulic R., Katalinic A. Antioxidative activity of propolis from Dalmatia (Croatia). *Acta Medica Croatica*. 2004;58:373-376.

[138] Zunini M. P., Rojas C., de Paula S., Elingold I., Migliaro E. A., Casanova M. B., Restuccia F. I., Morales S. A., Dubin M. Phenolic contents and antioxidant activity in Central-Southern Uruguayan propolis extracts. *Journal of the Chilean Chemical Society*. 2010;55:141-146.

[139] Mot A. C., Damian G., Sarbu C., Silaghi-Dumitrescu R. Redox reactivity in propolis: direct detection of free radicals in basic medium and interaction with hemoglobin. *Redox Report*. 2009;14:267-274.

[140] Jasprica I., Mornar A., Debeljak Z., Smolcic-Bubalo A., Medic-Saric M., Mayer L., Romic Z., Bucan K., Balog T., Sobocanec S., Sverko V. *In vivo* study of propolis supplementation effects on antioxidative status and red blood cells. *Journal of Ethnopharmacology*. 2007;110:548-554.

[141] Orsolic N., Terzic S., Sver L., Basic I. Polyphenolic compounds from propolis modulate immune responses and increase host resistance to tumour cells. *Food and Agricultural Immunology*. 2005;16:165-179.

[142] Grunberger D., Banerjee R., Eisinger K., Oltz E. M., Efros L., Caldwell M., Estevez V., Nakanishi K. Preferential cytotoxicity on tumor cells by caffeic acid phenethyl ester isolated from propolis. *Cellular and Molecular Life Sciences*. 1988;44:230-232.

[143] Borrelli F., Capasso F. CAPE, a constituent of propolis: a mini review. *Honeybee Science*. 2003;24:67-70.

[144] Bankova V. Chemical diversity of propolis makes it a valuable source of new biologically active compounds. *Journal of ApiProduct and ApiMedical Science*. 2009;1:23-28.

[145] Bankova V., Popova M., Bogdanov S., Sabatini A. G. Chemical composition of European propolis: expected and unexpected results. *Zeitschrift für Naturforschung*. 2002;57c:530-533.

[146] Popova M., Bankova V., Butovska D., Petkov V., Nikolova-Damyanova B., Sabatini A. G., Marcazzan G. L., Bogdanov S. Validated methods for the quantification of biologically active constituents of poplar type propolis. *Phytochemical Analysis*. 2004;15:235-240.

[147] Marostica Junior M. R., Daugsch A., Moraes C. S., Queiroga C. L., Pastore G. M., Park Y. K. Comparison of volatile and polyphenolic compounds in Brazilian green propolis and its botanical origin *Baccharis dracunculifolia*. *Ciencia e Tecnologia de Alimentos*. 2008;28:178-181.

[148] Marcucci M. C., Bankova V. S. Chemical composition, plant origin and biological activity of Brazilian propolis. *Current Topics in Phytochemistry*. 1999;2:115-123.

[149] Jorge R., Furtado N. A. J. C., Sousa J. P. B., da Silva A. A., Gregorio Jr. L. E., Martins C. H. G., Soares A. E. E., Bastos J. K., Cunha W. R., Silva M. L. A. Brazilian propolis: seasonal variation of the prenylated p-coumaric acids and antimicrobial activity. *Pharmaceutical Biology*. 2008;46:889-893.

[150] Salomao K., Pereira P. R. S., Campos L. C., Borba C. M., Cabello P. H., Marcucci M. C., de Castro S. L. Brazilian propolis: correlation between chemical composition and antimicrobial activity. *Evidence-Based Complementary and Alternative Medicine*. 2008;5:317–324.

[151] Neto T. M. S., Mota R. A., Silva L. B. G., Viana D. A., Lima-Filho J. Susceptibility of *Staphylococcus* spp. isolated from milk of goats with mastitis to antibiotics and green propolis extracts. *Letters in Drug Design and Discovery*. 2009;6:63-68.

[152] Oliveira A. P., Franca H. S., Kuster R. M., Teixeira L. A., Rocha L. M. Chemical composition and antibacterial activity of Brazilian propolis essential oil. *Journal of Venomous Animals and Toxins Including Tropical Diseases*. 2010;16:121-130.

[153] da Silva K. R., Mathias F. T., Dutra K. A., Kleinubing S. D., Santa H. S. D., da Rosa M. R., Buriol L., Torres Y. R., Monteiro M. C. Antimicrobial activity from a brazilian propolis oily extract compared with other propolis extracts. *Revista Ciencias Exatas e Naturais*. 2010;12: http://revistas.unicentro.br/index.php/RECEN/article/view/964/1099.

[154] Mello A. M., Gomes R. T., Lara S. R., Silva L. G., Alves J. B., Cortés M. E., Abreu S. L., Santos V. R. The effect of Brazilian propolis on the germ tube formation and cell wall of *Candida albicans*. *Pharmacologyonline*. 2006;3:352-358.

[155] Siqueira A. B. S., Gomes B. S., Cambuim I., Maia R., Abreu S., Souza-Motta C. M., de Queiroz L. A., Porto A. L. F. Trichophyton species susceptibility to green and red propolis from Brazil. *Letters in Applied Microbiology*. 2009;48:90-96.

[156] Fernandes F. F., Dias A. L., Ramos C. L., Ikegaki M., Siqueira A. M., Franco M. C. The "in vitro" antifungal activity evaluation of propolis G12 ethanol extract on *Cryptococcus neoformans*. *Revista do Instituto de Medicina Tropical de Sao Paulo*. 2007;49:93-95.

[157] Ioshida M. D. M., Young M. C. M., Lago J. H. G. Chemical composition and antifungal activity of essential oil from Brazilian propolis. *Journal of Essential Oil-Bearing Plants*. 2010;13:633-637.

[158] Banskota A. H., Tezuka Y., Adnyana I. K., Ishii E., Midorikawa K., Matsushige K., Kadota S. Hepatoprotective and anti-*Helicobacter pylori* activities of constituents from Brazilian propolis. *Phytomedicine*. 2001;8:16-23.

[159] Coelho L. G. V., Bastos E. M. F., Resende C. C., e Silva C. M. P., Sanches B. S. F., de Castro F. J., Moretzsohn L. D., Vieira W. L. D. S., Trindade O. R. Brazilian green propolis on *Helicobacter pylori* infection. A pilot clinical study. *Helicobacter*. 2007;12:572-574.

[160] Santos F. A., Bastos E. M. A., Uzeda M., Carvalho M. A. R., Farias L. M., Moreira E. S. A., Braga F. C. Antibacterial activity of Brazilian propolis and fractions against oral anaerobic bacteria. *Journal of Ethnopharmacology*. 2002;80:1-7.

[161] Santos. F. A., Bastos E. M. A. F., Maia A. B. R. A., Uzeda M., Carvalho M. A. R., Farias L. M., Moreira E. S. A. Brazilian propolis: physicochemical properties, plant origin and antibacterial activity on periodontopathogens. *Phytotherapy Research*. 2003;17:285–289.

[162] Hayacibara M. F., Koo H., Rosalen P. L., Duarte S., Franco E. M., Bowen W. H., Ikegaki M., Cury J. A. *In vitro* and *in vivo* effects of isolated fractions of Brazilian propolis on caries development. *Journal of Ethnopharmacology*. 2005;101:110-115.

[163] Costa E. M. M. B., Esmeraldo M. R. A., de Carvalho M. G. F., Daniel R. L. D. P., Pastro M. F., da Silva Jr. F. L. Evaluation of the antimicrobial action of propolis and substances used in endodontics against *Enterococcus faecalis*. *Pesquisa Brasileira em Odontopediatria e Clinica Integrada*. 2008;8:21-25.

[164] Santos VR, Pimenta FJ, Aguiar MC, do Carmo MA, Naves MD, Mesquita RA. Oral candidiasis treatment with Brazilian ethanol propolis extract. *Phytotherapy Research*. 2005;19:652-654.

[165] Do Amaral RC, Gomes RT, Rocha WMS, Abreu SLR, Santos VR. Periodontitis treatment with Brazilian green propolis gel. *Pharmacologyonline*. 2006;3:336-341.

[166] Santos V. R., Gomes R. T., Mesquita R. A., Moura M. D., França E. C., Aguiar E. G., Naves M. D., Abreu J. A., Abreu S. R. Efficacy of Brazilian propolis gel for the management of denture stomatitis: a pilot study. *Phytotherapy Research*. 2008;22:1544-1547.

[167] Valera M. C., da Rosa J. A., Maekawa L. E., de Oliveira L. D., Carvalho C. A., Koga-Ito C. Y., Jorge A. O. Action of propolis and medications against *Escherichia coli* and endotoxin in root canals. *Oral Surgery Oral Medicine Oral Pathology Oral Radiology and Endodontics*. 2010;110:70-74.

[168] Bastos E. M., Simone M., Jorge D. M., Soares A. E., Spivak M. *In vitro* study of the antimicrobial activity of Brazilian propolis against *Paenibacillus larvae*. *Journal of Invertebrate Pathology*. 2008;97:273-281.

[169] Pinto M. S., de Faria J. E., Message D., Cassini S. T. A., Pereira C. S., Gioso M. M. Effect of green propolis extracts on patogenic bacteria isolated from milk of cows with mastitis. *Brazilian Journal of Veterinary Research and Animal Science*. 2001;38:278-283.

[170] Da Silva J. F. M., De Souza M. C., Matta S. R., De Andrade M. R., Vidal F. V. N. Correlation analysis between phenolic levels of Brazilian propolis extracts and their antimicrobial and antioxidant activities. *Food Chemistry*. 2006;99:431-435.

[171] Nogueira M. A., Diaz M. G., Tagami P. M., Lorscheide J. Antimicrobial activity of essential oils and propolis against oral pathogens. *Journal of Basic and Applied Pharmaceutical Sciences*. 2007;28:93-97.

[172] Farnesi A. P., Aquino-Ferreira R., De Jong D., Bastos J. K., Soares A. E. Effects of stingless bee and honey bee propolis on four species of bacteria. *Genetics and Molecular Research*. 2009;8:635-640.

[173] Feresin G. E., Tapia A., Gimenez A., Ravelo A. G., Zacchino S., Sortino M., Schmeda-Hirschmann G. Constituents of the Argentinian medicinal plant *Baccharis grisebachii* and their antimicrobial activity. *Journal of Ethnopharmacology*. 2003;89:73-80.

[174] Dota K. F. D., Faria M. G., Bruschi M. L., Pelloso S. M., Lopes-Consolaro M. E., Svidzinski T. I. Antifungal activity of propolis extract against yeasts isolated from vaginal exudates. *Journal of Alternative and Complementary Medicine*. 2010;16:285-290.

[175] Dota K. F., Consolaro M. E., Svidzinski T. I., Bruschi M. L. Antifungal activity of Brazilian propolis microparticles against yeasts isolated from vulvovaginal candidiasis. *Evidence-Based Complementary and Alternative Medicine*. 2011;2011:201953.

[176] Shimizu T., Hino A., Tsutsumi A., Park Y. K., Watanabe W., Kurokawa M. Anti-influenza virus activity of propolis *in vitro* and its efficacy against influenza infection in mice. *Antiviral Chemistry and Chemotherapy*. 2008;19:7-13.

[177] Bufalo M. C., Figueiredo A. S., de Sousa J. P. B., Candeias J. M. G., Bastos J. K., Sforcin J. M. Anti-poliovirus activity of *Baccharis dracunculifolia* and propolis by cell viability determination and real-time PCR. *Journal of Applied Microbiology*. 2009;107:1669-1680.

[178] Shimizu T., Takeshita Y., Takamori Y., Kai H., Sawamura R., Yoshida H., Watanabe W., Tsutsumi A., Park Y.. K., Yasukawa K., Matsuno K., Shiraki K., Kurokawa M. Efficacy of Brazilian propolis against Herpes Simplex Virus Type 1 infection in mice and their modes of antiherpetic efficacies. *Evidence-Based Complementary and Alternative Medicine*. 2011;2011:976196.

[179] Urushisaki T., Takemura T., Tazawa S., Fukuoka M., Hosokawa-Muto J., Araki Y., Kuwata K. Caffeoylquinic acids are major constituents with potent anti-influenza effects in Brazilian green propolis water extract. *Evidence-Based Complementary and Alternative Medicine*. 2011;2011:254914.

[180] Ayres D. C., Marcucci M. C., Giorgio S. Effects of Brazilian propolis on *Leishmania amazonensis*. *Memorias do Instituto Oswaldo Cruz*. 2007;102:215-220.

[181] Pontin K., Filho A. A. S., Santos F. F., Silva M. L., Cunha W. R., Nanayakkara N. P., Bastos J. K., de Albuquerque S. *In vitro* and *in vivo* antileishmanial activities of a Brazilian green propolis extract. *Parasitology Research*. 2008;103:487-492.

[182] Salomao K., de Souza E. M., Barbosa H. S., de Castro S. L. Propolis and derivatives of megazol: *In vitro* and *in vivo* activity on *Trypanosoma cruzi*, mechanism of action and selectivity. *International Journal of Infectious Diseases*. 2010;14 Suppl 1:e441-e442.

[183] De Castro S. L., Salomao K., de Souza E. M., Henriques-Pons A., Barbosa H. S. Brazilian green propolis: effects *in vitro* and *in vivo* on *Trypanosoma cruzi*. *Evidence-Based Complementary and Alternative Medicine*. 2011;2011:185918.

[184] Banskota A. H., Tezuka Y., Midorikawa K., Matsushige K., Kadota S. Two novel cytotoxic benzofuran derivatives from Brazilian propolis. *Journal of Natural Products*. 2000;63:1277-1279.

[185] Kimoto T., Koya S., Hino K., Yamamoto Y., Nomura Y., Micallef M. J., Hanaya T., Arai S., Ikeda M., Kurimoto M. Renal carcinogenesis induced by ferric nitrilotriacetate in mice, and protection from it by Brazilian propolis and Artepillin C. *Pathology International*. 2000;50:679–689.
[186] Kimoto T., Aga M., Hino K., Koya-Miyata S., Yamamoto Y., Micallef M. J., Hanaya T., Arai S., Ikeda M., Kurimoto M. Apoptosis of human leukemia cells induced by Artepillin C, an active ingredient of Brazilian propolis. *Anticancer Research*. 2001;21:221-228.
[187] Kimoto T., Koya-Miyata S., Hino K., Micallef M. J., Hanaya T., Arai S., Ikeda M., Kurimoto M. Pulmonary carcinogenesis induced by ferric nitrilotriacetate in mice and protection from it by Brazilian propolis and artepillin C. *Virchows Archiv*. 2001;438:259-270.
[188] Luo J., Soh J. W., Xing W. Q., Mao Y., Matsuno T., Weinstein I. B. PM-3, a benzo-gamma-pyran derivative isolated from propolis, inhibits growth of MCF-7 human breast cancer cells. *Anticancer Research*. 2001;21:1665-1671.
[189] Mishima S., Inoh Y., Narita Y., Ohta S., Sakamoto T., Araki Y., Suzuki K. M., Akao Y., Nozawa Y. Identification of caffeoylquinic acid derivatives from Brazilian propolis as constituents involved in induction of granulocytic differentiation of HL-60 cells. *Bioorganic and Medicinal Chemistry*. 2005;13:5814-5818.
[190] Mishima S., Narita Y., Chikamatsu S., Inoh Y., Ohta S., Yoshida C., Araki Y., Akao Y., Suzuki K., Nozawa Y. Effects of propolis on cell growth and gene expression in HL-60 cells. *Journal of Ethnopharmacology*. 2005;99:5-11.
[191] Mishima S., Ono Y., Araki Y., Akao Y., Nozawa Y. Two related cinnamic acid derivatives from Brazilian honey bee propolis, baccharin and drupanin, induce growth inhibition in allografted sarcoma S-180 in mice. *Biological and Pharmaceutical Bulletin*. 2005;28:1025-1030.
[192] Shimizu K., Suzuki Y., Hashiguchi M., Hashiguchi T. Anti-tumor cell activity of water-dispersible propolis. *Journal of Tokyo Medical University*. 2006;64:153-158.
[193] Ahn M. R., Kunimasa K., Ohta T., Kumazawa S., Kamihira M., Kaji K., Uto Y., Hori H., Nagasawa H., Nakayama T. Suppression of tumor-induced angiogenesis by Brazilian propolis: Major component artepillin C inhibits in vitro tube formation and endothelial cell proliferation. *Cancer Letters*. 2007;252:235-243.
[194] Chen C. R., Lee Y. N., Chang C. M. J., Lee M. R., Wei I. C. Hot-pressurized fluid extraction of flavonoids and phenolic acids from Brazilian propolis and their cytotoxic assay in vitro. *Journal of the Chinese Institute of Chemical Engineers*. 2007;38:191-196.
[195] Li H., Kapur A., Yang J. X., Srivastava S., McLeod D. G., Paredes-Guzman J. F., Daugsch A., Park Y. K., Rhim J. S. Antiproliferation of human prostate cancer cells by ethanolic extracts of Brazilian propolis and its botanical origin. *International Journal of Oncology*. 2007;31:601-606.
[196] Yasui Y, Miyamoto S, Kim M, Kohno H, Sugie S, Tanaka T. Aqueous and ethanolic extract fractions from the Brazilian propolis suppress azoxymethane-induced aberrant crypt foci in rats. *Oncology Reports*. 2008;20:493-499.
[197] Buriol L., Finger D., Schmidt E. S., dos Santos J. M. T., da Rosa M. R., Quinaia S. P., Torres Y. R., Santa H. S. D., Pessoa C., de Moraes M. O., Costa-Lotufo L. V., Ferreira P. M. P., Sawaya A. C. H. F., Eberlin M. N. Chemical composition and biological

activity of oil propolis extract: an alternative to ethanolic extract. *Quimica Nova*. 2009;32:296-302.

[198] Chen C. R., Lee Y. N., Lee M. R., Chang C. M. J. Supercritical fluids extraction of cinnamic acid derivatives from Brazilian propolis and the effect on growth inhibition of colon cancer cells. *Journal of the Taiwan*. 2009;40:130-135.

[199] Messerli S. M., Ahn M. R., Kunimasa K., Yanagihara M., Tatefuji T., Hashimoto K., Mautner V., Uto Y., Hori H., Kumazawa S., Kaji K., Ohta T., Maruta H. Artepillin C (ARC) in Brazilian green propolis selectively blocks oncogenic PAK1 signaling and suppresses the growth of NF tumors in mice. *Phytotherapy Research*. 2009;23:423-427.

[200] Paulino N., Abreu S. R. L., Machado G., Silveira E. Scientific evidences to pharmacological anticancer action of *Baccharis dracunculifolia* Brazilian propolis. *Revista de Pesquisa e Inovacao Farmaceutica*. 2009;1:15-26.

[201] Wu J. J., Shen C. T., Jong T. T., Young, C. C., Yang H. L., Hsu S. L., Chang C. M. J., Shieh CJ. Supercritical carbon dioxide anti-solvent process for purification of micronized propolis particulates and associated anti-cancer activity. *Separation and Purification Technology*. 2009;70:190-198.

[202] Bufalo M. C., Candeias J. M., Sousa J. P., Bastos J. K., Sforcin J. M. In vitro cytotoxic activity of *Baccharis dracunculifolia* and propolis against HEp-2 cells. *Natural Products Research*. 2010;24:1710-1718.

[203] Moraes C. S., Daugsch A., Li H., Rhim J. S., Park Y. K. Comparative antiproliferation of human prostate cancer cells by ethanolic extracts of two groups of Brazilian propolis. *Ciencia e Tecnologia de Alimentos*. 2010;30:539-543.

[204] Carvalho A. A., Finger D., Machado C. S., Schmidt E. M., Costa P. M., Alves A. P. N. N., Morais T. M. F., Queiroz M. G. R., Quináia S. P., Rosa M. R., Santos J. M. T., Pessoa C., Moraes M.O., Costa-Lotufo L. V., Sawaya A. C. H. F., Eberlin M. N., Torres Y. R. *In vivo* antitumoural activity and composition of an oil extract of Brazilian propolis. *Food Chemistry*. 2011;126:1239-1245.

[205] Cavalcante D. R. R., de Oliveira P. S., Gois S. M., Soares A. F., Cardoso J. C., Padilha F. F., de Albuquerque Júnior RLC. Effect of green propolis on oral epithelial dysplasia in rats. *Brazilian Journal of Otorhynolaryngology*. 2011;77:278-284.

[206] Kunimasa K., Ahn M. R., Kobayashi T., Eguchi R., Kumazawa S., Fujimori Y., Nakano T., Nakayama T., Kaji K., Ohta T. Brazilian propolis suppresses angiogenesis by inducing apoptosis in tube-forming endothelial cells through inactivation of survival signal ERK1/2. *Evidence-Based Complementary and Alternative Medicine*. 2011;2011:870753.

[207] Szliszka E., Zydowicz G., Janoszka B., Dobosz C., Kowalczyk-Ziomek G., Krol W. Ethanolic extract of Brazilian green propolis sensitizes prostate cancer cells to TRAIL-induced apoptosis. *International Journal of Oncology*. 2011;38:941-953.

[208] Xuan H., Zhao J., Miao J., Li Y., Chu Y., Hu F. Effect of Brazilian propolis on human umbilical vein endothelial cell apoptosis. *Food and Chemical Toxicology*. 2011;49:78-85.

[209] Shinohara R., Ohta Y., Hayashi T., Ikeno T. Evaluation of antilipid peroxidative action of propolis ethanol extract. *Phytotherapy Research*. 2002;16:340–347.

[210] Nakanishi I., Uto Y., Ohkubo K., Miyazaki K., Yakumaru H., Urano S., Okuda H., Ueda J. I., Ozawa T., Fukuhara K., Fukuzumi S., Nagasawa H., Hori H., Ikota N.

Efficient radical scavenging ability of artepillin C, a major component of Brazilian propolis, and the mechanism. *Organic and Biomolecular Chemistry*. 2003;1:1452-1454.

[211] Simoes L. M., Gregorio L. E., Filho A. A. S., De Souza M. L., Azzolini A. E. C. S., Bastos J. K., Lucisano-Valim Y. M. Effect of Brazilian green propolis on the production of reactive oxygen species by stimulated neutrophils. *Journal of Ethnopharmacology*. 2004;94:59-65.

[212] Shimizu K., Ashida H., Matsuura Y., Kanazawa K. Antioxidative bioavailability of artepillin C in Brazilian propolis. *Archives of Biochemistry and Biophysics*. 2004;424:181-188.

[213] Marquele F. D., Di Mambro V. M., Georgetti S. R., Casagrande R., Valim Y. M. L., Fonseca M. J. V. Assessment of the antioxidant activities of Brazilian extracts of propolis alone and in topical pharmaceutical formulations. *Journal of Pharmaceutical and Biomedical Analysis*. 2005;39:455-462.

[214] Nakajima Y., Shimazawa M., Mishima S., Hara H. Water extract of propolis and its main constituents, caffeoylquinic acid derivatives, exert neuroprotective effects via antioxidant actions. *Life Sciences*. 2006;80:370-377.

[215] Sheng J., Zhou J., Wang L., Xu J., Hu Q. Antioxidant activity of ethanol and petroleum ether extracts from Brazilian propolis. *European Food Research and Technology*. 2007;225:249-253.

[216] Souza J. P. B., Tacon L. A., Correia C. C., Bastos J. K., Freitas L. A. P. Spray-dried propolis extract, II: Prenylated components of green propolis. *Pharmazie*. 2007;62:488–492.

[217] Nakanishi I., Uto Y., Ohkubo K., Kawashima T., Manda S., Matsumoto K., Hori H., Fukuhara K., Okuda H., Ikota N., Fukuzumi S., Ozawa T., Anzai K. Structure-activity relationship in radical-scavenging reactions of naturally-oriented Artepillin C derivatives. In: *Proceedings of the 14th Biennial Meeting of the Society for Free Radical Research International*. Beijing, China, 18-22 Oct 2008. 2008:125-128.

[218] Izuta H., Narahara Y., Shimazawa M., Mishima S., Kondo S., Hara H. 1,1-Diphenyl-2-picrylhydrazyl radical scavenging activity of bee products and their constituents determined by ESR. *Biological and Pharmaceutical Bulletin*. 2009;32:1947-1951.

[219] Simoes- Ambrosio L. M., Gregorio L. E., Sousa J. P., Figueiredo A. S., Azzolini A. E., Bastos J. K., Lucisano-Valim Y. M. The role of seasonality on the inhibitory effect of Brazilian green propolis on the oxidative metabolism of neutrophils. *Fitoterapia*. 2010;81:1102-1108.

[220] Teixeira E. W., Message D., Negri G., Salatino A., Stringheta P. C. Seasonal variation, chemical composition and antioxidant activity of Brazilian propolis samples. *Evidence-Based Complementary and Alternative Medicine*. 2010;7:307-315.

[221] Cottica S. M., Sawaya A. C. H. F., Eberlin M. N., Franco S. L., Zeoula L. M., Visentainer J. V. Antioxidant activity and composition of propolis obtained by different methods of extraction. *Journal of the Brazilian Chemical Society*. 2011;22:929-935.

[222] Rocha B. A., Rodrigues M. R., Bueno P. C. P., Costa-Machado A. R. M., Vaz M. M. O. L. L., Nascimento A. P., Barud H. S., Berretta-Silva A. A. Preparation and thermal characterization of inclusion complex of Brazilian green propolis and hydroxypropyl-β-cyclodextrin- Increased water solubility of the chemical constituents and antioxidant activity. *Journal of Thermal Analysis and Calorimetry*. 2011; DOI 10.1007/s10973-011-1713-4.

[223] Orsi RO, Sforcin JM, Funari SRC, Gomes JC. Effect of propolis extract on guinea pig lung mast cell. *Journal of Venomous Animals and Toxins including Tropical Deseases*. 2005;11:76-83.

[224] Paulino N., Teixeira C., Martins R., Scremin A,. Dirsch V. M., Vollmar A. M., Abreu S. R., de Castro S. L., Marcucci M. C. Evaluation of the analgesic and anti-inflammatory effects of a Brazilian green propolis. *Planta Medica*. 2006;72:899-906.

[225] Paulino N., Abreu S. R., Uto Y., Koyama D., Nagasawa H., Hori H., Dirsch V. M., Vollmar A. M., Scremin A., Bretz W. A. Anti-inflammatory effects of a bioavailable compound, Artepillin C, in Brazilian propolis. *European Journal of Pharmacology*. 2008;587:296-301.

[226] Orsatti C. L., Missima F., Pagliarone A. C., Sforcin J. M. Th1/Th 2 cytokines' expression and production by propolis-treated mice. *Journal of Ethnopharmacology*. 2010;129:314-318.

[227] Tani H., Hasumi K., Tatefuji T., Hashimoto K., Koshino H., Takahashi S. Inhibitory activity of Brazilian green propolis components and their derivatives on the release of cys-leukotrienes. *Bioorganic and Medicinal Chemistry*. 2010;18:151-157.

[228] Moura S. A. L., Ferreira M. A. N. D., Andrade S. P., Reis M. L. C., Noviello M. L., Cara D. C. Brazilian green propolis inhibits inflammatory angiogenesis in a murine sponge model. *Evidence-Based Complementary and Alternative Medicine*. 2011;2011:182703.

[229] Mezadri T. J., Leite M. F., Staack Jr. M. C., Colchon P. H., Balan A. B., Zanatta M. L., Costa I. C., Perin C., Tames D. R., Sousa J. P. B., Bastos J. K., Andrade S. F. Evaluation of the contraction of cutaneous wounds in Wistar rats treated with Brazilian green propolis gel. *Latin America*. 2009;28:762-767.

[230] Moura S. A. L., Negri G., Salatino A., Lima L. D. C., Dourado L. P. A., Mendes J. B., Andrade S. P., Ferreira M. A. N. D., Cara D. C. Aqueous extract of Brazilian green propolis: primary components, evaluation of inflammation and wound healing by using subcutaneous implanted sponges. *Evidence-Based Complementary and Alternative Medicine*. 2011;2011:748283.

[231] Staak Jr. M. C., Colchon P. H., Portes A. G., Mezadri T. J., Tames D. R., Andrade S. F. Histological evaluation on Brazilian green propolis effect in tissue repair of Wistar rats cutaneous wounds. *Latin American Journal of Pharmacy*. 2011;30:383-387.

[232] Reis G. S., Valadao A. F., Lima L. R. P., Moreira M. L. Preparation of a sunscreen and evaluation of the photoprotective action of the green propolis from Vale do Aço, Minas Gerais, Brazil. *Boletin Latinoamericano y del Caribe de Plantas Medicinales y Aromaticas*. 2009;8:282-288.

[233] Fonseca Y. M., Marquele-Oliveira F., Vicentini F. T., Furtado N. A., Sousa J. P., Lucisano-Valim Y. M., Fonseca M. J. Evaluation of the potential of Brazilian propolis against UV-induced oxidative stress. *Evidence-Based Complementary and Alternative Medicine*. 2011;2011:863917.

[234] Sa-Nunes A., Faccioli L. H., Sforcin J. M. Propolis: lymphocyte proliferation and IFN-γ production. *Journal of Ethnopharmacology*. 2003;87:93-97.

[235]Missima F., Sforcin J. M. Green Brazilian propolis action on macrophages and lymphoid organs of chronically stressed mice. *Evidence-Based Complementary and Alternative Medicine*. 2008;5:71-75.

[236] Pagliarone A. C., Missima F., Orsatti C. L., Bachiega T. F., Sforcin J. M. Propolis effect on Th1/Th2 cytokines production by acutely stressed mice. *Journal of Ethnopharmacology*. 2009;125:230-233.
[237] Pagliarone A. C., Orsatti C. L., Bufalo M. C., Missima F., Bachiega T. F., Junior J. P., Sforcin J. M. Propolis effects on pro-inflammatory cytokines production and Toll-like receptors 2 and 4 expression in stressed mice. *International Immunopharmacology*. 2009;9:1352-1356.
[238] Fischer G., Paulino N., Marcucci M. C., Siedler B. S., Munhoz L. S., Finger P. F., Vargas G. D., Hubner S. O., Vidor T., Roehe P. M. Green propolis phenolic compounds act as vaccine adjuvants, improving humoral and cellular responses in mice inoculated with inactivated vaccines. *Memorias do Instituto Oswaldo Cruz*. 2010;105:908-913.
[239] Orsatti C. L., Sforcin J. M. Propolis immunomodulatory activity on TLR-2 and TLR-4 expression by chronically stressed mice. *Natural Product Research*. 2011; DOI: 10.1080/14786419.2010.482049.
[240] Kubota Y., Umegaki K., Kobayashi K., Tanaka N., Kagota S., Nakamura K., Kunitomo M., Shinozuka K. Anti-hypertensive effects of brazilian propolis in spontaneously hypertensive rats. *Clinical and Experimental Pharmacology and Physiology*. 2004;31 Suppl 2:S29-30.
[241] Mishima S., Yoshida C., Akino S., Sakamoto T. Antihypertensive effects of Brazilian propolis: identification of caffeoylquinic acids as constituents involved in the hypotension in spontaneously hypertensive rats. *Biological and Pharmaceutical Bulletin*. 2005;28:1909-1914.
[242] Maruyama H., Sumitou Y., Sakamoto T., Araki Y., Hara H. Antihypertensive effects of flavonoids isolated from Brazilian green propolis in spontaneously hypertensive rats. *Biological and Pharmaceutical Bulletin*. 2009;32:1244-1250.
[243] Mesquita F. F., Rueda B. Z., Tardivo A. C., Alves M. J. Q. F. Effects of propolis flavonoids fraction on the cholesterol metabolism of rabbits with experimental hypercholesterolemia. *Revista Brasileira de Plantas Medicinais*. 2007;9:44-50.
[244] Alves M. J. Q. F., Mesquita F. F., Sakaguti M., Tardivo A. C. Hypocholesterolemic effect of propolis' caffeic acids. *Revista Brasileira de Plantas Medicinais*. 2008;10:100-105.
[245] Koya-Miyata S., Arai N., Mizote A., Taniguchi Y., Ushio S., Iwaki K., Fukuda S. Propolis prevents diet-induced hyperlipidemia and mitigates weight gain in diet-induced obesity in mice. *Biological and Pharmaceutical Bulletin*. 2009;32:2022-2028.
[246] El-Sayed S. M., Abo-Salem O. M., Aly H. A., Mansour A. M. Potential antidiabetic and hypolipidemic effects of propolis extract in streptozotocin-induced diabetic rats. *Pakistan Journal of Pharmaceutical Sciences*. 2009;22:168-174.
[247] Araki H., Jin C., Gomita Y., Doi S., Sugimoto H., Yamada H. The effect of Alecrim propolis on cyanide intoxication in mice. *Honeybee Science*. 2001;22:62-66.
[248] Fernandes A. A. H., Fernandes Jr. A., Novelli E. L. B. Effect of Brazilian propolis on experimental hepatotoxicity in rats. *Revista de Ciencias Farmaceuticas*. 2004;25:85-89.
[249] Park Y. K., Fukuda I., Ashida H., Nishiumi S., Yoshida K., Daugsch A., Sato H. H., Pastore G. M. Suppressive effects of ethanolic extracts from propolis and its main botanical origin on dioxin toxicity. *Journal of Agricultural and Food Chemistry*. 2005;53:10306-10309.

[250] Tavares D. C., Lira W. M., Santini C. B., Takahashi C. S., Bastos J..K. Effects of propolis crude hydroalcoholic extract on chromosomal aberrations induced by doxorubicin in rats. *Planta Medica*. 2007;73:1531-1536.

[251] Valadares B. L. B., Graf U., Spanó M. A. Inhibitory effects of water extract of propolis on doxorubicin-induced somatic mutation and recombination in *Drosophila melanogaster*. *Food and Chemical Toxicology*. 2008;46:1103-1110.

[252] Oliveira P. F., Neto M. A. B. M., Leandro L. F., Bastos J. K., Filho A. A. S., Tavares D. C. *In vivo* antigenotoxicity of baccharin, an important constituent of *Baccharis Dracunculifolia* DC (Asteraceae). *Basic and Clinical Pharmacology and Toxicology*. 2011;109:35-41.

[253] Shimazawa M., Chikamatsu S., Morimoto N., Mishima S., Nagai H., Hara H. Neuroprotection by Brazilian green propolis against *in vitro* and *in vivo* ischemic neuronal damage. *Evidence-Based Complementary and Alternative Medicine*. 2005;2:201-207.

[254] Inokuchi Y., Shimazawa M., Nakajima Y., Suemori S., Mishima S., Hara H. Brazilian green propolis protects against retinal damage *in vitro* and *in vivo*. *Evidence-Based Complementary and Alternative Medicicne*. 2006;3:71-77.

[255] Nakajima Y., Shimazawa M., Mishima S., Hara H. Neuroprotective effects of Brazilian green propolis and its main constituents against oxygen-glucose deprivation stress, with a gene-expression analysis. *Phytotherapy Research*. 2009;23:1431-1438.

[256] Barros M. P., Sousa J. P., Bastos J. K., de Andrade S. F. Effect of Brazilian green propolis on experimental gastric ulcers in rats. *Journal of Ethnopharmacology*. 2007;110:567-571.

[257] Lemos M., de Barros M. P., Sousa J. P., Filho A. A. S., Bastos J. K., de Andrade S. F. *Baccharis dracunculifolia*, the main botanical source of Brazilian green propolis, displays antiulcer activity. *Journal of Pharmacy and Pharmacology*. 2007;59:603-608.

[258] Barros M. P., Lemos M., Maistro E. L., Leite M. F., Sousa J. P., Bastos J. K., Andrade S. F. Evaluation of antiulcer activity of the main phenolic acids found in Brazilian green propolis. *Journal of Ethnopharmacology*. 2008;120:372-377.

[259] Nakamura T., Ohta Y., Tada M., Teruya A., Ohashi K., Ikeno K., Watanabe R., Tokunaga K., Harada N. Protective effect of Brazilian propolis ethanol extract against stress-induced gastric mucosal lesions in rats. Its evaluation using oxidative stress markers. *Journal of Analytical BioScience*. 2011;34:135–146.

[260] Eda M., Hayashi Y., Kinoshita K., Koyama K., Takahashi K., Akutu K. Anti-emetic principles of water extract of Brazilian propolis. P*harmaceutical Biology*. 2005;43:184-185.

[261] Paulino N., Scremin F. M., Raichaski L. B., Marcucci M. C., Scremin A., Calixto J. B. Mechanisms involved in the relaxant action of the ethanolic extract of propolis in the guinea-pig trachea in-vitro. *Journal of Pharmacy and Pharmacology*. 2002;54:845–852.

[262] Cestari S. H., Bastos J. K., Di Stasi L. C. Intestinal anti-inflammatory activity of *Baccharis dracunculifolia* in the trinitrobenzenesulphonic acid model of rat colitis. *Evidence-Based Complementary and Alternative Medicine*. 2011;2011:524349.

[263] Estrada G. O. D., da Silva J. F. M., Antunes O. A. C. Artepillin C: a review. *Letters in Drug Design and Discovery*. 2008;5:88-92.

[264] Li Y. J., Lin J. L., Yang C. W., Yu C. C. Acute renal failure induced by a Brazilian variety of propolis. *American Journal of Kidney Diseases*. 2005;46:125-129.

[265] Mani F., Damasceno H. C., Novelli E. L., Martins E. A., Sforcin J. M. Propolis: Effect of different concentrations, extracts and intake period on seric biochemical variables. *Journal of Ethnopharmacology*. 2006;105:95-98.

[266] Woisky R. G., Salatino A. Analysis of propolis: some parameters and procedures for chemical quality control. *Journal of Apicultural Research*. 1998;37:99-105.

[267] Funari C. S., Ferro V. O. Propolis analysis. *Ciencia e Tecnologia de Alimentos*. 2006;26:171-178.

[268] Ledon N., Casaco A., Gonzalez R., Merino N., Gonzalez A., Tolon Z. Efectos antipsoriásico, antiinflamatorio y analgésico del propoleo rojo colectado en Cuba. *Revista Cubana de Farmacia*. [online]. 1996;30:http://scielo.sld.cu/scielo.php?script =sci_arttext&pid=S0034-75151996000100008&lng=pt.

[269] Questa-Rubio O., Frontana-Uriba B., Perez J. C. Isoflavonoides en propoleos Cubanos. *Revista Cubana de Farmacia*. 2001;35 Suppl:58–61.

[270] Piccinelli A. L., Fernandez M. C., Cuesta-Rubio O., Hernandez I. M., De Simone F., Rastrelli L. Isoflavonoids isolated from Cuban propolis. *Journal of Agricultural and Food Chemistry*. 2005;53:9010-9016.

[271] Cuesta-Rubio O., Piccinelli A. L., Fernandez M. C., Hernandez I. M., Rosado A, Rastrelli L. Chemical characterization of Cuban propolis by HPLC-PDA, HPLC-MS, and NMR: the brown, red, and yellow Cuban varieties of propolis. *Journal of Agricultural & Food Chemistry*. 2007;55:7502-7509.

[273] Trusheva B., Popova M., Bankova V., Simova S., Marcucci M. C., Miorin P. L., Pasin F. D., Tsvetkova I. Bioactive constituents of Brazilian red propolis. *Evidence-Based Complementary and Alternative Medicine*. 2006;3:249-254.

[274] Da Luz CFP, Barth OM, Bacha Junior GL. Analise palinologica de propolis vermelha do Brasil: subsidios para a certificacao de sua origem botanica e geografica. *Mensagem Doce*. 2009;102:art. No 2.

[275] Daugsch A., Moraes C. S., Fort P., Park Y.K. Botanical origin of Brazilian reddish propolis and its major chemical constituents. *Honeybee Science*. 2007;27:55-62.

[276] Silva B. B., Rosalen P. L., Cury J. A., Ikegaki M., Souza V. C., Esteves A., Alencar S. M. Chemical composition and botanical origin of red propolis, a new type of Brazilian propolis. *Evidence-Based Complementary and Alternative Medicine*. 2008;5:313–316.

[277] Alencar S. M., Oldoni T. L. C., Castro M. L., Cabral I. S. R., Costa-Neto C. M., Cury J. A., Rosalen P. L., Ikegaki M. Chemical composition and biological activity of a new type of Brazilian propolis: Red propolis. *Journal of Ethnopharmacology*. 2007;113:278-283.

[278] Moraes C. S., Daugsch A., Fort P., Park Y. K. Extrações de própolis vermelha do nordeste brasileiro em diferentes concentrações alcoólicas, com diferentes solventes e suas atividades contra *Staphylococcus aureus*. *Mensagem Doce*. 2008;99:art. No 1.

[278] Cabral I. S. R., Oldoni T. L. C., Prado A., Bezerra R. M. N., Alencar S. M., Ikegaki M., Rosalen P. L. Phenolic composition, antibacterial and antioxidant activities of Brazilian red propolis. *Quimica Nova*. 2009;32:1523-1527.

[279] Maia-Araujo YLF, Mendonca LS, Orellana SC, Araujo ED. Comparação entre duas técnicas utilizadas no teste de sensibilidade antibacteriana do extrato hidroalcoólico de própolis vermelha. *Scientia Plena*. 2011;7:046201.

[280] Oldoni T. L. C., Cabral I. S. R., d'Arce M. A. B. R., Rosalen P. L., Ikegaki M., Nascimento A. M., Alencar S. M. Isolation and analysis of bioactive isoflavonoids and chalcone from a new type of Brazilian propolis. *Separation and Purification Technology*. 2011;77:208-213.

[281] Awale S., Li F., Onozuka H., Esumi H., Tezuka Y., Kadota S. Constituents of Brazilian red propolis and their preferential cytotoxic activity against human pancreatic PANC-1 cancer cell line in nutrient-deprived condition. *Bioorganic and Medicinal Chemistry*. 2008;16:181-189.

[282] Diaz-Carballo D., Freistuhler M., Malak S., Bardenheuer W., Reusch H. P. Mucronulatol from Caribbean propolis exerts cytotoxic effects on human tumor cell lines. *International Journal of Clinical Pharmacology and Therapeutics*. 2008;46:226-235.

[283] Li F., Awale S., Tezuka Y., Kadota S. Cytotoxic constituents from Brazilian red propolis and their structure-activity relationship. *Bioorganic and Medicinal Chemistry*. 2008;16:5434-5440.

[284] Albuquerque-Junior R. L. C., Barreto A. L. S., Pires J. A., Reis F. P., Lima S. O., Ribeiro M. A. G., Cardoso J. C. Effect of bovine type-I collagen-based films containing red propolis on dermal wound healing in rodent model. *International Journal of Morphology*. 2009;27:1105-1110.

[285] Iio A., Ohguchi K., Inoue H., Maruyama H., Araki Y., Nozawa Y., Ito M. Ethanolic extracts of Brazilian red propolis promote adipocyte differentiation through PPARγ activation. *Phytomedicine*. 2010;17:974-979.

[286] Rosalen P. L., Silva B. B., Falsetta M., Ikegaki M., Alencar S. M., Koo H. Influences of red propolis on *S. mutans*-transcriptome responses within biofilms (poster). On: *89$^{th}$ General Session and Exhibition of the IADR*. San Diego, USA: No 2772.

[287] Daleprane J. B., Dehne N., Ong T. P., Brune B., Abdalla D. S. P. Antiangiogenic properties of natural polyphenols from red propolis. *The FASEB Journal*. 2011;25:lb236.

[288] Righi A. A., Alves T. R., Negri G., Marques L. M., Breyer H., Salatino A. Brazilian red propolis: unreported substances, antioxidant and antimicrobial activities. *Journal of the Science of Food and Agriculture*. 2011;91:2363–2370.

[289] Tomas-Barberan F. A., Garcia-Viguera C., Vit-Olivier P., Ferreres F., Tomas-Lorente F. Phytochemical evidence for the botanical origin of tropical propolis from Venezuela. *Phytochemistry*. 1993;34:191-196.

[290] Trusheva B., Popova M., Naydenski H., Tsvetkova V., Rodriguez J. G., Bankova V. New polyisoprenylated benzophenones from Venezuelan propolis. *Fitoterapia*. 2004;75:683-689.

[291] Cuesta-Rubio O., Frontana-Uribe B. A., Ramirez-Apan T., Cardenas J. Polyisoprenylated benzophenones in Cuban propolis. Biological activity of nemorosone. *Zeitschrift für Naturforschung*. 2002;57c:372-378.

[292] Hernandez I. M., Fernandez M. C., Cuesta-Rubio O., Piccinelli A. L., Rastrelli L. Polyprenylated benzophenone derivatives from Cuban propolis. *Journal of Natural Products*. 2005;68:931–934.

[293] Castro M. L., Nascimento A. M., Ikegaki M., Costa-Neto C. M., Alencar S. M., Rosalen P. L. Identification of a bioactive compound isolated from Brazilian propolis type 6. *Bioorganic and Medicinal Chemistry*. 2009;17:5332-5335.

[294] Ishida V. F. C., Negri G., Salatino A., Bandeira M. F. C. L. A new type of Brazilian propolis: Prenylated benzophenones in propolis from Amazon and effects against cariogenic bacteria. *Food Chemistry*. 2011;125:966–972.

[295] Duarte S., Koo H., Bowen W. H., Hayacibara M. F., Cury J. A., Ikegaki M., Rosalen P. L. Effect of a novel type of propolis and its chemical fractions on glucosyltransferases and on growth and adherence of mutans Streptococci. *Biological and Pharmaceutical Bulletin*. 2003;26:527-531.

[296] Duarte S., Rosalen P. L., Hayacibara M. F., Cury J. A., Bowen W. H., Marquis R. E., Rehder V. L., Sartoratto A., Ikegaki M., Koo H. The influence of a novel propolis on mutans streptococci biofilms and caries development in rats. *Archives of Oral Biology*. 2006;51:15-22.

[297] Castro M. L., Vilela W. R., Zauli R. C., Ikegaki M., Redher V. L., Foglio M. A., Alencar S. M., Rosalen P. L. Bioassay guided purification of the antimicrobial fraction of a Brazilian propolis from Bahia state. *BMC Complementary Alternative Medicine*. 2009;9:25.

[298] Diaz-Carballo D., Ueberla K., Kleff V., Ergun S., Malak S., Freistuehler M., Somogyi S., Kucherer C., Bardenheuer W., Strumberg D. Antiretroviral activity of two polyisoprenylated acylphloroglucinols, 7-epi-nemorosone and plukenetione A, isolated from Caribbean propolis. *International Journal of Clinical Pharmacology and Therapeutics*. 2010;48:670-677.

[299] Diaz-Carballo D., Malak S., Bardenheuer W., Freistuehler M., Reusch H. P. The contribution of plukenetione A to the anti-tumoral activity of Cuban propolis. *Bioorganic and Medicinal Chemistry*. 2008;16:9635-9643.

[300] Popolo A., Piccinelli L. A., Morello S., Cuesta-Rubio O., Sorrentino R., Rastrelli L., Pinto A. Antiproliferative activity of brown Cuban propolis extract on human breast cancer cells. *Natural Product Communications*. 2009;4:1711-1716.

[301] Popolo A., Piccinelli A. L., Morello S., Sorrentino R., Osmany C. R., Rastrelli L., Aldo P. Cytotoxic activity of nemorosone in human MCF-7 breast cancer cells. *Canadian Journal of Physiology and Pharmacology*. 2011;89:50-57.

[302] Melliou E., Stratis E., Chinou I. Volatile constituents of propolis from various regions of Greece– Antimicrobial activity. *Food Chemistry*. 2007;103:375-380.

[303] Kalogeropoulos N., Konteles S. J., Troullidou E., Mourtzinos I., Karathanos V.T. Chemical composition, antioxidant activity and antimicrobial properties of propolis extracts from Greece and Cyprus. *Food Chemistry*. 2009;116:452-461.

[304] Popova M. P., Chinou I. B., Marekov I. N., Bankova VS. Terpenes with antimicrobial activity from Cretan propolis. *Phytochemistry*. 2009;70:1262-1271.

[305] Popova M., Trusheva B., Antonova D., Cutajar S., Mifsud D., Farrugia C., Tsvetkova I., Najdenski H., Bankova V., The specific chemical profile of Mediterranean propolis from Malta. *Food Chemistry*. 2011;126:1431-1435.

[306] Pratsinis H., Kletsas D., Melliou E., Chinou I. Antiproliferative activity of Greek propolis. *Journal of Medicinal Food*. 2010;13:286-290.

[307] Lu L. C., Chen Y. W., Chou C. C. Antibacterial activity of propolis against *Staphylococcus aureus*. *International Journal of Food Microbiology*. 2005;102:213-220.

[308] Yang H. Y., Ho W. L., Chang C. M., Chou C. C. Antibacterial activity of propolis ethanol extract against *Streptococcus mutans* as influenced by concentration, temperature, pH and cell age. *Journal of Food and Drug Analysis*. 2007;15:75-81.

[309] ChenY. W., Wu S. W., Ho K. K., Lin S. B., Huang C. Y., Chen C. N. Characterisation of Taiwanese propolis collected from different locations and seasons. *Journal of the Science of Food and Agriculture*. 2008;88:412-419.

[310] El-Bassuony A., AbouZid S. A new prenylated flavanoid with antibacterial activity from propolis collected in Egypt. *Natural Product Communications*. 2010;5:43-45.

[311] Raghukumar R., Vali L., Watson D., Fearnley J., Seidel V. Antimethicillin-resistant *Staphylococcus aureus* (MRSA) activity of 'pacific propolis' and isolated prenylflavanones. *Phytotherapy Research*. 2010;24:1181-1187.

[312] Chen C. N., Wu C. L., Shy H. S., Lin J. K. Cytotoxic prenylflavanones from Taiwanese propolis. *Journal of Natural Products*. 2003;66:503–506.

[313] Kumazawa S., Ueda R., Hamasaka T., Fukumoto S., Fujimoto T., Nakayama T. Antioxidant prenylated flavonoids from propolis collected in Okinawa, Japan. *Journal of Agricultural and Food Chemistry*. 2007;55:7722–7725.

[314] Huang W. J., Huang C. H., Wu C. L., Lin J. K., Chen Y. W., Lin C. L., Chuang S. E., Huang C. Y., Chen C. N. Propolin G, a prenylflavanone, isolated from Taiwanese propolis, induces caspase-dependent apoptosis in brain cancer cells. *Journal of Agricultural and Food Chemistry*. 2007;55:7366-7376.

[315] Weng M. S., Liao C. H., Chen C. N., Wu C. L., Lin J. K. Propolin H from Taiwanese propolis induces G1 arrest in human lung carcinoma cells. *Journal of Agricultural and Food Chemistry*. 2007;55:5289-5298.

[316] Aguero M. B., Svetaz L., Sanchez M., Luna L., Lima B., Lopez M. L., Zacchino S., Palermo J., Wunderlin D., Feresin G. E., Tapia A. Argentinean Andean propolis associated with the medicinal plant *Larrea nitida* Cav. (Zygophyllaceae). HPLC–MS and GC–MS characterization and antifungal activity. *Food and Chemical Toxicology*. 2011;49:1970-1978.

[317] Nieva Moreno M. I., Zampini I. C., Ordonez R. M., Jaime G. S., Vattuone M. A., Isla M.I. Evaluation of the cytotoxicity, genotoxicity, mutagenicity, and antimutagenicity of propolis from Tucuman. Argentina. *Journal of Agricultural and Food Chemistry*. 2005;53:8957-8962.

[318] Aguero M. B., Gonzalez M., Lima B., Svetaz L., Sanchez M., Zacchino S., Feresin G. E., Schmeda-Hirschmann G., Palermo J., Wunderlin D., Tapia A. Argentinean propolis from *Zuccagnia punctata* Cav. (Caesalpinieae) exudates: phytochemical characterization and antifungal activity. *Journal of Agricultural and Food Chemistry*. 2010;58:194-201.

[319] Vera N., Solorzano E., Ordonez R., Maldonado L., Bedascarrasbure E., Isla M. I. Chemical composition of Argentinean propolis collected in extreme regions and its relation with antimicrobial and antioxidant activities. *Natural Product Communications*. 2011;6:823-827.

[320] Awale S., Shrestha S. P., Tezuka Y., Ueda J., Matsushige K., Kadota S. Neoflavonoids and related constituents from Nepalese propolis and their nitric oxide production inhibitory activity. *Journal of Natural Products*. 2005;68:858–864.

[321] Li F., Awale S., Tezuka Y., Kadota S. Cytotoxicity of constituents from Mexican propolis against a panel of six different cancer cell lines. *Natural Product Communications*. 2010;5:1601-1606.
[322] Murase M., Kato M., Sun A., Ono T., Nakamura J., Sato T., Kumazawa S. *Rhus javanica* var. *chinensis* as a new plant origin of propolis from Okayama, Japan. *Bioscience Biotechnology and Biochemistry*. 2008;72:2782-2784.
[323] Silva M. S. S., de Lima S. G., Oliveira E. H., Lopes J. A. D., Chaves M. H., Reis F. A. M., Citó A. M. G. L. Anacardic acid derivatives from Brazilian propolis and their antibacterial activity. *Ecletica Quimica*. 2008;33:53-58.
[324] Ito J., Chang F. R., Wang H. K., Park Y. K., Ikegaki M., Kilgore N., Lee K. H. Anti-AIDS agents. 48.1 anti-HIV activity of moronic acid derivatives and the new melliferone-related triterpenoid isolated from Brazilian propolis. *Journal of Natural Products*. 2001;64:1278–1281.
[325] Li F., Awale S., Tezuka Y., Kadota S. Cytotoxic constituents of propolis from Myanmar and their structure-activity relationship. *Biological and Pharmaceutical Bulletin*. 2009;32:2075-2078.
[326] Li F., Awale S., Zhang H., Tezuka Y., Esumi H., Kadota S. Chemical constituents of propolis from Myanmar and their preferential cytotoxicity against a human pancreatic cancer cell line. *Journal of Natural Products*. 2009;72:1283-1287.
[327] Segueni N., Magid A. A., Decarme M., Rhouati S., Lahouel M., Antonicelli F., Lavaud C., Hornebeck W. Inhibition of stromelysin-1 by caffeic acid derivatives from a propolis sample from Algeria. *Planta Medica*. 2011;77:999-1004.
[328] Sha N., Guan S. H., Lu Z. Q., Chen G. T., Huang H. L., Xie F. B., Yue Q. X., Liu X., Guo D. A. Cytotoxic constituents of Chinese propolis. *Journal of Natural Products*. 2009;72:799-801.
[329] Kumazawa S., Suzuki S., Ahn M. R., Kamihira M., Udagawa Y., Bang K. S., Nakayama T. A new chalcone from propolis collected on Jeju Island, Korea. *Food Science and Technology Research*. 2006;12:67-69.
[330] Ophori E. A., Eriagbonye B. N., Ugbodaga P. Antimicrobial activity of propolis against *Streptococcus mutans*. *African Journal of Biotechnology*. 2010;9:4966-4969.
[331] Petrova A., Popova M., Kuzmanova C., Tsvetkova I., Naydenski H., Muli E, Bankova V. New biologically active compounds from Kenyan propolis. *Fitoterapia*. 2010;81:509-514.
[332] Trusheva B., Popova M., Koendhori E. B., Tsvetkova I., Naydenski H., Bankova V. Indonesian propolis: chemical composition, biological activity and botanical origin. *Natural Product Research*. 2011;25:606-613.
[333] Trusheva B., Popova M., Kortenska V., Totseva I., Rodriguez J.G., Bankova V. Chemical composition and antioxidant activity of propolis from Venezuela. *Oxidation Communications*. 2005;28:490-496.
[334] Kumazawa S., Goto H., Hamasaka T., Fukumoto S., Fujimoto T., Nakayama T. A new prenylated flavonoid from propolis collected in Okinawa, Japan. *Bioscience Biotechnology and Biochemistry*. 2004;68:260-262.
[335] Huang W. J., Lin C. W., Lee C. Y., Chi L. L., Chao Y. C., Wang H. N., Chiou B. L., Chen T.J., Huang C.Y., Chen C.N. NBM-HD-3, a novel histone deacetylase inhibitor with anticancer activity through modulation of PTEN and AKT in brain cancer cells. *Journal of Ethnopharmacology*. 2011;136:156-167.

In: Beneficial Effects of Propolis on Human Health ... ISBN: 978-1- 62081-440-6
Editors: Tahira Farooqui and Akhlaq A. Farooqui 

*Chapter 2*

# Propolis: A Complex Product with Mixed Origin

***Antonio Salatino*** [*] ***and Maria Luiza Faria Salatino***
Department of Botany, Institute of Biosciences,
University of São Paulo, São Paulo, SP, Brazil

## Abstract

Among the hive products, propolis has recently been the object of intense investigation. Many papers have been published about the chemical analysis of propolis from several regions of the world. Propolis contains minor constituents and two main components: beeswax and resins. Minor propolis constituents are sugars, amino acids, pollen and minerals. Propolis resin derives from plants, a fact that turns propolis into a product with two origins: animal and plant. Most studies about propolis chemistry deal with resin constituents. Propolis may be characterized botanically, chemically and geographically. Propolis from certain parts of the world has typical chemical characteristics: European propolis derives from poplars (*Populus* spp.) and contains esters of caffeic acid and flavonoids such as chrysin, galangin and pinocembrin; Southeastern Brazilian propolis derives from *Baccharis dracunculifolia* and contains caffeoylquinic acids and prenylated phenylpropanoids; Cuban and Venezuelan propolis contains resin of *Clusia* spp. and polyprenylated benzophenones; Okinawan, Taiwan and Kenyan propolis contains resin of *Macaranga* spp. and geranyl flavonoids. Mediterranean propolis contains sugars and terpenoids. Many new compounds from distinct parts of the world have recently been isolated and their biological activities determined. The chemical composition of propolis resin is variable and may be derived from several plant sources. Determination of plant origin and standardization of propolis are priorities in propolis research. Little has been done about several aspects of propolis chemistry, for example, wax analysis for characterization of bee lineages. Propolis is regarded as a complementary food, in addition to alternative medicine. However, little work has been carried out aiming the determination of nutrients, such as sugar, pollen, amino acids, vitamins and minerals.

[*] Corresponding author: asalatin@ib.usp.br.

**Keywords**: propolis, flavonoids, terpenoids, phenolic substances, artepillin C, caffeic acid phenethyl ester, *Populus*, *Baccharis*, *Macaranga*.

## INTRODUCTION

Up until 1980, propolis was viewed in most apiaries as a nuisance in the process of honey production. At best, it was assumed as a honeybee byproduct. Presently, in contrast, propolis is ranked among the chief products, if not the main one, in apiaries of many countries. This quick change in the appreciation of propolis has followed a growing interest in the product by the population of both eastern and western worlds as an alternative and complementary food and medicine.

Starting in the 1960's, the first scientific evidences were published, giving support to some of the alleged properties of propolis, mainly antibacterial (Lavie 1968, Schneidewinde et al. 1979, Vanhaelen and Vanhaelenfastre 1979a,b). In the 1980's, propolis started becoming popular in several western countries. Since then, the market demand for propolis increased steadily. In consequence, increasing profits derived from propolis production have been noted. In 2010, the mean value of honey and propolis shipped from Brazil were, respectively, US $2.95 and US $87.21 (Belmiro et al. 2011). Propolis turned out as an important focus of scientific research. In the last 20 years, numerous patent proposals involving propolis have been deposited (see e.g. patent number CN 102132810-A, published 27 Jul 2011, inventor: Bai, W.).

Much has been published about biological activities of propolis, such as antimicrobial, anti-inflammatory, anti-tumor, antihepatotoxic, wound-healing, anti-HIV and enhancement of the immune system, among others (for reviews, see Marcucci 1995, Burdock 1998, Banskota et al. 2001, Ramos and Miranda 2007, Sforcin 2007, Sforcin and Bankova 2011).

Propolis is used by the bee communities for several purposes, e.g. to close holes and crevices in the hive, reduce the size of the hive entrance and embalm bodies of small invading animals (Ghisalberti 1979). Other uses involve gluing insect enemies, (e.g. ants) (dos Santos et al. 2010) and enhancing the immunity of the hive (Simone-Finstrom and Spivak 2010).

Propolis is assumed to contain several minor or infrequent components, such as vitamins, minerals, amino acids, pollen, enzymes and sugars (Marcucci 1995). The main components of propolis are wax and resin. The former is assumed to derive from material secreted by the bees and the latter is originated from plants. The resin is collected by worker bees from shoot apices or plant exudates. Propolis resin contains the substances which have been pointed out as possessing biological activity (Salatino et al. 2011).

The present paper aims to present an overview and an update about propolis chemical composition. It also aims to point out perspectives and topics understudied in propolis chemistry.

## MINOR OR INFREQUENT COMPONENTS

Vitamins and minerals have been detected in propolis samples (Marcucci 1995). Vitamins $B_1$, $B_2$, $B_6$, C and E, and minerals containing Ag, Al, Ca, Ce, Hg, La, Mg, Sb, Va and silicon have been reported for propolis (Deblock-Bostyn 1982). Nikolaev (1978; cited by Ahmed G. Hegazi, available at www.apinetla.com.ar/congreso/c05.pdf) mentioned the presence in propolis of Ca, Cu, Fe, I, K, Mg, Mn, Na, Zn, along with vitamins $B_1$, $B_2$, $B_6$, C, E and fatty acids. Vitamins $B_1$, $B_2$ and tocopherol were found in Brazilian propolis (Moreira 1986).

Amino acids have been reported as propolis constituents (Gabrys et al. 1986, Moreira 1986). Marcucci et al. (1996) analyzed the contents of amino acids of four samples of Brazilian propolis. Total amino acid contents were in the range 13.56-87.04 μg/g, with the main representatives in all samples being aspartic and glutamic acids, leucine and lysine. The authors suggested that the sources of amino acids could be plants, pollen or material secreted by the bees.

Pollen is invariably present in propolis. Analysis of pollen is useful for geographical characterization of the product (Barth 1998). Early palynological studies were carried out for determination of plant sources of resin (Junkunz 1932, d'Albore 1979) and some relatively recent works in this thread have been published (e.g. Barth and da Luz 2009). However, it is now clear that pollen analysis of propolis for the determination of propolis plant source is misleading, because sources of honey and pollen, on one hand, and of propolis, on the other hand, correspond, in general, to distinct plant species. For example, pollen from *Dalbergia ecastophyllum* was not detected in Brazilian red propolis, although it has been well established that the mentioned legume tree is its resin source (see text below). Pollen in propolis is now viewed as a contaminant originated from previous visits of bees to plant sources of nectar and pollen. It may contribute with nutritious substances found in propolis, such as sugars, amino acids and protein, as well as with functional substances, e.g. flavonoids and carotenoids. Most available works on propolis pollen convey the identification of plant species, but give no data about the amount of pollen in the samples analyzed.

Enzymes, probably stemming from bee saliva, have been reported in propolis. One of them is β-glucosidase, whose activity has been shown to be high in fresh material and barely detected in stored propolis (Zhang et al. 2011).

Sugars have received little attention as propolis components. Sucrose, glucose and fructose are expected to be present as contaminants derived from nectar. These and some other sugars may also derive from pollen present in propolis. Bankova et al. (1998) found relatively high amounts of sugars and polyols, such as ribose, xylose, mannose, sorbose, fructose, galactose, glucose, sucrose, lactose, maltose, melibiose, erytritol, xylitol, inositol in propolis from the Canary Islands. Quan et al. (2008) determined contents of sucrose, glucose and fructose in the range 0.04%-1.15% in most samples of propolis from Europe (Bulgaria), Asia (Solomon Islands, India) and Africa (Kenya, Tanzania and Zambia). They put forward the hypothesis that some sugars present in propolis derive from glycosides which have been hydrolyzed by bee enzymes (e.g. glucosidases). Popova et al. (2011) analyzed 17 samples of Maltese propolis by GC/MS. Quantitatively, sugars and sugar derivatives were either the main (3 samples) or the second main constituents (14 samples), corresponding to mono- and disaccharides, sugar alcohols and uronic acids. According to Popova et al. (2010a), similar chemical profile characterizes also other Mediterranean propolis, such as Greek propolis. This claim is strengthened by the finding of considerable amounts of sugars in samples from several continental areas of Greece, the Greek islands and Crete (Kalogeropoulos et al. 2009). It is interesting that sugars might turn out as chemical markers of propolis from the Greek region of the Mediterranean; in general, only phenolic compounds and terpenoids have so far been indicated as markers of propolis types. It has been argued that a likely origin of such substances is mucilage (Popova et al. 2010a), as earlier suggested by Crane (1988). Species of *Ferula* (Apiaceae) have been pointed out as propolis sources of Maltese and Iranian propolis (see below Section 'Propolis Plant Sources'). It is suggestive that species of that genus have schizogenous ducts with gums, a potential source of propolis (Trusheva et al. 2010). Several species of *Ferula* are known to possess polysaccharides, some of them economically important, such as Barijh gum from *F. gumosa* (Mohammadzadeh et al. 2007). In addition, high contents of monosaccharides, pectinic substances and water-soluble polysaccharides have been determined in the aerial parts of *Ferula kuhistanica* and *F. tenuisecta* (Erkulov et al. 2011).

## PROPOLIS WAX

Wax is assumed to be biologically inert. Commercially, it is an undesirable propolis component, not only because it adds weight and no biological properties to the product, but also because it may cause turbidity in alcohol extracts maintained at low temperatures, as in the winter months or in extracts kept in refrigerators. For these reasons, it is important to include the determination of wax content among the parameters for standardization and quality control of propolis. Propolis wax may be determined by exhaust extraction with chloroform, evaporation of the solvent, treatment of the residue with hot alcohol and cooling the extract at freezer temperature; the wax precipitates and is then weighed (Woisky & Salatino, 1998). The proportion of wax in propolis varies widely. Contents of wax propolis determined between 1900 and 1950, presumably from European propolis and quoted by Ghisalberti (1979), range from 14.8% to 40%. Contents of Brazilian propolis have been reported in the range 3.1% - 16.4% (Negri et al. 1998; Woisky and Salatino 1998).

Relatively little has been done regarding the chemical composition of propolis wax. The main constituents of Brazilian propolis wax are monoesters, followed by hydrocarbons. The proportion of monoesters in 23 samples of Brazilian propolis lay in the range 88.5% - 58.0%, and of hydrocarbons in the range 1.2% - 37.5% (Negri et al. 1998). The wax contents of carboxylic acids and alcohols of the esters, and also of the hydrocarbons, vary widely from one sample to another. The main carboxylic acid residues in the monoesters are chiefly palmitic ($C_{16}$) followed by stearic ($C_{18}$) and oleic ($C_{18:1}$) acids; the main alcohol residues correspond to primary alcohols with carbon chains in the range $C_{24}$ – $C_{32}$. The main hydrocarbons of the same propolis samples are $C_{27}$, $C_{29}$ and $C_{31}$. Although far from predominant, unsaturated hydrocarbons are commonly detected. Such a chemical profile is similar to the composition of beeswax (Tulloch 1980; Nelson & Blomquist 1995). Plant waxes rarely contain unsaturated constituents (Bianchi 1995). The results suggest that propolis wax is produced by bees, probably in the same way as comb wax. Suggestively, comparison of the composition of comb and propolis waxes from the same hives did not detect expressive differences in the distribution of carboxylic acids, primary alcohols and hydrocarbons, showing again that the waxes of both comb and Brazilian propolis virtually have the same composition and hence the same origin (Negri et al. 2000).

Certain constituents of propolis, such as triterpenoids, have solubility similar to substances of wax. For this reason, triterpenoids are extracted along with the fatty esters and hydrocarbons typical of natural waxes (Negri et al. 2000). This represents a factor that may lead to overestimations of propolis wax contents.

## PROPOLIS RESIN

Among propolis constituents, the resin has been object of the greatest attention, both chemically or pharmacologically. In general, the resin accounts for the color, smell and biological properties of propolis. Bees often collect resin from plant exudates or shoot apices. For this reason, many propolis substances, chiefly those with biological activity, are resin constituents. The importance of the determination of the plant origin of propolis has long been recognized. It is viewed as fundamental for propolis characterization and standardization, thus assuming a high relevance in propolis research.

### Propolis Plant Sources

Ghisalberti (1979) commented that as early as 1908, Helfenberg stated that bees obtained propolis from birch, ash, elm and balsam trees and thus the composition of propolis varied with its origin. Ghisalberti commented also that in 1926, Jaubert isolated chrysin (the substance responsible for the color of beeswax) and was already aware that bees obtained propolis from *Populus nigra* var. *pyramidalis*. Catorini (1963) described the details of the collection of resin from bud exudates of poplars (*Populus nigra*). In his review about the plant origin of propolis, König (1986) commented that in temperate regions, poplar plants (genus *Populus*, Salicaceae) predominate as propolis sources; alder (*Alnus*, Betulaceae), birch (*Betula*, Betulaceae), hazel (*Corylus*, Betulaceae), oak (*Quercus*, Fagaceae) and willow (*Salix*, Salicaceae) would be secondary sources, although in central Russia, birch predominated over poplar. König (1986) mentioned other possible sources of propolis, such as *Acacia* (Leguminosae, Mimosoideae), *Eucalyptus*, *Plumeria* (Apocynaceae), *Psidium* (Myrtaceae) and *Schinus* (Anacardiaceae). Bankova et al. (2000) comments that many plant species have been pointed out as possible sources of propolis based only on bee behavior; such species should be regarded only as preliminary information, because chemical comparative data (from plants and propolis) is needed for reliable determination of plant sources.

Determination of plant sources of propolis have been made on the basis of several observations: bee behavior, histological analysis, collection and observation of material attached to the hind legs and comparative chemistry. The latter approach has involved analyses of propolis and of the plant part assumed as the source (buds, young leaves, exudates); in some cases, chemical analyses were done also of material recently collected and attached to the hind legs of bees or inside their corbicula (e.g. Kumazawa et al. 2008). Chemotaxonomy, i.e. the study of the distribution of secondary metabolites among plant groups (Harborne and Turner 1984), and plant geography have been important for the recognition of plant sources. Once the identification of propolis resin is done, it is often possible to limit the possibilities of assignment of plant sources to a small group of species growing in the neighborhood of the hive, sometimes to only one species. Since chemical composition of propolis is dependent on the plant source, and plant species have definite areas of distribution in the world, geographic patterns are recognized of several important types of propolis (Salatino et al. 2011).

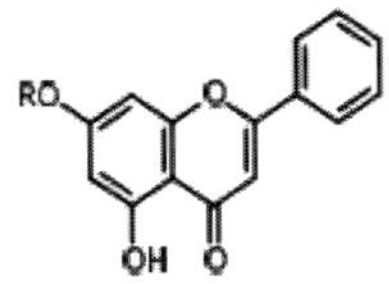

1 $R_1$ = H CHRYSIN

2 $R_2$ = $CH_3$ TECTOCHRYSIN

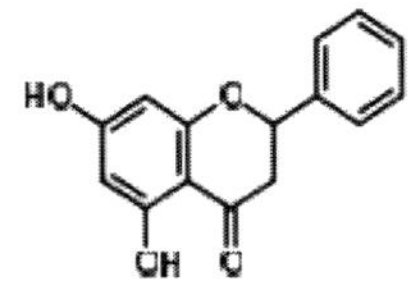

3 PINOCEMBRIN

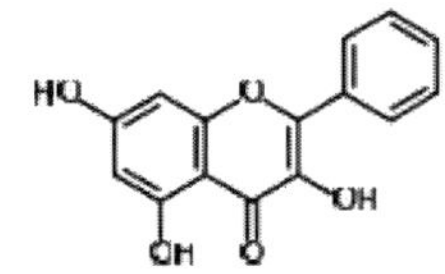

4 GALANGIN

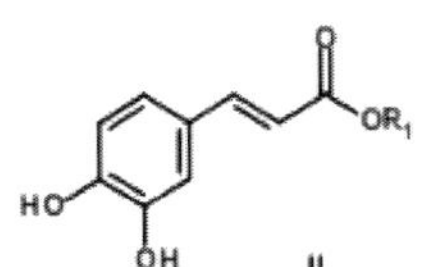

5 $R_1$ = 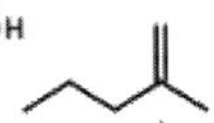

6 R2 = 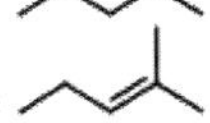

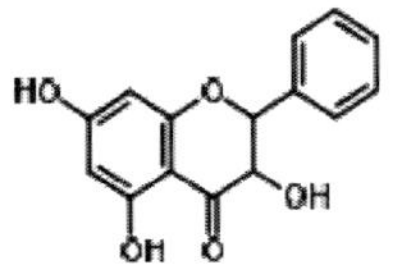

3 PINOBANKSIN

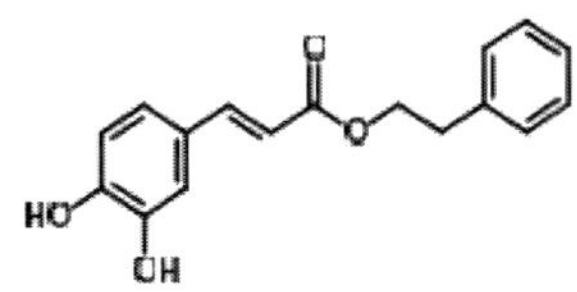

8 CAFFEIC ACID PHENETHYL ESTER (CAPE)

Figure 1. Propolis constituents of temperate propolis derived of poplar (*Populus* spp., Salicaceae).

Several reviews have been published on plant species which have been recognized as propolis sources (Bankova et al. 2000, Bankova 2005, Salatino et al. 2011). Table 1 provides a list of propolis types, corresponding plant sources and characteristic compounds. More detailed comments about the chemical composition of the propolis types will be given in the next section. Poplars are widely cultivated in temperate regions, in both New and Old Worlds, as well as either the Northern or the Southern Hemispheres. Honeybees have a marked preference for certain plant species and poplars are among them. They are recognized as the main source of propolis in temperate regions of both Northern and Southern hemispheres. The characteristic compounds of poplar propolis are flavonoids with no B-ring substituents (chrysin, pinocembrin, galangin, pinobanksin; (Figure 1). But in certain temperate areas, other plant species have been pointed out as propolis sources. In the Andean regions of Argentina, poplars are not cultivated; in one of these areas, *Larrea nitida* was recognized as propolis source, with lignans and related substances (Agüero et al. 2011, Table 1). In Tucumán, also in Argentina, trees of the endemic *Zuccagnia punctata* (Ceasalpinioideae), was established as resin source (Agüero et al. 2010, Table 1); in the propolis samples and in the plant resin, chrysin and galangin and pinocembrin (characteristic poplar flavonoids) were found, but no chrysin, pinobanksin and esters of caffeic acid; in addition, other substances were detected, including chalcones, not present in proplar resin. However, from the family Leguminosae, species of Faboideae have more often found to be propolis sources, mainly from genus *Dalbergia*. Such are the cases of red propolis from Northeast Brazil, Cuba and Mexico, and also from the Nepalese propolis; all of these propolis types contain isoflavonoids (Table 1, Figure 2), compounds highly characteristic of the subfamily Faboideae (Papilionoideae).

Flowers of species of *Clusia* are sources of material for production of propolis in several parts of the New World: Brazilian Amazon, Cuba and Venezuela (Table 1). They contain complex polyisoprenylated benzophenones (Figure 3). *Macaranga* is a genus with widespread distribution, from the Pacific through the Indian Ocean to West Africa (Matsubayashi et al. 2006). Substances on the surface of *M. tanarius* are used in Okinawa by honeybees as propolis sources (Kumazawa et al. 2008, Table 1). Characteristic constituents of *Macaranga* species and of propolis from Taiwan, Egypt and Kenya are geranyl flavonoids (Table 1, Figure 4). Diterpenes from conifers, chiefly Cupressaceae, are frequent constituents of propolis from the Mediterranean, in regions such as Sicily, Greece and Cyprus (Table 1, Figure 5). But propolis from Malta, as well as from Iran, has mono-, sesqui- and diterpene esters of benzoic acids, substances characteristic of *Ferula* species (Table 1, Figure 6). It was commented above (Section Minor Components) that relatively high contents of sugars is another chemical characteristic of propolis derived from *Ferula* species.

## Chemical Composition of Propolis Resin

Due to the recognized biological and pharmacological importance of the constituents derived from plants, the chemical composition of propolis resin has been extensively studied. Several reviews covering the subject have been published (Ghisalberti 1979, Marcucci 1995, Bankova et al. 2000, Bankova 2005). Many new compounds have been reported for propolis. Some of them have been detected in plants, but many others remain exclusively as propolis components, although it is reasonable to assume that they are derived from a plant source.

Constituents most commonly detected as resin constituents of propolis belong to one of two wide diverse classes of secondary metabolites: phenolic compounds and terpenoids. Among the former, relevant representatives are flavonoids and phenylpropanoids, often combined, forming esters. Terpenoids from propolis resin frequently are triterpenoids, but diterpenoids are characteristic of some geographical areas. Propolis often contains relatively low amounts of volatile terpenoids; they are responsible for the aroma, contribute with biological activity and may be valuable for the organoleptical characterization of the propolis type. Among volatile monoterpenes, α- and β-pinenes, geraniol and linalyl propionate have been reported in propolis; ledol, spatulenol and palustrol are some of the sesquiterpenes reported as propolis constituents (Bankova et al. 2000).

The resins collected by honeybees are often plant exudates. They comprise substances with low polarity. For this reason, glycosides, frequently found in plants, are rarely found in propolis. The first glycosides isolated from propolis (diterpene rhamnosides) were announced as a rarity (Popova et al. 2001). The possibility that glucosidases, known to be one of the minor constituents of propolis (see above, in section Minor or Infrequent Components), may promote hydrolysis of glucosides cannot be ruled out. Most comparisons between chromatographic profiles of extracts of propolis samples and plant sources have shown great similarities (see, e.g. Silva et al. 2008, regarding the origin of Brazilian red propolis). Thus it has been assumed that the substances stemming from the plants are not changed after incorporation in propolis. However, propolis glucosidases do promote some changes in plant substances, at least in poplar propolis: due to the activity of propolis glucosidases, salicin from the poplar bud is not detected in propolis (Zhang et al. 2011). Nitrogenous compounds, e.g. alkaloids, are frequent in plant secondary metabolism, but have so far not been detected in propolis.

**Table 1. Propolis types, corresponding geographic areas, resin plant sources and characteristic constituent compounds**

| Geographic area | Main plant sources - Species (family, common name) | Characteristic constituents | References |
|---|---|---|---|
| *Temperate regions* | | | |
| North and South Hemispheres | *Populus* spp., mainly *P. nigra* (Salicaceae, poplars) | Flavonoids with no B-ring substituents, esters of caffeic acid | Bankova et al. (2000), Bankova (2005) |
| *South America* | | | |
| Southeast Brazil | *Baccharis dracunculifolia* (Asteraceae, alecrim-do campo) | Prenylated phenylpropanoids, caffeoylquinic acids | Bankova et al. (1999), Park et al. (2002), Kumazawa et al. (2003), Teixeira et al. (2005) |
| Northeast Brazil | *Dalbergia ecastophyllum* (Leguminosae, Faboideae, rabo-de-bugio) | Isoflavonoids | Daugsch et al. (2008), Silva et al. (2008) |
| North-Central Brazil | *Mangifera indica* (Anacardiaceae) | Cycloartane triterpenoids | da Silva et al. (2005) |
| Amazonian Brazil | *Clusia* spp. (Clusiaceae) | Polyisoprenylated benzophenones | Ishida et al. (2011) |
| Argentina, Andean region | *Larrea nitida* (Zygophyllaceae) | Lignans | Agüero et al. (2011) |
| Argentina, Tucumán | *Zuccagnia punctata* (Leguminosae, Caesalpinioideae) | Flavonoids with no B-ring substituents, chalkones | Agüero et al. (2010) |
| Venezuela | *Clusia* spp. (Clusiaceae) | Polyisoprenylated benzophenones | Tomás-Barberán et al. (1993), Trusheva et al., 2004) |
| *Central and North America* | | | |
| Cuba | *Dalbergia ecastophyllum* (Leguminosae, Faboideae) | Isoflavonoids | Piccinelli et al. (2011) |
| Cuba | *Clusia* spp. (Clusiaceae) | Polyisoprenylated benzophenones | Cuesta-Rubio et al. (1999), Hernández et al. (2005) |
| Mexico | Leguminosae, Faboideae, probably *Dalgergia* spp. | Isoflavonoids | Lotti et al. (2010) |
| *Europe* | | | |
| Mediterranean (Sicily, Greece, Crete, Cyprus) | Conifers (probably Cupressus sempervirens, Cupressaceae) | Flavonoids with no B-ring substituents, diterpenes | Kalogeropoulos et al. (2009), Popova et al. (2010a) |

| Geographic area | Main plant sources - Species (family, common name) | Characteristic constituents | References |
|---|---|---|---|
| Malta | *Ferula communis* (Apiaceae) | Sugars, terpenyl esters of benzoic acids | Popova et al. (2011) |
| *Asia* | | | |
| Indonesia | *Macaranga tanarius* (Euphorbiaceae), *Mangifera indica* (Anacardiaceae) | Geranyl flavanones, cycloartane triterpenoids | Trusheva et al. (2011) |
| Iran | *Populus* spp. (Salicaceae), *Ferula* spp. (Apiaceae) | Flavonoids with no B-ring substituents, caffeoyl esters, terpene esters of bezoic acids | Trusheva et al. (2010) |
| Korea | *Populus* spp. (Salicaceae) | Flavonoids with no B-ring substituents, caffeoyl esters | Ahn et al. (2004) |
| Myanmar | *Mangifera indica* (Anacardiaceae) | Cycloartane triterpenoids | Li et al. (2009) |
| Okinawa | *Macaranga tanarius* (Euphorbiaceae) | Geranyl flavanones | Kumazawa et al. (2008) |
| Nepal | *Dalbergia* spp. (Leguminosae, Faboideae) | Isoflavonoids | Awale et al. (2005), |
| Taiwan | *Macaranga* spp. (Euphorbiaceae) | Geranyl flavanones | Huang et al. (2007) |
| *Africa* | | | |
| Egypt | *Macaranga* spp. (Euphorbiaceae) | Geranyl flavanones | El-Bassuony (2009) AbouZid and El-Bassuony (2010) |
| Kenya | *Macaranga schweinfurthii* (Euphorbiaceae) | Geranyl flavonols, geranyl stilbenes | Petrova et al. (2010) |

In continuation, an overview and update are given about the composition of types of propolis from several parts of the world.

## Temperate Poplar Propolis

Compounds virtually universal in poplar propolis are flavonoids without substituents at the B-ring, such as flavones (e.g. chrysin, **1**, tectochrysin, **2**), flavanones (e.g. pinocembrin, **3**), flavonols (e.g. galangin, **4**) and flavanonols (e.g. pinobanksin, **5**) (Figure 1). Esters of caffeic acid are also frequently reported constituents of poplar propolis. Examples are the prenyl esters **6** and **7** and the caffeic acid phenethyl ester (**8**, Figure 1), commonly designated by the abbreviation CAPE.

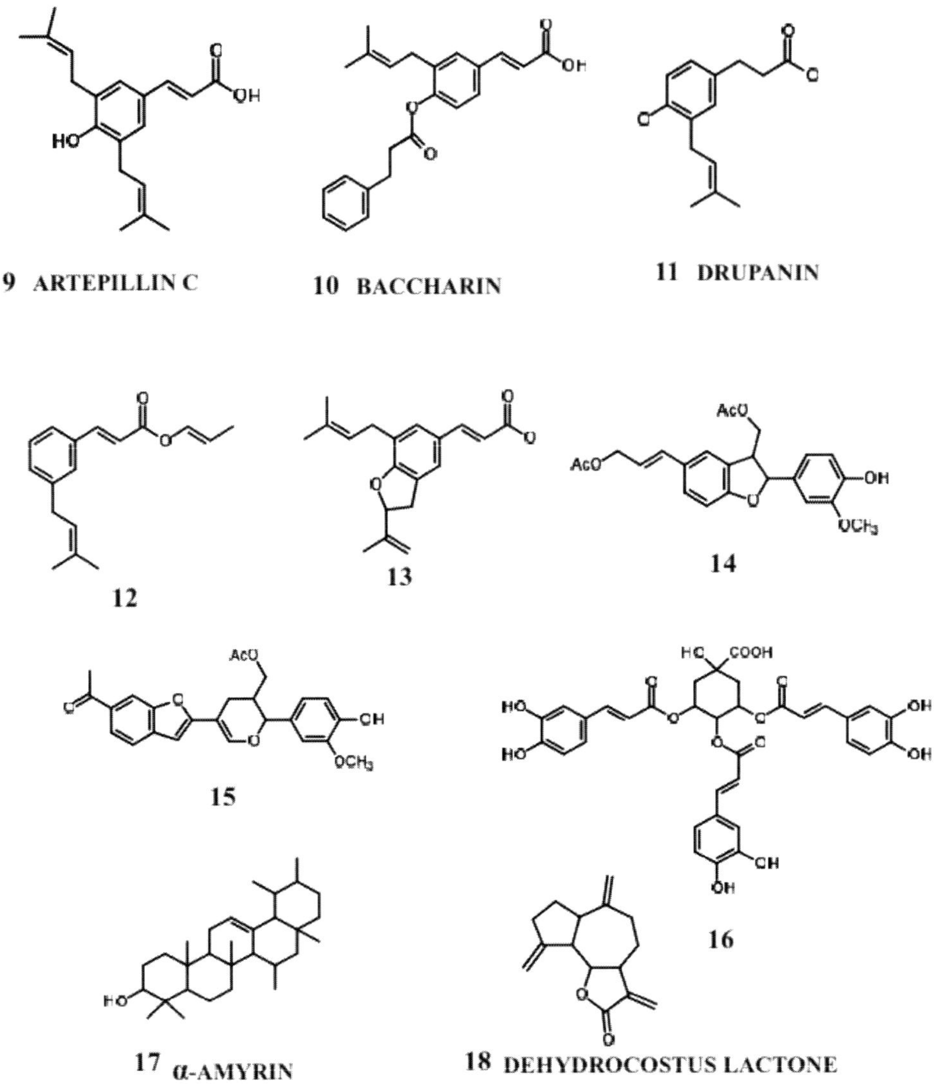


Figure 2. Propolis constituents of Brazilian alecrim (*Baccharis dracunculifolia*, Asteraceae) propolis, from the Southeastern and Central regions.

## Brazilian Propolis

### *a. Alecrim or Green Propolis*

Several types of propolis are produced in Brazil (Table 1). The type of propolis mostly consumed in Brazil and exported (mainly to Japan) is the alecrim or green propolis, from the Southeast and Central region of the country. Two classes of substances predominate: prenylated phenylpropanoids (Bankova et al. 2000, Salatino et al. 2005) and caffeoylquinic acids (Tatefuji et al. 1996) (Figure 2). More attention was initially given to the former class of constituents, probably because chemical composition was then preferentially based on alcohol extracts. Artepillin C (**9**) is the best known prenylated phenylpropanoid. Baccharin (**10**) and drupanin (**11**) (Akao et al. 2003) and the allyl ester of 3-prenyl-cinnamic acid (**12**) (Negri et al. 2003a) are other examples of prenylated phenylpropanoids. In some of these compounds, one the prenyl groups is involved in the formation of a heterocycle, as in compound **13** (Tazawa et al. 1999, Figure 2). Alcohol extracts of alecrim propolis have yielded other complex phenolic compounds, such as **14** (Banskota et al. 1998) and **15** (Banskota et al. 2000). More recently, attention has been directed to aqueous extracts, from which caffeoylquinic acids are obtained (Mishima et al. 2005a,b; Nakajima et al. 2007, 2009; Chikaraishi et al. 2010; Urushisaki et al. 2011; de Moura et al. 2011). Several pharmacological effects have been reported for these phenolic substances, e.g. anti-hyperglycemic effect by tri-*O*-caffeoylquinic acid (**16**, Figure 2) (Matsui et al. 2004). Lower polar solvents have also been used in chemical analysis of Brazilian propolis (Negri et al. 2003b). Among the constituents detected in chloroform extracts are triterpenes (e.g. α-amyrin, **17**) and sesquiterpenes (e.g. dehydrocostus lactone, **18**, Figure 2). The plant source of triterpenes in propolis from Southeastern Brazil remain undetermined. Triterpenoids may be abundant in some samples and absent in others from the same region (Teixeira et al. 2006, 2010).

***b. Southern Brazilian Propolis***

There are types of Brazilian propolis other than alecrim propolis. Poplars are cultivated in the south of the country. Pinocembrin and related flavonoids were detected in poplar buds and propolis from the state of Paraná (Adelmann et al. 2007). Propolis from the extreme south of Brazil yielded moronic acid (a triterpenoid with anti-HIV action) and other structurally related compounds as major components (Ito et al. 2001).

***c. Northeastern and Central-Northern Brazilian Propolis***

The red resin of the legume tree *Dalbergia ecastophyllum* is the major source of propolis from northeast Brazil (Table 1). In addition to simple phenylpropanoids, the isoflavonoids isosativan (**19**) and medicarpin (**20**, Figure 3) are constituents of Brazilian red propolis (Trusheva et al. 2006). Other constituent classes of red propolis are neoflavonoids, lignans and chalcones; also, new pterocarpans and related substances, such as compounds **21** and **22** (Figure 3), have been isolated from red propolis (Awale et al 2008). The contribution of plant sources other than *D. ecastophyllum* is likely, because a polyisoprenylated benzophenone, a class of metabolites typical of *Clusia* (Clusiaceae) was isolated from a sample of Brazilian red propolis (Trusheva et al. 2006). Hyperibone (**23**, Figure 4), also a poplyprenylated benzophenone, is a constituent of a Northeastern non-red propolis from the state of Bahia (Castro et al. 2009). A propolis sample from Ceará state contains flavonoid aglycones and triterpenoids, including the rare canaric acid (**24**, Figure 4) (Albuquerque et al. 2007). Propolis from the state of Piauí (Brazilian Central-Northern region) contains cycloartane triterpenoids (e.g. **25**, Figure 4), compounds characteristic of *Mangifera indica* (Anacardiaceae, the mango tree) (da Silva et al. 2005). A *C*-glycoflavone was detected in this type of propolis (Righi et al. 2011).

***d. Amazonian Propolis***

Two chemical profiles were determined for propolis samples collected in the municipality of Manaus (Brazilian Amazon): predominance of either triterpenoids (lupeol, lupenone, β-amyrin, β-amyrenone) or polyisoprenylated benzophenones, such as 7-*epi*-nemorosone and 7-*epi*-clusianone (**26**, Figure 3) (Ishida et al. 2011).

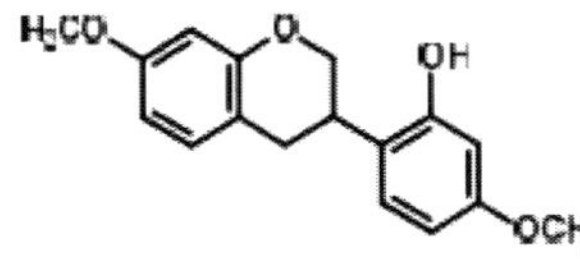

**19 ISOSATIVAN**

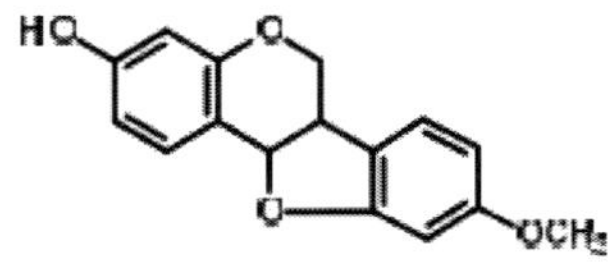

**20 MEDICARPIN**

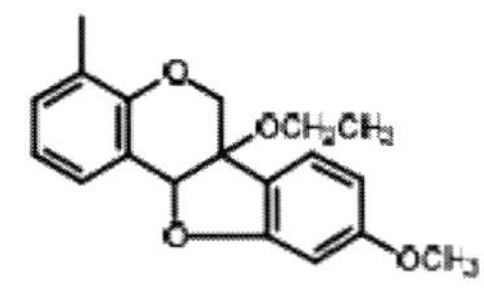

**21**

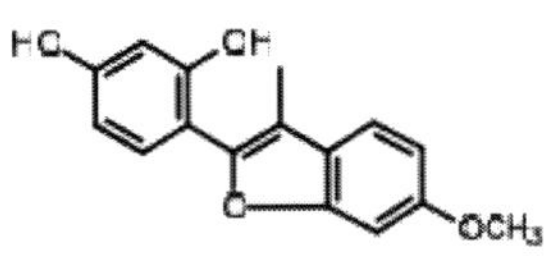

**22**

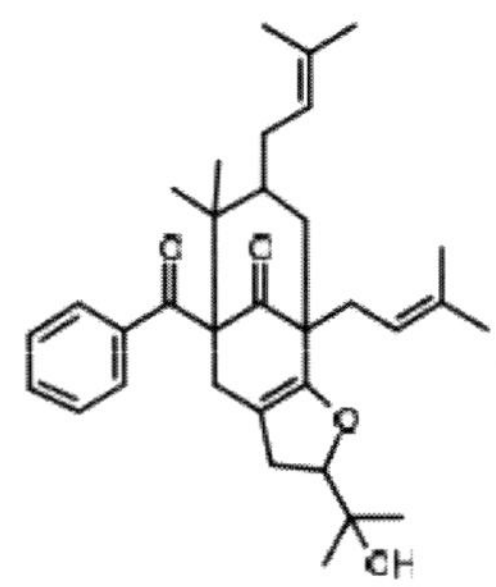

**23 HYPERIBONE**

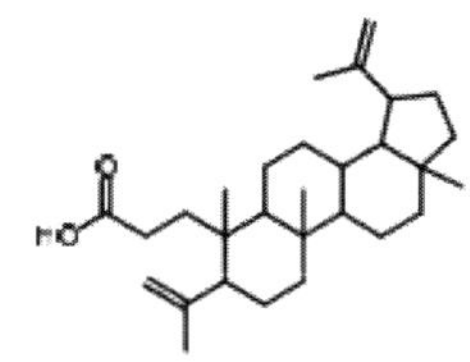

**24 CANARIC ACID**

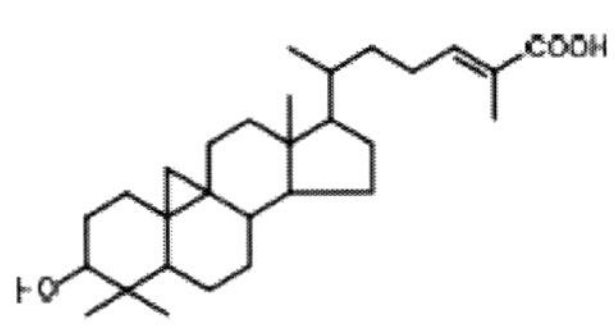

**25**

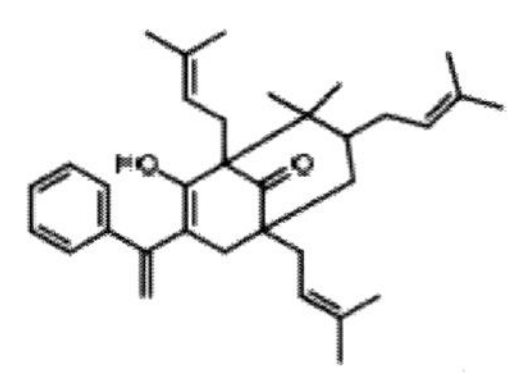

**26 7-*EPI*-CLUSIANONE**

Figure 3. Propolis constituents of Brazilian propolis from the Northeast (red propolis, **19**-**23**), Ceará (**24**), Piauí (**25**) and Amazon (**26**).

## Argentinean, Chilean and Uruguayan Propolis

In addition to poplar, different types of propolis have been reported from these countries. Major compounds of propolis from Tucumán (Argentina) are flavonols (e.g. isalpinin, galangin and rhamnocitrin), flavanones (e.g. 7-hydroxyflavanone and pinocembrin) and chalcones (e.g. 2',4'-dihydroxychalcone). The substances were shown to be derived from *Zuccagnia punctata* (Leguminosae, Caesalpinioideae) (Table 1, Agüero et al. 2010). Dimers of phenylpropanoids, including epoxylignans (e.g. **27**, Figure 4) are components of propolis from Andean regions of Argentina, which is derived from *Larrea nitida* (Zygophyllaceae) (Table 1, Agüero et al. 2011). Chilean propolis from a semi-arid region with Mediterranean climate and devoid of cultivated poplars, contains lignans, e.g. **28** (Figure 4) among its main constituents; some phenolic compounds in this propolis types contain up to three residues of phenylpropanoids (e.g. **29**, Figure 4) (Valcic et al. 1998). Propolis from a still more arid region in Chile contains other phenolic substances, such as viscidone, vanillin, methylenedioxy-acetophenone, ethoxymethoxy-benzaldehyde and cinnamic acid-3-methoxy-4-hydroxy methyl ester (Muñoz et al. 2001). From a propolis sample from the Chilean region in the Western Andean Maule region, typical poplar flavonoids, such as chrysin, galangin and pinocembrin were isolated (Astudillo et al. 2000). Propolis from Uruguay probably is also derived from poplars (Kumazawa et al. 2002).

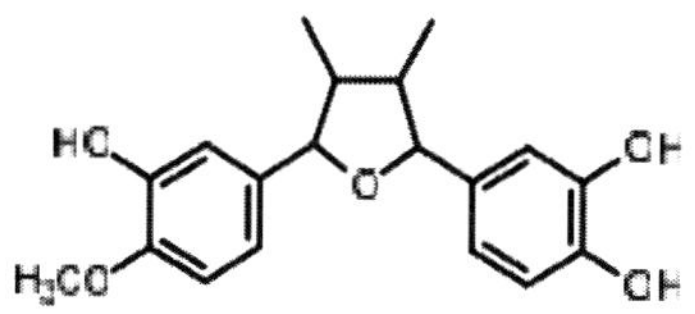

27

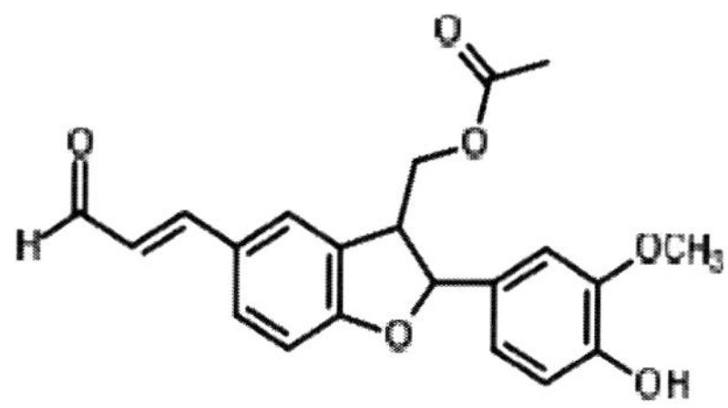

28

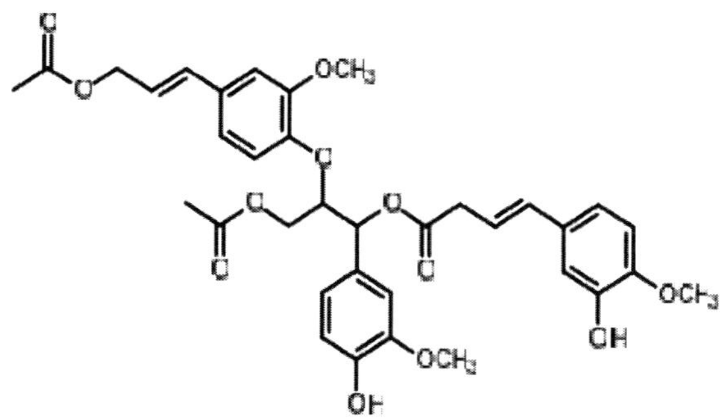

29

Figure 4. Propolis constituents from Argentinean (**27** and **28**) and Chilean (**29**) propolis.

## Venezuelan Propolis

From tropical regions, Venezuelan propolis was the first type to be object of analysis for identification of its components. The first report about its constituents was the paper by Tomás-Barberán et al. (1993). They showed that the chemical profile of propolis of *Apis mellifera* from several regions of Venezuela and propolis of native bees had compounds also found in exudates of flowers of *Clusia*, including *C. minor* (Clusiaceae). The main substances were polyisoprenylated benzophenones, e.g. nemorosonol. New polyisoprenylated benzophenones were isolated from a sample of Venezuelan propolis (Trusheva et al. 2004), along with scrobiculatones A and B (**30**, Figure 5).

## Cuban, Salvadoran and Mexican Propolis

There are at least three types of Cuban propolis: brown, red, and yellow. The brown type is probably the most common in the island and contains nemorosone as main constituent, a polyisoprenylated benzophenone which is also abundant in the flower resin of *Clusia rosea* (Cuesta-Rubio et al. 2002) and recognized as having several biological activities (Camargo et al. 2011). New polyisoprenylated benzophenones have been isolated from Cuban propolis (e.g. **31**, Figure 5) (Cuesta-Rubio et al. 1998, Hernández et al. 2005). The red Cuban propolis contains, among other substances, medicarpin (**20**) and other isoflavonoids (Piccinelly et al. 2005); it shares several characteristics with red Brazilian propolis, such as color, constituent substances and plant origin (*Dalbergia ecastophyllum*; Piccinelli et al. 2011). The intense red color of the plant resin, which is transferred to both red Brazilian and Cuban propolis, is accounted for rare substances, such as retusapurpurin (**32**, Figure 5), biosynthetically produced by the condensation of an isoflavan and a chalcone. Two types of yellow Cuban propolis are recognized: type A, containing mainly triterpenic acids and low contents of polymethoxylated flavones and flavonols, and type B, with predominance of acetyl triterpenes (Hernández et al. 2010). Plant sources of the yellow types A and B of yellow Cuban propolis remain unknown.

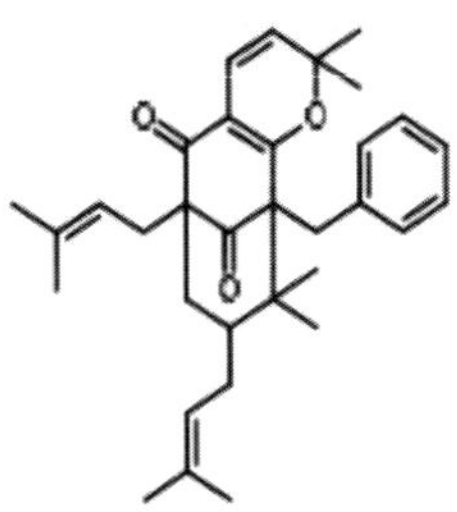

**30 SCROBICULATONE B**

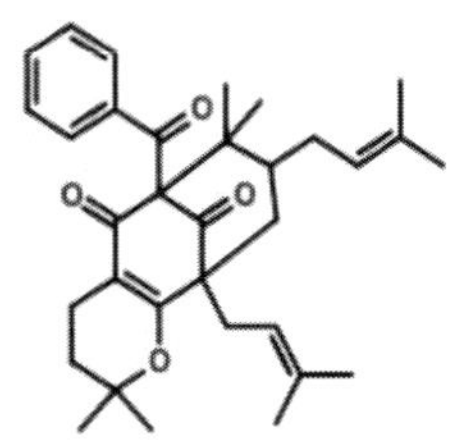

**31**

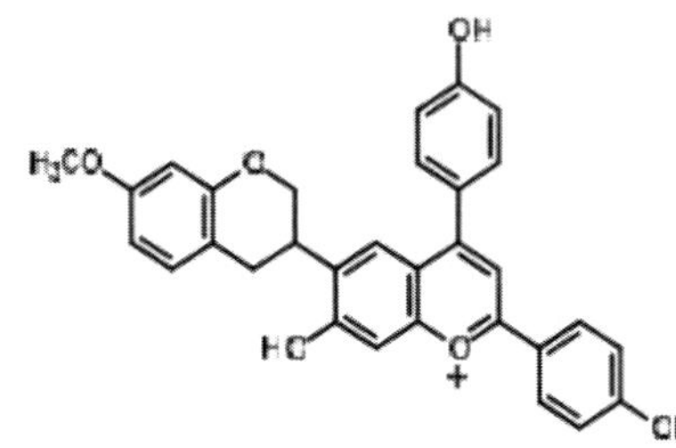

**32 RETUSAPURPURIN**

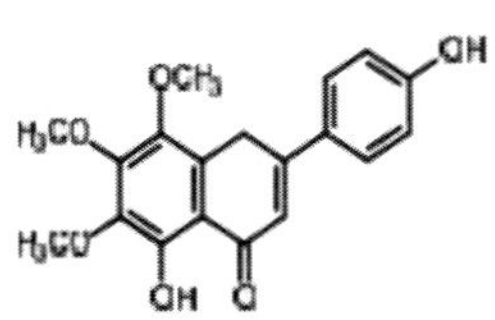

**33 XANTHOMICROL**

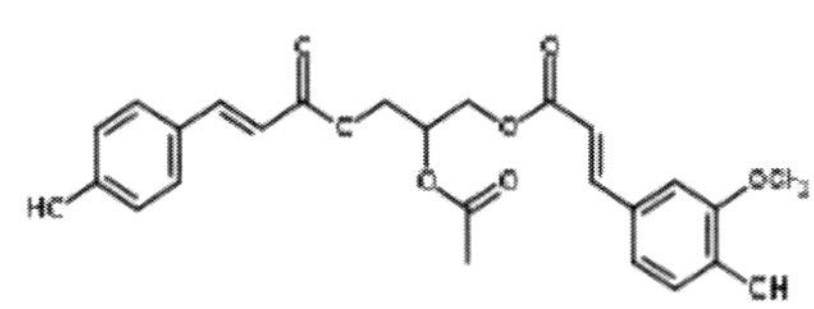

**34**

Figure 5. Propolis constituents from Venezuelan (**30**), Cuban (**31** and **32**) and Mexican (**33** and **34**) propolis.

Also, three types of propolis have been reported from Mexico. A sample from Champoton revealed a chemical profile suggesting an origin from *Dalbergia* (Leguminosae, Faboideae); it is a red propolis containing diphenyl propanes, flavanones, flavanes, isoflavans and pterocarpanes (Lotti et al., 2010). A sample from the Sonoran desert contains typical poplar flavonoids (e.g. CAPE, chrysin, pinocembrin, galangin), but also flavonoids probably derived from an additional plant source. Examples of the latter substances are naringenin, hesperetin and xanthomicrol (**33**, Figure 5) (Hernandez et al. 2007). A sample from the Sonora state yielded also flavonoids typical of *Populus nigra* and substances characterizing other species of *Populus*, e.g. 2-acetyl-1-*p*-coumaroyl-3-feruloylglycerol (**34**, Figure 5) (Li et al. 2010). It has been suggested that the source of this type of triglyceride is *Populus tremula* (Bankova et al. 2002). New cytotoxic phenylallylflavanones have been isolated from another sample from Sonoran Mexican propolis (Li et al. 2011).

Analysis of a propolis sample from El Salvador led to the isolation of two new chalcones, 2',3'-dihydroxy-4,4'-dimethoxychalcone and 2',3',4-trihydroxy-4'-methoxy chalcone (Popova et al. 2001). No suggestion has been given regarding the corresponding plant source.

## European Propolis

### *a. Temperate Continental Propolis*

Most of the propolis produced in Europe has long been known to contain components derived from poplars (Bankova et al. 1992). A sample of propolis from Rutten, the Netherlands, yielded flavonoids and caffeic acid esters typical of *Populus nigra*, a species of section *Aigeiros* (Greenaway et al. 1991). Netherland propolis contains also glycerol triesters (Banskota et al. 2002), such as **34** (Figure 5), present also in Mexican propolis (see above) and probably derived from other *Populus* species. A similar chemical profile characterizes propolis from Austria, France and Germany (Hegazi et al. 2000) and from Bulgaria, Italy and Switzerland (Banskota et al. 2002).

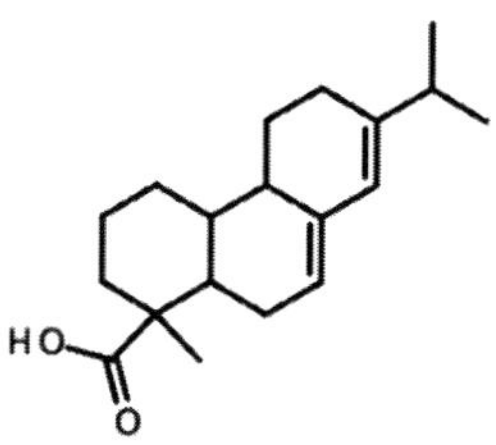


**35 ABIETIC ACID**

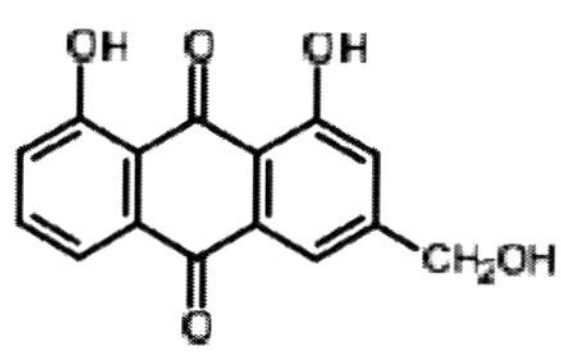


**36 EMODIN**

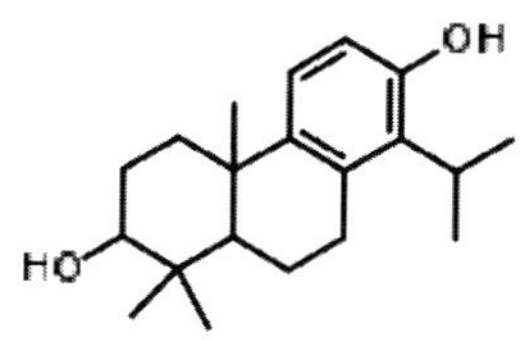


**37 TOTAROL**

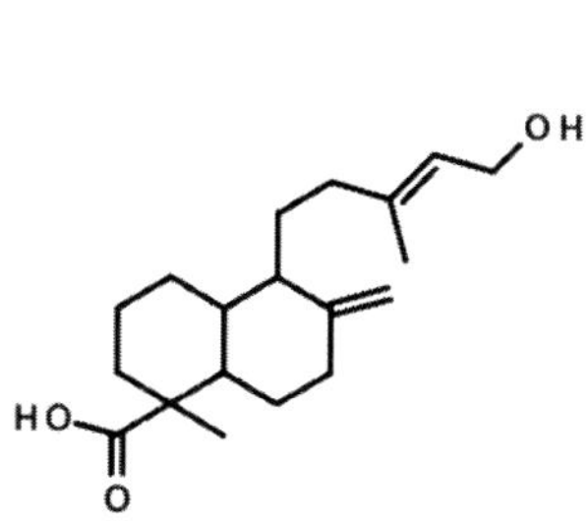


**38 ISOCUPRESSIC ACID**

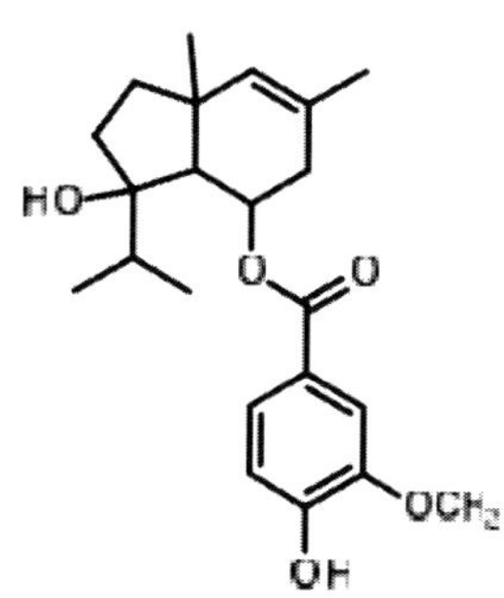


**39 TEFERIN**

Figure 6. Propolis constituents from Mediterranean propolis.

### *b. Mediterranean Propolis*

Propolis from the islands and the region bordering the Mediterranean has been shown to have a distinctive composition. It has been commented above that this type of propolis contains relatively high contents of sugars (see Section Minor or Infrequent Components). Along with sugars, flavonoids and esters typical of poplars are present, but at lower concentration, while other classes of components may occur with relatively higher abundance, such as diterpenes (Melliou and Chinou 2004). Complex composition of propolis from several locations of Greece and Cyprus was reported by Kalogeropoulos et al. (2009), including the diterpene abietic acid (**35**) and anthraquinones, e.g. emodin (**36**, Figure 6). A wide diversity of diterpenes was reported from several propolis samples from continental Greece and the Greek islands, including Crete (Popova et al. 2009, 2010a); examples of these diterpenoids are totarol (**37**) and isocupressic acid (**38**, Figure 6). Likely plant sources of these diterpenes are conifers widely cultivated in the regions, such as plants of species of *Pinus* and *Cupressus*. No suggestion has been given regarding the plant origin of the anthraquinones. Diterpenes are abundant also in propolis form Sicily and Malta (Popova et al. 2011). In Maltese propolis, in addition to poplar compounds, benzoic esters of sesquiterpene alcohols (e.g. teferin, **39** Figure 6) have been reported. The source of these esters is probably *Ferula communis* (Apiaceae), an herb common in Malta (Popova et al. 2011). Species of *Ferula* are probably also secondary sources of the same substances from Iranian propolis (Trusheva et al. 2010).

## Asian Propolis

As in other temperate parts of the world, Chinese and Japanese propolis has substances derived from poplars as main components. New flavonoids have been reported from Chinese propolis (Usia et al. 2002). Among these substances, compound **40** (Figure 7) stands out for having a residue of phenylpropene *C*-attached to ring A (Figure 7). It is a new compound derived of chrysin and hence is probably derived from poplar. Substances of propolis from several Korean regions (Ahn et al. 2004) are also typical components of poplar exudate buds.

Propolis from Okinawa and Taiwan, both Pacific islands, contain rare flavonanones, bearing prenyl and/or geranyl substituents (Kumazawa et al. 2004, 2008; Huang et al. 2007). Compound **41** (Figure 7), called either propolin G (Huang et al. 2007) or nymphaeol C (Kumazawa et al. 2008), bears both a prenyl and a geranyl group attached to the flavanone nucleus. The plant source of these compounds in Okinawan propolis is *Macaranga tanarius* (Euphorbiaceae) (Table 1, Kumazawa et al. 2008). *Macaranga* species are likely sources of geranyl-flavonoids from propolis samples in all other parts of the world; as yet, no other plant group is known to produce such substances. Geranyl flavanones are constituents also of Indonesian propolis, indicating that *Macaranga tanarius* contributes as plant source propolis production. Other classes of substances, namely alkyl resorcinols (e.g. **42**, Figure 7) and cycloartene triterpenes, were isolated from the same propolis samples. These substances are components of *Mangifera indica* (mango tree, Anacardiaceae), and thus Indonesian propolis has at least two plant origins (Trusheva et al. 2011). Mango trees are cultivated widely in tropical regions; it was mentioned above that a Brazilian propolis from Piauí has been reported as bearing cycloartane triterpenoids (see Northeastern and Central-Northern Brazilian propolis).

Propolis from Chitwan (Nepal) yielded new and known isoflavonoids and flavanones (Shrestha et al. 2007a,b). From another sample of propolis from the same region, these substances and several others were isolated. The propolis sample was shown to contain flavonoids, isoflavonoids (isoflavan, pterocarpans), chalcones and open-chain neoflavonoids (e.g. **43**, Figure 7) (Awale et al. 2005). Given the structures of the substances obtained from

Nepalese propolis, it was suggested that a probable plant source might be a species of *Dalbergia*, possibly trees of *D. sissoo*, which are abundant in the region (Awale et al. 2005).

## African Propolis

Few works have been done about propolis from Africa. Some investigations have dealt with activities of propolis, but did not include chemical analysis (e.g. El-Rahman 2010). Northern Africa, especially the region bordering the Mediterranean, probably produces propolis with characteristics mentioned above, relative poplar propolis and Mediterranean propolis. GC/MS analysis of propolis samples from Algeria and European countries, such as Bulgaria, Greece and Turkey, detected compounds typical of bud exudates of *Populus* section *Aigeiros*. However, certain regions of the north of Africa have been regarded as border areas of poplar cultivation, and thus poplars may not be always available. Thus, although poplar substances were present in a propolis sample from Tunisia, it showed composition distinct from a sample from Spain, because the former had relatively high amounts of myricetin 3,7,3'-trimethyl ether, and in the latter, the mentioned flavonol was not detected (Martos et al. 1997).

In Egypt there seems to be a wide variation of propolis composition. Hegazi and Abd El Hardy (2001) reported distinct composition for proplis from three Egyptian locations, only one of them with a chemical profile resembling that of bud poplars (presence of caffeate esters). Propolis from three other regions again had distinct compositions, only one with a typical poplar profile (El Hady and Hegazi (2002). Propolis from the Canary Islands has its own chemical characteristics, which include an abundance of sugars and sugar alcohols and furofuran lignans, e.g. compound **44** (Figure 8) (Bankova et al. 1998). Compounds typical of *Macaranga* (Euphorbiaceae), i.e. geranyl flavanones, were isolated from Egyptian propolis; among the compounds obtained, three are new flavonoids, e.g. compound **45** (Figure 8) (El-Bassuony 2009; AbouZid and El-Bassuony 2010).

Very little has been done about propolis in Africa south of the Sahara. An interesting report involves two samples from Kenya, one from the Mwingi district (Eastern region) and another from Voi (in the South) (Petrova et al. 2010). The chemical composition of the samples is very distinct. From the Mwingi sample, lactone lignans were isolated, among them, a new compound (tetrahydrojusticidin B, **46**, Figure 8). Other constituents of Mwingi propolis are triterpenes (e.g. alcohols of the amyrin type) and sugars. The plant source of this propolis type is still unknown. From the Voi sample, compounds typical of *Macaranga* (Euphorbiaceae), namely geranyl flavonoids were isolated. However, unlike the geranyl flavanones reported for propolis from Okinawa (Kumazawa et al. 2008), Taiwan (Huang et al. 2007) and Egypt (El-Bassuony 2009), the substances from Kenyan propolis are geranyl-flavonols (**47**, Figure 8). Complex geranyl stilbenes were also isolated from the Voi propolis, such as schweinfurthin A (**48**, Figure 8). Since these geranyl-stilbenes are known exclusively from *Macaranga schweinfurthii*, with populations spreading from the Northwest to the Northeast and East Africa, Petrova et al. (2010) put forward the suggestion that individuals of this plant species are sources of the Voi propolis.

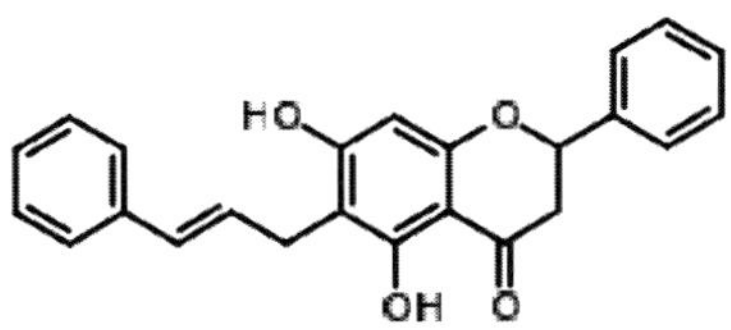


**40**

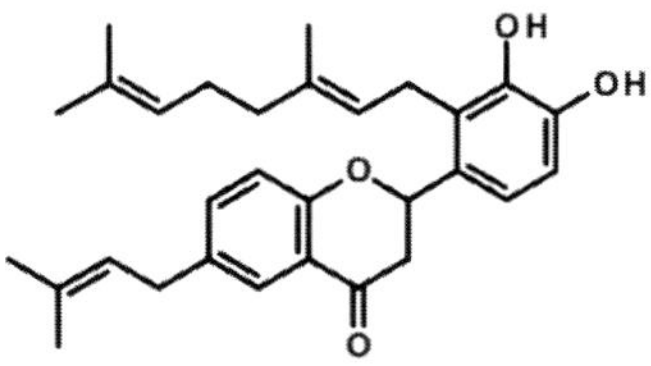


**41 NYMPHAEOLC**

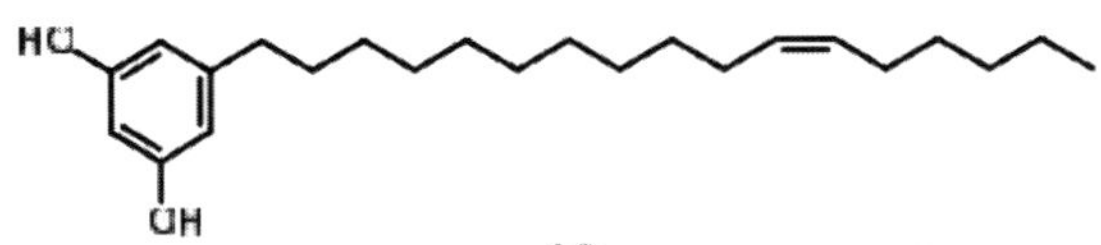


**42**

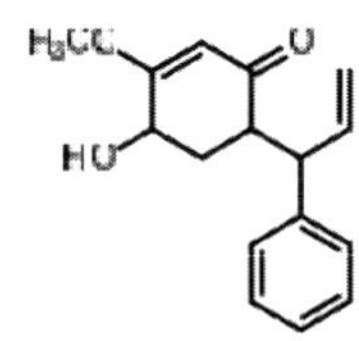


**43**

Figure 7. Constituents from Asian propolis: Chinese (**40**), Okinawan (41), Indonesian (**42**) and Nepalese (**43**).

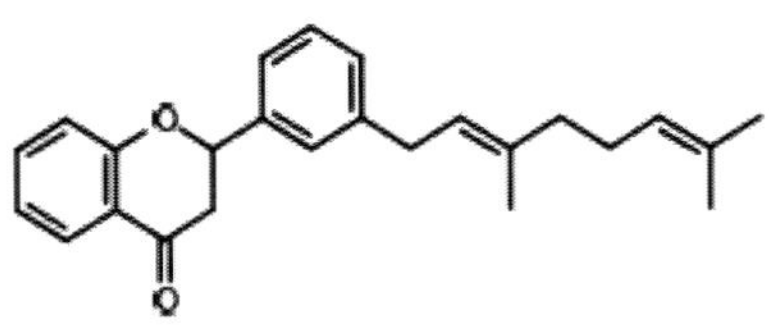

**44**

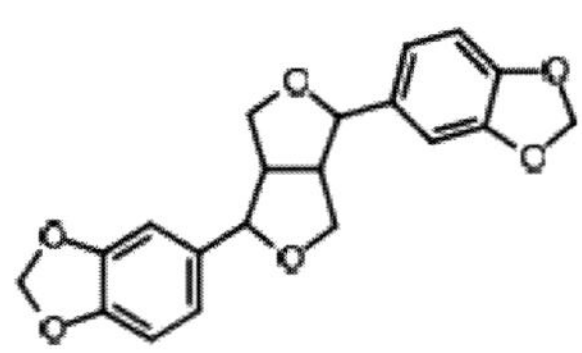

**45**

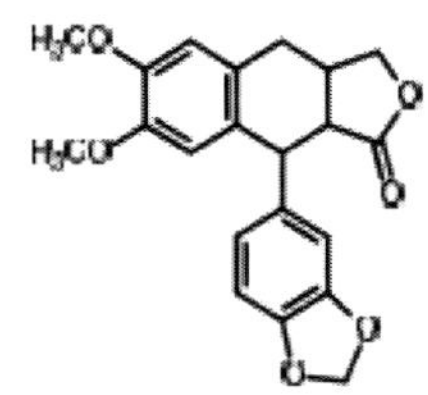

**46**

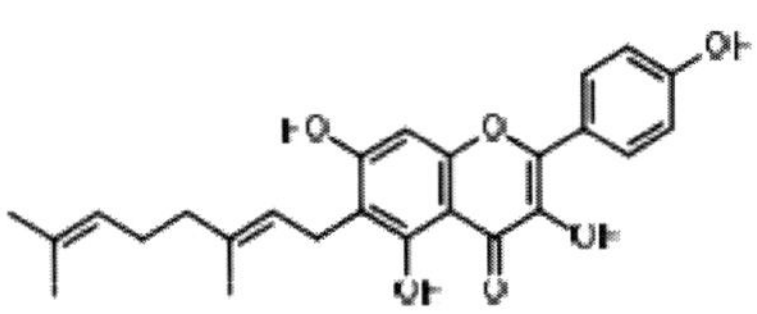

**47**

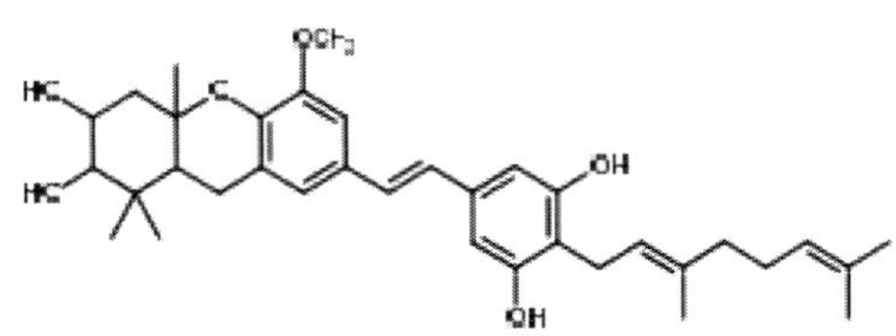


**47 SCHWEINFURTHIN A**

Figure 8. Constituents from African propolis: Canary Islands (44), Egyptian (45) and Kenyan (46, from Mwingi region, and 47, from Voi region).

## Chemical Variation of Propolis Composition

From the data presented in the previous sections, it is possible to evaluate the enormous diversity of propolis chemistry. Propolis composition, mainly of its resin, is completely dependent on the corresponding plant sources. The chemical composition of plant parts is not constant; it is influenced by factors such as season, organ development and plant phenology, all factors that may account for the variability of propolis composition along the year (see e.g. Teixeira et al. 2010). In the same region, distinct plant species may contribute to propolis production, so that completely distinct compositions may characterize propolis samples from nearby locations. It is doubtful whether genetic factors linked to honeybees might influence the choice of plant sources, as has been suggested (Silici and Kutluca 2005). It is possible to evaluate how variable may be the composition of propolis in a definite geographical area by the observation of the geographic distribution of brown, red, and yellow Cuban propolis (Figure 9; Cuesta-Rubio et al. 2007). In some Cuban provinces, such as Guantánamo and Holguín, only one type of propolis (brown) seems to occur (Figure 9). But brown and yellow types are produced in Matanzas, while mixed types (red + yellow, brown + red + yellow) were characterized in several locations (e.g. Villa Clara, Figure 9), indicating the contribution of several plant sources.

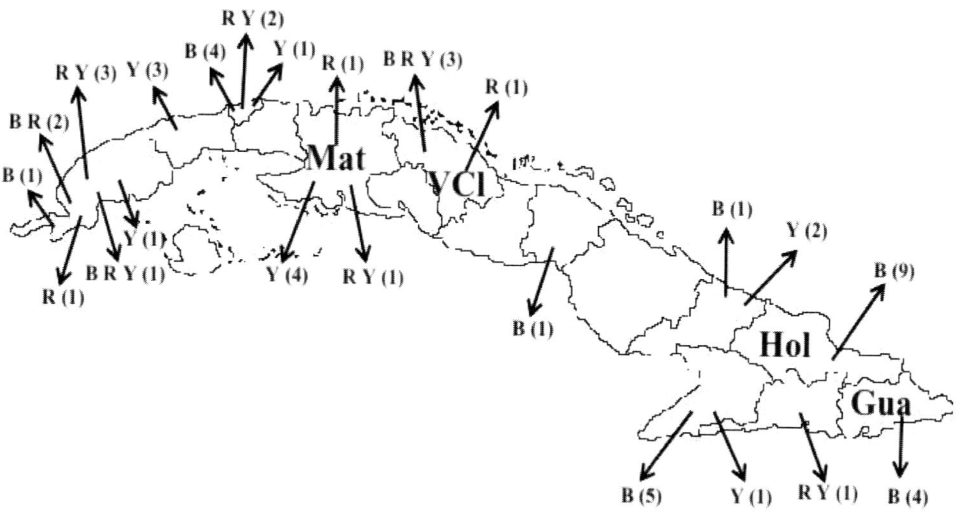


Figure 9. Distribution of brown (B), red (R), and yellow (Y) propolis in Cuban provinces. BR: mixed brown and red; RY: mixed red and yellow; BRY: mixed brown, red and yellow; Gua: Guantánamo province; Hol: Holguín province; Mat: Matanzas province; VCl: Villa Clara province. Digits within parentheses indicate numbers of propolis samples analyzed in the locality.

## PROPOLIS STANDARDIZATION

### *a. Parameters and Methods*

The wide variation in chemical composition, even within the borders of a small location, is a serious constraint regarding the use of propolis and its derivatives. From the past 20 years until now, standardization of propolis has been a theme persistently aimed at in propolis research (Volpert and Elstner 1993; Woisky and Salatino 1998, Bankova et al. 2000; Bankova 2005a,b; Hubicka et al. 2006; Popova et al. 2007; Lozina et al. 2010). Parameters and relatively fast and inexpensive procedures have been proposed for chemical characterization of propolis. Most procedures do not allow the identification of individual chemical constituents, but they intend to make sure that biological active classes of substances are present in acceptable amounts. Some papers propose the quantification of propolis components, such as waxes, which do not add biological properties, but contribute to increase the volume and mass of the product. Contents of total volatile substances and ash are other recommended parameters. Standardization is important also for detection of counterfeits in propolis commercialization. Proposals from several papers converge to some common parameters, such as total phenolics and total flavonoids (Woisky and Salatino 1998; Bankova 2005b, Popova et al. 2007). Other proposals include biological assays, such as tests for evaluation of antimicrobial activity (Popova et al. 2007).

***b. Chemical Markers of Propolis Types***

Marker substances are useful for the chemical characterization of propolis samples, giving reliance relative the plant origin of the product and hence to its chemical composition. A marker compound is assumed to be relatively abundant and always present in the propolis type under consideration. In addition, fast laboratory procedures have to be available for its detection. Two types of propolis have been the focus of more studies: poplar (from temperate regions) and alecrim, or green, propolis (from Southeast and Central Brazil). The substance of poplar propolis receiving more attention lately is caffeic acid phenethyl ester, commonly abbreviated as CAPE (**8**, Figure 1). Many pharmacological activities have been ascribed to CAPE (Aviello et al. 2010). It was reported for the first time as a propolis constituent (Bankova et al. 1987) and later in bud exudates of *Populus nigra*. It is one of the most abundant caffeic esters of poplar propolis. Two marker compounds have been proposed for Brazilian alecrim propolis: artepillin C (**9**) and the allyl ester of 3-prenylcinnamate (**12**, Figure 2). A wide diversity of biological properties have been assigned to artepillin C (for review, see Duque-Estrada et al. 2008). The substance is relatively abundant in alcohol extracts. The allyl ester of 3-prenylcinnamate is obtained in higher amounts from chloroform extracts (Negri et al. 2003a) of alecrim propolis and apical buds of the plant (Nascimento et al. 2008).

## CONCLUSION AND PERSPECTIVES ON THE CHEMISTRY OF PROPOLIS

Propolis chemistry is still an emerging field of research. But its contribution to natural products chemistry and, more specifically, to plant chemistry is undisputed (Salatino et al. 2011). For a long time to come, a continuation or an intensification of the presently observed rhythm of publications about new propolis types and propolis chemical constituents is expected.

Proposals for standardization of propolis samples require refining. Probably, some parameters and procedures may be adequate to some types of propolis, but not to others. Thus, an adequate strategy may possibly be the establishment of parameters and procedures specifically oriented toward a certain type of propolis, as has been recommended for the standardization of poplar (Popova et al. 2007) and Taiwan propolis (Popova et al. 2010b). The identification of propolis plant sources is fundamental for propolis type characterization, as is also the establishment of geographic delimitation of propolis types. Geographic limits are expected to widen, as occurred with propolis containing geranyl flavonoids (Salatino et al. 2011). The establishment of marker substances for specific propolis types is another fundamental step toward characterization and standardization. So far, markers have been suggested only for the two most studied types of propolis (alecrim and poplar propolis).

Propolis wax has been given little attention, probably because it is a biologically inert component. Several basic aspects of propolis wax remain unclear. Propolis wax likely has an origin similar to the comb wax, which means that it is essentially a bee product (Negri et al. 2000). Instead of stemming from exudates, the resin of alecrim propolis is originated from whole apical buds and young leaves. These plant parts have surface waxes, and they are expected to be part of propolis wax. What are the proportions of plant wax and beeswax in alecrim propolis? Do poplar bud exudates and *Clusia* flower exudates have wax? Undoubtedly, the impermeable material on the surface of fruits of *Macaranga tanarius*, which bees collect to produce Okinawan propolis (Table 1), contains wax, and it seems reasonable to assume that they are part of the propolis wax. The waxes of the Brazilian comb and propolis seem to have fatty acids, primary alcohols and hydrocarbons with distribution that vary according to the geographic location; it has been suggested that such distribution reflects the genetic of the bees, or the degree of bee Africanization in Brazil (Custodio et al. 2003). The relationship of chemical characteristics of the waxes with the genetic and taxonomy of the bees is an aspect that possibly deserves consideration.

Sugars have been pointed out as quantitatively relevant for only a few types of propolis, mainly from the Mediterranean region. It is not clear if sugars are really absent or irrelevant in other types of propolis or if not, adequate methods have been applied for their detection in propolis analysis from other regions. Propolis is commercialized worldwide as a complementary food, although it has been widely used in popular medicine. However, contrary to what has been observed regarding chemical analysis of honey, very little has been done about propolis contents of vitamins, amino acids and minerals. It seems clear that much more research on these propolis constituents are needed for a wider understanding of propolis chemistry and origin. Pollen in propolis is a likely source of several nutrients, such as amino acids and vitamins. Pollen analysis is not adequate toward the determination of the origin of the propolis resin, but it may be useful as additional information about the geographic region where the propolis was produced. Hence, pollen analysis may turn out as an item to be recommended for propolis standardization.

## ACKNOWLEDGMENTS

The authors are fellow researchers of CNPq (Conselho Nacional do Desenvolvimento Científico e Tecnológico, Brazil).

## REFERENCES

AbouZid, S., El-Bassuony, A. 2010. A new prenylated flavanoid with antibacterial activity from propolis collected in Egypt. *Natural Product Communications*5: 43-45.

Adelmann, J., Passos, M., Breyer, D.H., dos Santos, M. H. R., Lenz, C., Leite, N. F., Lanças, F. M., Fontana, J. D. 2007. Exotic flora dependence of an unsual Brazilian propolis: the pinocembrin biomarker by capillary techniques. *Journal of Pharmaceutical and Biomedical Analysis* 43: 174-178.

Agüero, M.B., Gonzales, MB. L., Svetaz, L., Sánchez, M., Zacchino, S., Feresin, G. E., Schmeda-Hirschmann, G., Palermo, J., Wunderlin, D., Tapia, A. 2010. Argentinean propolis from *Zuccagnia punctata* Cav. (Ceasalpinioideae) exudates: phytochemical characterization and antifungal activity. *Journal of Agricultural and Food Chemistry* 58: 194-201.

Agüero, M.B., Svetaz, L., Sánchez, M., Luna, L., Lima, B., López, M.L., Zacchino, S., Palermo, J., Wunderlin, D., Feresin, G. E., Tapia, A. 2011. Argentinean Andean propolis associated with the medicinal plant *Larrea nitida* Cav. (Zygophyllaceae). HPLC-MS and GC-MS characterization and antifungal activity. *Food and Chemical Toxicology* 49: 1970-1978.

Ahn, M.-R., Kumazawa, S., Hamasaka, T., Bang, K.-S., Nakayama, T. 2004. Antioxidant activity and constituents of propolis collected in various areas of Korea. *Food Chemistry* 52: 7286-7292.

Akao, Y., Maruyama, H., Matsumoto, K., Ohguchi, K., Nishizawa, K., Sakamoto, T., Araki, Y., Mishima, S., Nozawa, Y. 2003. Cell growth inhibitory effect of cinnamic acid derivatives from proplis on human tumor cell lines. *Biological & Pharmaceutical Bulletin* 26: 1057-1059.

Albuquerque, I.L., Alves, L.A., Lemos, T.L.G., Monte, F.J.Q., Braz-Filho, R.B. 2007. Ácido canárico (3,4-*seco*-derivado do lupano) em própolis do Ceará. *Química Nova* 30: 828-831.

Astudillo, L, Avila, F., Morrison, R., Gutierrez, M. J., Bastida, J., Codina, C., Schmeda-Hirschmann, G. 2000. Biologically active compounds from Chilean propolis. *Boletin de la Sociedad Chilena de Química* 45: 577-581.

Aviello, G., Scalisi, C., Fileccia, R., Capasso, R., Romano, B., Izzo, A.A., Borrelli, F. 2010. Inhibitory effect of caffeic acid phanethyl ester, a plant derived compound, on rat intestinal contractility. *European Journal of Pharmacology* 640: 163-170.

Awale, S., Li, F., Onozuka, H., Esumi, H., Tezuka, Y., Kadota, S. 2008. Constituents of Brazilian red propolis and their preferential cytotoxic activity against human pancreatic PANC-1 cancer cell line in nutrient-deprived condition. *Bioorganic & Medicinal Chemistry* 16: 181-189.

Awale, S., Shrestha, S.P., Tezuka, Y., Ueda, J., Matsushige, K., Kadota, S. 2005. Neoflavonoids and related constituents from Nepalese propolis and their nitric oxide production inhibitory activity. *Journal of Natural Products* 68: 858-864.

Bankova, V. 2005a. Recent trends and important developments in propolis research. *Evidence-Based Complementary and Alternative Medicine* 2: 29-32.

Bankova, V. 2005b. Chemical diversity of propolis and the problem of standardization. *Journal of Ethnopharmacology* 100: 114-117.

Bankova, V., Boudourova-Krasteva, G., Sforcin, J.M., Frete, X., Kujumgiev, A. Maimoni-Rodella, R., Popov, S. 1999. Phytochemical evidence for the origin of Brazilian propolis from São Paulo state. *Zeitschrift für Naturforschung* C 54: 5-6.

Bankova, V.S., Christov, R.S., Tejera, A.D. 1998. Lignans and other constituents of propolis from the Canary Islands. *Phytochemistry* 49: 1411-1415.

Bankova, V, de Castro, S.L., Marcucci, M. C. 2000. Propolis: recent advances in chemistry and plant origin. *Apidologie* 31: 3-15.

Bankova, V., Dyulgerov, A., Popov, S., Evstatieva, L., Kuleva, L., Pureb, O., Zamjansan, Z. 1992. Propolis produced in Bulgaria and Mongolia: phenolic compounds and plant origin. *Apidologie* 23: 79-85.

Bankova, V., Dyulgerov, A., Popov, S.S., Marekov, N.L. 1987. A GC/MS study of the propolis phenolic constituents. *Zeitschrift für Naturforschung* C 42: 147-151.

Bankova, V., Popova, M., Bogdanov, S., Sabatini, A.G. 2002. Chemical composition of European propolis: expected and unexpected results. *Zeitschift für Naturforschung* C 57: 530-533.

Banskota, A.H., Nagaoka, T., Sumioka, L.Y., Tezuka, Y., Awale, S., Midorikawa, K., Matsushige, K., Kadota, S. 2002. Antiproliferative activity of the Netherland propolis and its active principles in cancer cell lines. *Journal of Ethnopharmacology* 80: 67-73.

Banskota, A.H., Tezuka, Y., Kadota, S. 2001. Recent progress in pharmacological research of propolis. *Phytotherapy Research* 15: 561-571.

Banskota, A.H., Tezuka, Y., Midorikawa, K., Matsushige, K., Kadota, S. 2000. Two novel cytotoxic benzofuran derivatives from Brazilian propolis. *Journal of Natural Products* 63: 1277-1279.

Banskota, A.H., Tezuka, T., Prasain, J.K., Matsushige, K., Saiki, I., Kadota, S. 1998. Chemical constituents of Brazilian propolis and their cytotoxic activities. *Journal of Natural Products* 61: 896-900.

Barth, O.M. 1998. Pollen analysis of Brazilian propolis. *Granja* 37: 97-101.

Barth, O.M., da Luz C.F.P. 2009. Palynological analysis of Brazilian red própolis samples. *Journal of Apicultural Research and the Bee World* 48: 181-188.

Belmiro, M.S., Oki, Y., Fernandes, G.W. 2011. Propolis: nosso tesouro. *Mensagem Doce* 112: 9.

Bianchi, G. 1995. Plant waxes. *In* Hamilton, R. J. (ed.) *Waxes: Chemistry, Molecular Biology and Functions.* The Oily Press, Dundee, p. 175-222.

Burdock, G.A. 1998. Review of the biological properties and toxicity of bee propolis (propolis). *Food and Chemical Toxicology* 36: 347-363.

Camargo, M.S., Varela, S.D., Oliveira, A.P.S., Resende, F.A., Cuesta-Rubio, O., Vilegas, W., Varanda, E.A. 2011. Assessment of estrogenic, mutagenic and antimutagenic activity of nemorosone. *Revista Brasileira de Farmacognosia* 21: 921-927.

Castro, M.L., Nascimento, A.M., Ikegaki, M., Costa-Neto, C.M., Alencar, S.M., Rosalen, P.L. 2009. Identification of a bioactive compound isolated from Brazilian proplis type 6. *Bio-organic & Medicinal Chemistry* 17: 5332-5335.

Catorini, P.E. 1963. Le api e gli uomini. *Fitoterapia* 34: 85-93.

Chikaraishi, Y., Izuta, H., Shimazawa, M., Mishima, S., Hara, H. 2010. Angiostatic effects of Brazilian green propolis and its chemical constituents. *Molecular Nutrition & Food Research* 54: 566-575.

Crane, E. 1988. *Beekeeping: science, practice and world resources.* Heinemann, London.

Cuesta-Rubio, O., Cuellar, A.C., Rojas, N., Castro, H.V., Rastrelli, L., Aquino, R. 1999. A polyisoprenylated benzophenone from Cuban propolis. *Journal of Natural Products* 62: 1013-1015.

Cuesta-Rubio, O. Frontana-Uribe, B.A., Ramírez-Apan, T., Cárdenaz, J. 2002. Polyisoprenylated benzophenones in Cuban propolis. *Zeitschrift für Naturforschung* C 57: 372-378.

Cuesta-Rubio, O., Piccinelli, A.L., Fernandez, M.C., Hernandez, I.M., Rosado, A., Rastrelli, L. 2007. Chemical characterization of Cuban propolis by HPLC-PDA, HPLC-MS and NMR: the brown, red, and yellow Cuban varieties of propolis. *Journal of Agricultural and Food Chemistry* 55: 7502-7509.

Custodio, A.R., Ferreira, M.M.C., Negri, G., Salatino, A. 2003. Clustering of comb and propolis waxes based on the distribution of aliphatic constituents. *Journal of the Brazilian Chemistry Society* 14: 354-357.

d'Albore, G.R. 1979. L'origine géographique de la propolis. *Apidologie* 10: 241-267.

da Silva, M.S.S., Citó, A.M.G.L., Chaves, M.H., Lopes, J.A.D. 2005. Triterpenoides tipo cicloartano de própolis de Teresina – Piauí. *Química Nova* 28: 801-804.

Daugsch, A., Moraes, C.S., Fort, P., Park, Y.K. 2008. Brazilian red propolis – chemical composition and botanical origin. *Evidence-Based Complementary and Alternative Medicine* 5: 435-441.

Deblock-Bostyn, G. 1982. L'Abeille et ses produits. *Bulletin de la Societé Pharmaceutique de Lille* 38: 181-203.

de Moura, S.A.L., Negri, G., Salatino, A., Lima, L.D.C., Dourado, L.P.A., Mendes, J.B., Andrade, S.P., Ferreira, M.A.N.D., Cara, D.C. 2011. Aqueous extract of Brazilian green propolis: primary componentes, evaluation of inflammation and wound healing by using subcutaneous implanted sponges. *Evidence-Based Complementary and Alternative Medicine* (available on-line, DOI: 10.1093/ecam;nep112.

dos Santos, C.G., Blochtein, B., Megiolaro, F.L., Imperatriz-Fonseca, V.L. 2010. Age polyethism in *Plebeia emerina* (Friese) (Hymenoptera: Apidae) colonies related to propolis handling. *Neotropical Entomology* 39: 691-696.

Duque-Estrada, G.O., da Silva, J.F.M., Antunes, O.A.C. 2008. Artepillin C: a review. *Letters in Drug Design & Discovery* 5: 88-92.

El-Bassuony, A.A. 2009. New prenylated compound from Egyptian propolis with antimicrobial activity. *Revista Latinoamericana de Química* 37: 85-90.

El Hady, F.K.A., Hegazi, A.G. 2002. Egyptian propolis: 2. Chemical composition, antiviral and antimicrobial activities of East Nile Delta propolis. *Zeitschrift für Naturforschung* C 57: 386-394.

El-Rahman, S.S.A. 2010. West-Libyan propolis and rosemary have synergistic anti-tumor effect against 12-*O*-tetradecoylphorbol-13-acetate-induced skin tumor in BULB/C mice previously initiated with 7,12-dimethylbenz[*a*]anthracene. *Basic and Applied Pathology* 3: 46-51.

Erkulov, Z.E., Malikova, M. Kh., Rakhmanberdyeva, R.K. 2011. Carbohydrates from the aerial part of *Ferula kuhistanica* and *F. tenuisera*. *Chemistry of Natural Compounds* 47: 182-184.

Gabrys, J., Konecki, J., Krol, W., Scheller, S., Shani, J. 1986. Free amino acids identified and quantified by gas-liquid chromatography. *Pharmaceutical Research Communications* 18: 513-518.

Ghisalbelti, E.L. (1970). Propolis: a review. *Bee World* 60: 59-84.

Greenaway, W., English, S., Whatley, F.R., Rood, S.B. 1991. Inter-relationships of poplars in a hybrid swarm as studied by gas-chromatography-mass spectrometry. *Canadian Journal of Botany* 69: 203-208.

Harborne, J.B., Turner, B.L. 1984. *Plant chemosystematics*. Academic Press, London.

Hegazi, A.G., El Hady, A., Abd Allah, F.A. 2000. Chemical composition and antimicrobial activity of European propolis. *Zeitschrift für Naturforschung* C 55: 70-75.

Hegazi, A.G., Abd El Hardy. 2001. Egyptian propolis: 1. Antimicrobial activity and chemical composition of Upper Egypt propolis. *Zeitschrift für Naturforschung* C 56: 82-88.

Hernández, I.M., Fernandez, M.C., Cuesta-Rubio, O., Piccinelli, A.L., Rastrelli, L. 2005. Polyprenylated benzophenone derivatives from Cuban propolis. *Journal of Natural Products* 68: 931-934.

Hernández, I.M., Cuesta-Rubio, O., Fernández, M.C., Pérez, R., Porto, R.M., Piccinelli, A.L., Rastrelli, L. 2010. Studies on the constituents of yellow Cuban propolis: GC-MS determination of triterpenoids and flavonoids. *Journal of Agricultural and Food Chemistry* 58: 4725-4730.

Hernandez, J., Goycoolea, F.M., Quintero, J., Acosta, A., Castañeda, M., Dominguez, Z., Robles, R., Vazquez-Moreno, L., Velazquez, E.F., Astiazaraan, H., Lugo, E., Velazquez, C. 2007. *Planta Medica* 73: 1469-1474.

Huang, W.-J., Huang, C.H., Wu, C.-L., Lin, J.-K., Chen, Y.-W., Lin, C.-L., Chuang, S.-E., Huang, C.-Y., Chen, C.-N. 2007. Propolin G, a prenylflavanone, isolated from Taiwanese propolis, induces caspase-dependent apoptosis in brain cancer cells. *Journal of Agricultural and Food Chemistry* 55: 7366-7376.

Hubicka, U., Krzek, J., Kaleta, J., Niedzwiedz, A. 2006. Evaluation of densitometric TLC quantitative analysis of selected phenolic acids for standardization of propolis concentrates. *JPC - Journal of Planar Chromatography- Modern TLC* 19: 449-453.

Ishida, V.F.C., Negri, G., Salatino, A., Bandeira, M.F.C.L. 2011.A new type of Brazilian propolis: prenylated benzophenones in propolis from Amazon and effects against cariogenic bacteria. *Food Chemistry* 125: 966-972.

Ito, J., Chang, F.R., Wang, H.K., Park, Y.K., Ikegaki, M., Kilgore, N., Lee, K.H. 2001. Anti-AIDS agents. 48. Anti-HIV activity of moronic acid derivatives and the new melliferone-related triterpenoid isolated from Brazilian propolis. *Journal of Natural Products* 64: 1278-1281.

Junkunz, B. 1932. Über das Biennen Harz (Propolis). *Chemisches Umschau* 39: 30-33.

Kalogeropoulos, N., Konteles, S.J., Troullidou, E., Ioannis, M., Karathanos, V.T. 2009. Chemical composition, antioxidant activity and antimicrobial properties of propolis extracts from Greece and Cyprus. *Food Chemistry* 116: 452-461.

Kumazawa, S., Goto, H., Hamasaka, T., Fukumoto, S., Fujimoto, T., Nakayama, T. 2004. A new prenylated flavonoid from propolis collected in Okinawa, Japan. *Bioscience, Biotechnology and Biochemistry* 68: 260-262.

Kumazawa, S., Hayashi, K., Kajiya, K., Ishii, T., Hamasaka, T., Nakayama, T. 2002. Studies of the constituents of Uruguayan propolis. *Journal of the Agricultural and Food Chemistry* 50: 4777-4782.

Kumazawa, S., Nakamura, J., Murase, M., Miyagawa, M., Ahn, M.-R., Fukumoto, S. 2008. Plant origin of Okinawan propolis: honeybee behavior observation and phytochemical analysis. *Naturwissenschaften* 95: 781-786.

Kumazawa, S., Yoneda, M., Shibata, I., Kanaeda, J., Hamasaka, T., Hakayama, T. Direct evidence for the plant origin of Brazilian propolis by the observation of honeybee behavior and phytochemical analysis. *Chemical & Pharmaceutical Bulletin* 51: 740-742.

Lavie, P. 1968. Les substances antibiotiques dans la colonie d'abeilles. *In* R. Chauvin (ed.) *Traité de biologie de l'abeille*. Masson et Cie., Paris, v. 3, 1-115.

Li, F., Awale, S., Tezuka, Y., Esumi, H., Kadota, S. 2010. Study on the constituents of Mexican propolis and their cytotoxic activity against PANC-1 human pancreatic cancer cells. *Journal of Natural Products* 73: 623-627.

Li, F., Awale, S., Zhang, H., Tezuka, Y., Esumi, H., Kadota, S. 2009. Chemical constituents of propolis from Myanmar and their preferential cytotoxicity against a human pancreatic cancer cell line. *Journal of Natural Products* 72: 1283-1287.

Li, F., He, Y.M., Awale, S., Kadota, S., Tezuka, Y. 2011. Two new cytotoxic phenylallylflavanones from Mexican propolis. *Chemical & Pharmaceutical Bulletin* 59: 1194-1196.

Lotti, C., Fernandez, M.C., Piccinelli, A.L., Cuesta-Rubio, O., Hernández, I.M., Rastrelli, L. 2010. Chemical constituents of red Mexican propolis. *Journal of Agricultural and Food Chemistry* 58: 2209-2213.

Lozina, L.A., Peichoto, M.E., Acosta, O.C., Granero, G. E. 2010. Standardization and organoleptic and physicochemical characterization of 15 Argentinean propolis. *Latin American Journal of Pharmacy* 29: 102-110.

Marcucci, M.C. 1995. Propolis: chemical composition, biological properties and therapeutic activity. *Apidologie* 26: 83-99.

Martos, I., Cossentini, M., Ferreres, F., Tomás-Barberán, F.A. 1997. Flavonoid composition of Tunisian honeys and propolis. *Journal of Agriculture and Food Chemistry* 45: 2814-2829.

Matsubayashi, H., Lagan, P., Sukor, J.R.A. 2006. Utilization of *Macaranga* trees by the Asian elephants (*Elephas maximus*) in Borneo. *Mammal Study* 31: 115-118.

Matsui, T., Ebuchi, S., Fujise, T., Abesundara, K.J.M., Doi, S., Yamada, H., Matsumoto, K. 2004. Strong anti-hyperglycemic effects of water-soluble fraction of Brazilian propolis and its bioactive constituents, 3,4,5-tri-*O*-caffeoylquinic acid. *Biological & Pharmaceutical Bulletin* 27: 1797-1803.

Melliou, E., Chinou, I. 2004. Chemical analysis and antimicrobial activity of Greek propolis. *Planta Medica* 70: 515-519.

Mishima, S., Yoshida, C., Akino, S., Sakamoto, T. 2005. Anti-hypertensive effects of Brazilian propolis: identification of caffeoylquinic acids as constituents involved in the hypotension in spontaneously hypertensive rats. *Biological & Pharmaceutical Bulletin* 28: 1909-1914.

Mishima, S., Inoh, Y., Narita, Y., Ohta, S., Sakamoto, T., Araki, Y., Suzuki, K.M., Akao, Y., Nozawa, Y. 2005. Identification of caffeoylquinic acid derivatives from Brazilian propolis as constituents involved in induction of granulocytic differentiation of HL-60 cells. *Bio-organic & Medicinal Chemistry* 13: 5814-5818.

Mohammadzadeh, M.J., Emam-Djomeh, Z., Safari, M., Mousavi, M., Ghanbarzadeh, B., Philips, G.O. 2007. Physicochemical and emulsifying properties of Barijeh (*Ferula gumosa*) gum. *Iranian Journal of Chemistry & Chemical Engineering – International English Edition* 26: 81-88.

Muñoz, O., Peña, R.C., Ureta, E., Montenegro, G., Timmermann, B.N. 2001. Propolis from Chilean matorral hives. *Zeitschrift für Naturforschung* C 56: 269-272.

Nakajima, Y., Shimazawa, M., Mishina, S., Hara, H. 2007. Water extract of propolis and its main constituents, caffeoylquinic acid derivatives, exert neuroprotective effects *via* antioxidant actions. *Life Sciences* 80: 370-377.

Nakajima, Y., Shimazawa, M., Mishina, S., Hara, H. 2009. Neuroprotective effects of Brazilian green propolis and its main constituents against oxygen-glucose deprivation stress, with gene-expression analysis. *Phytotherapy Research* 23: 1431-1438.

Nascimento, E.A., Chang, R., Morais, S.A.L., Piló-Veloso, D., Reis, D.C. 2008. Um marcador químico de fácil detecção para a própolis de alecrim-do-campo (*Baccharis dracunculifolia*). *Revista Brasileira de Farmacognosia* 18: 379-386.

Negri, G., Marcucci, M.C., Salatino, A., Salatino, M.L. 2000. Comb and propolis waxes from Brazil (states of São Paulo and Paraná). *Journal of Brazilian Chemical Society* 11: 453-457.

Negri, G., Marcucci, M.C., Salatino, A., Salatino, M.L. 2000. Comb and propolis waxes from Brazil: triterpenoids in propolis waxes. *Journal of Apicultural Research* 39: 86-88.

Negri, G., Marcucci, M.C., Salatino, A., Salatino, M.L.F. 1998. Hydrocarbons and monoesters of propolis waxes from Brazil. *Apidologie* 29: 305-314.

Negri, G., Salatino, M.L.F., Salatino, A. 2003a. 'Green propolis': unreported constituents and a novel compound from chloroform extracts. *Journal of Apicultural Research* 42: 39-41.

Negri, G. Salatino, M.L.F., Salatino, A. 2003b. Unusual chemical composition of a sample of Brazilian propolis, as assessed by analysis of a chloroform extract. *Journal of Apicultural Research* 42: 53-56.

Nelson, D.R., Blomquist, G. J. 1995. Insect waxes. *In* Hamilton, R. J. (ed.) *Waxes: Chemistry, Molecular Biology and Functions*. The Oily Press, Dundee, pp. 1-90.

Park, Y.K., Alencar, S.M., Aguiar, C.L. 2002. Botanical origin and chemical composition of Brazilian propolis. *Journal of Agricultural and Food Chemistry* 50: 2502-2506.

Peña, R.C. 2008. Propolis standardization: a chemical and biological review. *Ciencia e Investigacion Agraria* 35: 17-26.

Pereira, A. dos Santos, Seixas, F.R.M.S., de Aquino-Neto, R. 2002. Própolis: 100 anos de pesquisa e suas perspectivas futuras. *Quimica Nova* 25: 321-326.

Petrova, A., Popva, M., Kuzmanova, C., Tsevetkova, I., Naydenski, H., Muli, E., Bankova, V. 2010. New biologically active compounds from Kenyan propolis. *Fitoterapia* 81: 509-514.

Piccinelli, A.L., Fernández, M.C., Cuesta-Rubio, O., Hernández, I.M., De Simone, F., Rastrelli, L. 2005. Isoflavonoids isolated from Cuban propolis. *Journal of Agricultural and Food Chemistry* 53: 9010-9016.

Piccinelli, A.L., Lottit, C., Camponet, L., Cuesta-Rubio, O., Fernández, M.C., Rastrelli, L. 2011. Cuban and Brazilian red propolis: botanical origin and comparative analyzes by high-performance liquid chromatography-photodiode array detection/electrospray ionization tandem mass spectrometry. *Journal of Agricultural and Food Chemistry* 59: 6484-6491.

Popova, M.P., Bankova, V.S., Bogdanov, S., Tsvetkova, I., Naydenski, C., Marcazzan, G.L., Sabatini, A.G. 2007. Chemical characteristics of poplar-type propolis of different geographic origin. *Apidologie* 38: 306-311.

Popova, M., Bankova, V., Spassov, S., Tsvetkova, I., Naydenski, C., Silva, M.V., Tsartarova, M. 2001. New bioactive chalcones in propolis from El Salvador. *Zeitschrift für Naturforschung* C 56: 593-596.

Popova, M., Bankova, V., Tsvetkova, I., Naydenski, C., Silva, M.V. 2001. The first glycosides isolated from propolis: diterpene rhamnosides. *Zeitschrift für Naturforschung* C 56: 1108-1111.

Popova, M., Chen, C.N., Chen, P.Y., Huang, C.Y., Bankova, V. 2010b. A validated spectrophotometric method for quantification of prenylated flavanones in Pacific propolis from Taiwan. *Phytochemical Analysis* 21: 186-191.

Popova, M., Chinou, I., Marekov, I., Bankova, V. 2009. Terpenes with antimicrobial activity from Cretan propolis. *Phytochemistry* 70: 1262-1271.

Popova, M., Graikou, K., Chinou, I., Bankova, V. 2010a.GC-MS profiling of diterpene compounds in Mediterranean propolis from Greece. *Journal of Agricultural and Food Chemistry* 58: 3167-3176.

Popova, M., Trusheva, B., Antonova, D., Simone, C., Mifsud, D., Farrugia, C., Tsvetokova, I., Najdenski, H., Bankova, V. 2011.The specific chemical profile of Mediterranean propolis from Malta. *Food Chemistry* 126: 1431-1435.

Quan, W.L., Khan, Z., Watson, D.G., Fearnley, J. 2008. Analysis of sugars in bee pollen and propolis by ligand exchange chromatography in combination with pulsed amperometric detection and mass spectrometry. *Journal of Food Composition and Analysis* 21: 78-83.

Ramos, A.F.N., Miranda, J.L. 2007. Propolis: a review of its anti-inflammatory and healing actions. *Journal of Venomous Animals and Toxins Including Tropical Dieseases* 13: 697-710.

Rapta, P., Misik, V., Stasko, A., Vrábel, I., 1995. Redox intermediates of flavonoids and caffeic acid esters from propolis: an EPR spectroscopic and cyclic voltammetry study. *Free Radical Biology & Medicine* 18: 901-908.

Righi, A.A., Alves, T.R., Negri, G., Marques, L.M., Breyer, H., Salatino, A. 2011. Brazilian red propolis: unreported substances, antioxidants and antimicrobial activities. *Journal of the Science of Food and Agriculture* 13: 2363-2370.

Salatino, A., Fernandes-Silva, C.C., Righi, A.A., Salatino, M.L.F. 2011. Propolis research and the chemistry of plant products. *Natural Products Reports* 28: 925-936.

Salatino, A., Teixeira, E.W., Negri, G., Message, D. 2005. Origin and chemical variation of Brazilian propolis. *Evidence-Based Complementary and Alternative Medicine* 2: 33-38.

Sforcin, J.M., Bankova, V. 2011. Is there a potential for the development of new drugs? *Journal of Ethnopharmacology* 133: 253-260.

Silva, B.B., Rosalen, P.L., Cury, J.A., Ikegaki, M., Souza, V.C., Esteves, A., Alencar, S.M. 2008. Chemical composition and botanical origin of red propolis, a new type of Brazilian propolis. *Evidence-Based Complementary and Alternative Medicine* 5: 313-316.

Shrestha, S.P., Narukawa, Y., Takeda, T. 2007a. Chemical constituents of Nepalese propolis: isolation of new dalbergiones and related compounds. *Journal of Natural Medicines* 61: 73-76.

Shrestha, S.P., Narukawa, Y., Takeda, T. 2007b. Chemical constituents of Nepalese propolis (II). *Chemical & Pharmaceutical Bulletin* 55: 926-929.

Schneidewinde, E.M., Buge, A., Kala, H., Metzner, J., Zschunke, A. 1979. Identification of an anti-microbially active constituent isolated from propolis. *Pharmazie* 34: 103-106.

Silici, S., Kutluca, W. 2005. Chemical composition and antibacterial activity of propolis collected by three different races of honeybees in the same region. *Journal of Ethnopharmacology* 99: 69-73.

Simone-Finstrom, M., Spivak, M. 2010. Propolis and bee health: the natural history and significance of resin use by honey bees. *Apidologie* 41: 295-311.

Tatefuji, T., Izumi, N., Ohta, T., Arai, s., Ikeda, M., Kurimoto, M. 1996. Isolation and identification of compounds from Brazilian propolis which enhance macrophage spreading and mobility. *Biological & Pharmaceutical Bulletin* 19: 966-970.

Tazawa, S., Tsutomu, W., Noro. 1999. Studies on the constituents of Brazilian própolis. II. *Chemical & Pharmaceutical Bulletin* 47: 1388-1392.

Teixeira, E.W., Message, D., Negri, G., Salatino, A., Stringheta, P. C. 2010. Seasonal variation, chemical composition and antioxidant activity of Brazilian propolis samples. *Evidence-Based Complementary and Alternative Medicine* 7: 307-315.

Teixeira, E.W., Message, D., Negri, G., Salatino, A. 2006. Bauer-7-en-3β-yl acetate: a major constituent of unusual samples of Brazilian propolis. *Química Nova* 29: 245-246.

Teixeira, E.W., Negri, G., Meira, R.M.S.A., Message, D., Salatino, A. 2005. Plant origin of green propolis: bee behavior, plant anatomy and chemistry. *Evidence-Based Complementary and Alternative Medicine* 2: 85-92.

Tomás-Barberán, A., García-Veiguera, C., Vit-Olivier, P., Ferreres, F., Tomás-Lorente, F. 1993. Phytochemical evidence for the botanical origin of tropical propolis from Venezuela. *Phytochemistry* 34: 191-196.

Trusheva, B., Popova, M., Bankova, V., Simona, S., Marcucci, M.C., Miorin, P.L., Pasin, F.R., Tsvetkova, I. 2006. Bioactive constituents of Brazilian red propolis. *Evidence-Based Complementary and Alternative Medicine* 3: 249-254.

Trusheva, B., Popova, M., Koendhori, E.B., Tsvetkova, I., Najdenski, H., Bankova, V. 2011. Indonesian propolis: chemical composition, biological activity and botanical origin. *Natural Product Research* 25: 606-613.

Trusheva, B., Popova, M., Naydensky, H., Tsvetkova, I., Rodriguez, G., Bankova, V. 2004. New poyisoprenylated benzophenones from Venezuelan propolis. *Fitoterapia* 75: 683-689.

Trusheva, B., Todorov, I., Ninova, M., Najdenski, H., Daneshmand, A., Bankova, V. 2010. Antibacterial mono- and sesquiterpene esters of benzoic acids from Iranian propolis. *Chemistry Central Journal* 4: 8.

Tulloch, A.P. 1980. Beeswax: composition and analysis. *Bee World* 6: 47-62.

Urushisaki, T., Takemura, T., Tazawa, S., Mayuko, F., Hosokawa-Muto, J., Araki, Y., Kuwata, K. 2011. Caffeoylquinic acids are major constituents with potent anti-influenza effects in Brazilian green propolis water extract. *Evidence-Based Complementary and Alternative Medicine* (available on-line, doi: 10.1155/2011/254914).

Usia, T., Banskota, A.H., Midorikawa, K., Matsushige, K., Kadota, S. 2002. Constituents of Chinese propolis and their antiproliferative activities. *Journal of Natural Products* 65: 673-676.

Valcic, S., Montenegro, G., Timmermann, B. 1998. Lignans from Chilean propolis. *Journal of Natural Products* 61: 771-775.

In: Beneficial Effects of Propolis on Human Health ... ISBN: 978-1- 62081-440-6
Editors: Tahira Farooqui and Akhlaq A. Farooqui 

*Chapter 3*

# SEASONAL VARIATION IN THE COMPOSITION AND THE ANTIMICROBIAL AND ANTIOXIDANT ACTIVITIES OF PROPOLIS

***Eduardo Morgado Schmidt*[1] *and Alexandra Christine Helena Frankland Sawaya*[2,*]**

[1]Thomson Mass Spectrometry Laboratory, Institute of Chemistry
[2]Plant Biology Department, Institute of Biology, State University of Campinas, UNICAMP, Campinas, Brazil

## ABSTRACT

Propolis is a resin collected by bees from many parts of plants, such as leaf and flower buds, bark and resinous tree exudates. It is used by worker bees to protect the hive against insects and microorganisms as well as to seal cracks and reinforce the combs. A thin layer is applied to the hive entrance and in the combs before the queen lays eggs, to maintain these areas aseptic. However the amounts of resins collected and of propolis used in these activities can vary with the seasons. Propolis has been used by mankind for its many therapeutic properties since ancient times. Over 300 compounds have been identified in samples of propolis from different origins. Several pharmacological properties of propolis have been attributed to phenolic compounds (phenylpropanoids and flavonoids) and the concentration of these compounds in propolis is often used to evaluate sample quality. More recently, the possibility of using propolis for its antioxidant properties has come under study, as the phenolic compounds in its composition are known for their antioxidant activity. Propolis can also be used to evaluate the environmental pollution in a region or along the year, by assessing the metal contents in the resins that make up its compositions. These metals may be vital, non-essential or toxic to humans.

One of the main problems towards the standardization of propolis is its variable chemical composition and this is possibly the main obstacle to its routine use in therapy. Propolis composition varies according to the regional flora, place and time of collection, type of collector employed and genetic characteristics (species of bee). This set of factors

* Corresponding author: E-mail: franksawaya@terra.com.br.

determines the composition of the propolis sample as well as its physical, chemical and biological properties. However, it has been observed that a reduction in the concentration of some biologically active compounds in one season is frequently accompanied by the increase of another class of active compounds. Therefore the resultant activity remains constant throughout the year. This applies mainly to antimicrobial activities which are important to the survival of the hive. Other biological activities, such as antioxidant activity, were not quite as constant throughout the year.

**Keywords:** Propolis, seasonal variation, phenolic compounds, flavonoids, antioxidant activity, metal contents, antimicrobial activity

## 1. INTRODUCTION

The Word *propolis* comes from the Greek words *pro,* meaning before, and *polis*, meaning city. This reflects an observation made by beekeepers, since ancient times, that bees construct a barrier of propolis (Figure 1) to protect the entrance of their hives from insects and predators as well as to seal cracks and reinforce the combs. A thin layer is applied to the hive entrance and also in the combs, to protect against microorganisms [1].

Although propolis is considered to be an apicultural product, along with honey and royal jelly, it is not actually produced by the bees themselves. It is basically a resin collected by bees from many parts of plants, such as leaf and flower buds, bark and resinous tree exudates. Within the hive these resins are mixed with different proportions of beeswax and other components. Therefore the chemical composition of propolis varies, qualitatively and quantitatively, according to the vegetation in the region of the hive. Different species of bees also gather resins from different plants within the same region, so the chemical composition of propolis also varies according to the species of bee [2] [3].

In countries within the temperate zone of the Northern Hemisphere, the climatic conditions only allow the bees to collect propolis resins during a few months, ranging from late spring to early autumn; the preferred plant sources are species of *Populus,* so not much seasonal variation between samples is expected [4]. However in countries lying in tropical and sub-tropical regions such as Brazil, bees collect resins all year round. As the composition of plant resins can also vary throughout the year, the amount and composition of propolis can vary with the seasons.

Propolis from *Apis mellifera* bees, commonly known as honeybees, usually contains between 50-60% of resins and balsamic components, 30-40% of beeswax, 5-10% of essential oils and 5% of pollen, along with micro-elements such as aluminum, calcium, strontium, iron, copper, manganese and small amounts of vitamins (B1, B2, B6, C and E). Balsamic substances, soluble in hydro-alcoholic solvents, such as the phenolic compounds in propolis, are responsible for most of the known therapeutic effects of propolis [5]. As these properties are directly linked to the composition of propolis, they may also vary seasonally.

The metal contents of propolis, on the other hand, can be used to evaluate the environmental pollution in a region throughout the year. Some metals can be considered vital, and their presence in propolis is a bonus, others are non-essential and finally, some are toxic. The presence of heavy metals such as lead, cadmium, mercury and others, may be incorporated from environmental sources, and can be toxic when present above specific reference values[6] [7].

Studies of the multiple therapeutic properties of propolis have confirmed its antimicrobial, anti-inflammatory, anesthetic, anticancer, anti HIV and anticariogenic activities [8]. Due to these multiple properties, propolis is used in numerous pharmaceutical and nutritional products [9]. As propolis composition can vary according to the regional flora, place and time of collection, type of collector employed and species of bee, the standardization of propolis is possibly the main obstacle to its routine use in therapy.

This review focuses on studies that have determined how the composition of propolis varies in composition due to factors such as: age, seasonality and form of collection. Studies analyzing the way its biological activities, mainly its antimicrobial and antioxidant activities, are affected by this seasonal variation will also be discussed.

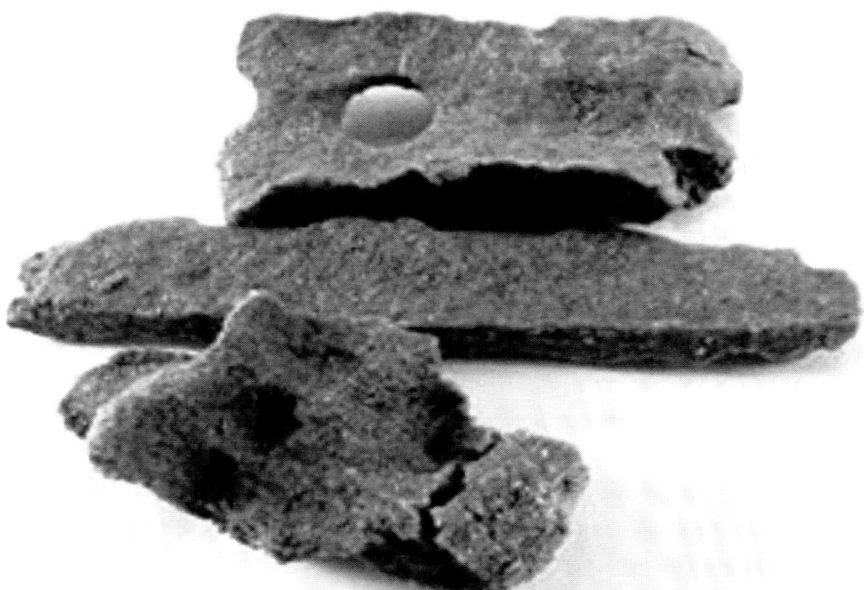

Figure 1. Crude propolis.

## 2. Variation in the Amount of Propolis Produced and its Chemical Composition

A study was carried out to evaluate if the amount of propolis is affected by the way it is collected. Three different procedures for propolis collection, that is: scraping the hive walls, plastic screen and CPI (from Portuguese "Coletor de Propolis Inteligente") were tested. Five hives of Africanized *Apis mellifera* bees were used for each type of collection. No statistical differences in the amount of propolis collected by either method and throughout the seasons were found. No correlation could be observed between the average monthly temperatures, precipitation, relative air humidity, hours of sunlight or wind speed, with the amount of propolis collected. However the authors observed that the greatest amount of propolis was collected in the spring with the plastic screen and in the fall with the CPI, but no explanation for this phenomenon was proposed, and the composition of the propolis samples was not analyzed [10].

Due to the importance of metals in the chemical composition of propolis, a study compared qualitatively and quantitatively the metal content of green Brazilian propolis samples using atomic absorption spectrophotometry. Only aluminum, calcium and manganese were found in all the samples, with aluminum levels higher that the other two elements. The aluminum levels varied, but were all below limits considered tolerable for the human adult. When aged samples (remained in the hive for over 180 days) were compared to fresh samples (remained for approximately one month), the aluminum concentration in the fresh samples was higher, but there were no significant differences in the levels of calcium and manganese. The authors proposed that rainwater may have washed out some of the aluminum content of the aged samples. There was also a positive correlation between aluminum content and organic compounds, mainly total phenolic content, as some phenolic compounds may also be washed by rainwater or degraded due to climatic conditions [11]. This is in agreement with a previous study of Chinese and Uruguayan propolis in which aged propolis was found to have approximately 20% less flavonoids than fresh propolis [12].

Since propolis composition is known to vary due to the regional flora, place and time of collection, type of collector employed and genetic characteristics of the bees, several physical and chemical tests are used to evaluate its composition and quality. The parameters of what constitutes good quality propolis are not easy to define, for quality propolis from different regions may be chemically different. However some simple tests are routinely employed to this end. In sum: sensorial evaluation (color, taste and consistency), total phenolics and flavonoids, levels of wax, ashes and dry residue of extracts, are routinely analyzed. The Brazilian Ministry of Agriculture has determined the limits of ashes, loss on drying, insoluble residues and wax which are considered acceptable for Brazilian propolis [13].

The determination of total phenolics and flavonoids in a propolis sample requires a simple spectrophotometric analysis. Total flavonoid concentration is based on the stable complexation of these compounds with aluminum in methanol, allowing quantification by absorption UV-VIS spectrophotometry at 425nm [9]. Total phenolic compounds are quantified in a similar manner, using the Folin – Ciocalteau reagent and correlating with absorption at 700 nm or 760 nm, although other compounds such as sugars and aromatic amines may interfere in this analysis [9].

The form of extraction of crude propolis, by maceration or Soxhlet extractor, the concentration and type of solvent, as well as the length of extraction time affects the yield of propolis extracts. Although the total phenolic compounds of the propolis extracts varied between 6.41 and 15.24%, no correlation could be found between these concentrations and any of the factors that varied in the experiment [5]. However, other studies have also shown the importance of these parameters on propolis composition [14]. Therefore it is difficult to compare results of studies using different extraction methods. This variation in composition due to the use of diverse extraction procedures may be even greater than the variation caused by changes in the plant resins used, leading to biased results. Much care must be taken to delimit a specific extraction procedure before comparing propolis sample composition.

Other more sophisticated spectrometric tests are applied by producers and researchers alike. Mass spectrometry, coupled or not to chromatographic methods, may be used. For the more volatile and semi-volatile compounds, gas chromatography – mass spectrometry (GC-

MS) has frequently been used. However many of the active components of propolis are not volatile, and cannot be adequately analyzed by this method. Therefore modern techniques such as electrospray ionization mass spectrometry (ESI-MS) may be used directly to obtain sample profiles, also known as fingerprints, but may also be coupled to high ( and ultra high) performance liquid chromatography (HPLC and UPLC) for more detailed qualitative and quantitative sample analysis. The effect of geographic origin on propolis composition was clearly shown in studies comparing the fingerprints of propolis samples from all the continents by mass spectrometry [2] [15]. The variation in composition between propolis of different species of bees was also characterized in this way [3] [16]. However, more recent studies have shown that the composition of propolis from stingless bees varies monthly, probably due to the offer of resins from different species of plants in different seasons. This was observed in *Scaptotrigona* colonies located in state of São Paulo (with the sub-tropical climate) and in the state of Maranhão (in a tropical-equatorial climate) [17].

Two colonies of *Apis mellifera* bees, one Africanized and one not, in Botucatu (state of São Paulo, Brazil) were selected and the propolis collected monthly for one year; then grouped according to the season. The samples were extracted in ethanol and analyzed by GC-MS. Differences in composition were observed between the two colonies and also seasonally. However, it was observed that a reduction in the concentration of some biologically active compounds (such as phenolics) in one season was frequently accompanied by the increase of another class of active compounds (such as terpenes). The authors proposed that the bees used resins mainly from one preferred plant source, but other plants, one of which produce more resins in the autumn, were also used. These plant sources were proposed to be species of *Baccharis* and of *Araucaria* [4].

Red colored propolis from a different region in Brazil, in the state of Pernambuco (Northeastern Brazil), was collected in February, June and October 2006; that is in the summer, winter and spring. The volatile composition of the crude propolis samples was evaluated by GC-MS. The methanolic extracts of the same samples were compared by thin layer chromatography (TLC). Although trans-anethole was the main volatile compound in all three samples, the other volatiles varied qualitatively and quantitatively. The methanolic extract showed the same profile in all three months, and the main constituents were phenolic compounds, terpenes and sugars [18].

In another study of the seasonal variation on the composition of red propolis, samples from the state of Alagoas in the Northeast of Brazil were collected every two months, throughout one year. The TLC and HPLC of these samples showed a similar chromatographic profile, with differences only in the quantity of the compounds, determined by the area of peaks by HPLC [19].

Although European propolis is not expected to vary seasonally, samples collected in three different areas in Central Algarve during the winter and the spring were analyzed. The total phenolic components and flavonoids were determined; the highest amounts of total phenols and flavanones and dihydroflavonols were observed for the samples collected in the spring, but no such significant difference was observed for the flavones and flavonols. The increase in and the flavanones and dihydroflavonols, may partly explain the increase of the content of total phenols in the spring. As this is the southernmost region of Portugal, the mild winter weather may allow bees to collect propolis during the winter or these winter samples may be aged samples, with resins collected by bees in the autumn [20].

Diverse samples of propolis from different geographic areas, and from different types of bees, all showed antimicrobial activity, in spite of their different chemical composition [21]. This is logical considering the importance of this activity for the survival of the hive, but will this pattern be present for other activities of propolis, such as the antioxidant activity?

## 3. Variation in the Antimicrobial and Biological Activity of Propolis

In Brazil, propolis is produced all year long, so seasonal variations in its composition are expected. The studies that have observed this phenomenon in propolis from native stingless bees and honeybees have already been discussed earlier in this chapter. However, other studies are needed to determine if and how these variations affect the biological activities of propolis.

The antimicrobial action of propolis has been widely investigated, but reports dealing with seasonal effect on propolis activity are not common. Two studies were carried out by Sforcin and collaborators to evaluate the antimicrobial activity of propolis collected throughout the year: one to evaluate the effect of propolis samples on strains of *Candida* yeast and another on bacteria. The material was produced by Africanized honeybees in Botucatu, São Paulo State and pooled by season. It appears that this is the same propolis that was analyzed by Bankova et al. [4], where chemical variation in the composition of the samples pooled by seasons was observed.

The *in vitro* antimicrobial activity of the propolis samples, collected during the four seasons, was tested on the following strains of bacteria isolated from human infections: *Staphylococcus aureus, Escherichia coli, Pseudomonas aeruginosa* and *Salmonella typhimurium*. Dilutions of ethanolic extract of propolis (EEP) in agar were used, and the survival curve of each bacterial strain was plotted. Although Gram-positive bacteria were inhibited by low propolis concentrations (0.4%), Gram-negative bacteria were less susceptible to this substance, the minimal inhibitory concentration ranging from 4.5 to 8.0%. But there was no significant difference with regards to the seasonal effect on the survival curve of *Staphylococcus aureus* and *Escherichia coli* [22].

In the second study, the activity of the propolis extracts on yeast pathogens isolated from human infections was determined. Hydro-alcoholic solutions of propolis were prepared with each pool and diluted in agar, using serial concentrations of propolis from each pool and the minimal inhibitory concentration (MIC) was determined. The results showed that the strains of *Candida* albicans used were slightly more susceptible than the strains of *Candida tropicalis,* but both were susceptible to low concentrations of propolis. No differences were seen, however, in relation to seasonal effects in the minimal inhibitory concentration of propolis [23]. Furthermore, no seasonal variations were observed in the effect of these propolis samples, neither on natural killer cells nor on blood biochemical parameters [24] [25].

Red propolis, collected by *Apis mellifera* bees in the northeast of Brazil, is reported to have a different plant source: *Dalbergia ecastophyllum.* A study evaluating the effect of seasonal periods on the antibacterial activity of the Brazilian red propolis against the following bacteria *Streptococcus mutans* UA159, *Streptococcus sobrinus* 6715,

*Staphylococcus aureus* ATCC 25923 and *Actinomyces naeslundii ATCC 12104;* was carried out. The minimal inhibitory and bactericidal concentrations (MIC and MBC) were determined. A variation in their values was observed for *S. mutans, S.sobrinus* and *S. aureus,* but not for *A. naeslundii* [26].

On the whole, the antimicrobial activity of propolis varied little, throughout the year. This is not surprising, in light of the importance of this activity for hive survival. It would seem that if the bees cannot find their preferred source of resins in one season; they will search of another source of antimicrobial resins.

## 4. Antioxidant Activity of Propolis

In the human body, oxidation is linked to ageing and tissue degradation, mainly due to free radical formation. There are many natural substances that fight these radicals, vitamins C and E, among others. As antioxidants are defined as substances that, in low concentrations, retard or prevent the oxidation of other substances, antioxidant capacity is not an exact value but depends on the source of stress or oxidation and the substrate. Therefore different methods result in different values of antioxidant capacity for the same substances [27]. The methods that determine antioxidant activity function are based on two main mechanisms; one that involves a hydrogen atom transfer (HAT) and one that involves an electron transfer (ET) [27] [28].

Propolis has been used by mankind for its many therapeutic properties since ancient times. Over 300 compounds have been identified in samples of propolis from different origins. These substances belong to several chemical classes, such as flavonoids, phenolics, terpenes and others. As several illnesses are caused or induced by tissue oxidation, it is not surprising that several pharmacological activities of propolis are related to antioxidant and radical-scavenging activity. Several pharmacological properties of propolis have been attributed to phenolic compounds (phenylpropanoids and flavonoids) and the concentration of these compounds in propolis is often used to evaluate sample quality. The antioxidant biological activity of phenolic compounds is mainly due to their capacity to capture free radicals [29] and to chelate transition metal-ions like iron, copper, manganese, cobalt and chromium [30]. For these reasons, the possibility of using propolis for its antioxidant properties has come under study.

Artepillin C (Figure 2) is one of the compounds found in green Brazilian propolis that presents a strong radical quenching activity. It also shows macrophage stimulating activity, antibacterial and antitumor activity [31].

Several diseases are linked to reactive oxygen species (ROS) produced by neutrophils. The intake of antioxidants, such as propolis, could benefit patients either as a prophylactic or therapeutic treatment; however its chemical composition may vary under the influence of seasonality, affecting the biological effect. To verify this, the effect of green propolis samples produced monthly from November 2001 through October 2002 in São Paulo state, on the oxidative metabolism of stimulated neutrophils, by using both luminol and lucigenin to produce chemiluminescence, was evaluated. This green propolis is found in the southeast region of Brazil, and the chemical of its main botanical source, *Baccharis dracunculifolia*, is thought to vary along the year. Although all the propolis samples produced during a one-year period displayed antioxidant activity the level of activity varied. [32]

Aged and fresh propolis from Prudentopolis in the state of Paraná, Brazil, was analyzed. The level of total phenolic compounds was determined by the Folin-Ciocalteau method and the amount of flavonoids by $AlCl_3$ in methanol [14]. The antiradical activity was determined by two unrelated methods: first of all by the assay based on chemiluminescence of luminol in micellar environment, adapted to complex extracts by Silva and colaborators [27]. As a way of comparison, antiradical capacity was evaluated by the well-known assay which employs the DPPH radical. Total phenolic levels were all statistically different with a trend toward higher amounts of total phenolic acids in fresh propolis, but the amount of flavonoids was slightly higher in aged propolis. All extracts obtained from fresh propolis had higher radical scavenging activity [11].

It is important to bear in mind that different compounds may correlate better with one antioxidant evaluation method than another. For example, in a study of the antioxidant activity of samples of Brazilian propolis, two essays were used: DPPH and Ferric reducing ability power (FRAP). Although all samples presented the antioxidant compound, Artepillin C, in their composition, variation in the antioxidant activity of the samples was observed. The results of both antioxidant essays were well correlated to the phenolic contents; but the correlation between the FRAP essay and flavonoids was poor. Therefore the flavonoids showed antioxidant activity by the DPPH free radical scavenging method, but not the reducing power observed by the FRAP method [33].

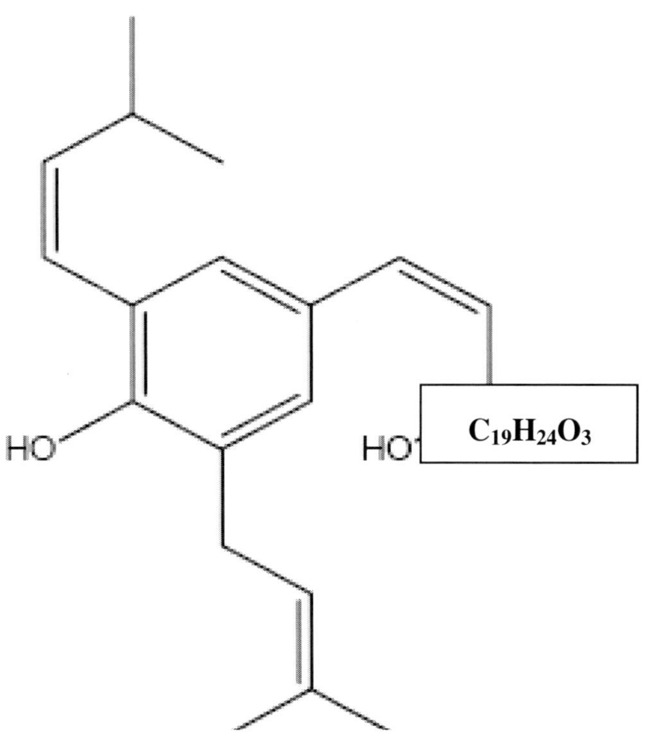


Figure 2. Structural and molecular formulas of Artepillin-C.

Samples collected in Central Algarve during the winter and the spring were analyzed by different evaluation methods and showed variation in their composition and in the antioxidant activity. The DPPH method and chelating metal ions showed significant differences between collection seasons, but not the ABTS+ free radical-scavenging activity. Samples obtained in winter were better to scavenger DPPH, but samples from spring were better to chelate iron ions. Once again, the result was dependent on the method used. The methods for evaluating the capacity for inhibiting the superoxide radical anion formation and for chelating metal ions are different from those that evaluate DPPH or ABTS radical scavenging (which are based on the electron transfer). The chemical structure of the phenol is determinant on the antioxidant activity [34].

Stingless bee propolis is not as studied as honeybee propolis. However samples of propolis were collected monthly over the period of one year from colonies of native Brazilian stingless *Scaptotrigona* bees: in the state of Maranhão in the Northeastern and in state of São Paulo in the southeastern region of Brazil between 2006 and 2007, their antioxidant activity determined by the DPPH radical scavenging assay. For each species, the highest antioxidant activity was observed in propolis collected in October and November (spring months), As the composition of the samples varied along the year, the effect of the seasons on the availability of resins, the composition of propolis and the antioxidant activity was observed [35].

## CONCLUSION

The chemical composition of propolis from regions with tropical and subtropical climates (such as Brazil) and Mediterranean climates (such as south Portugal) were found to vary throughout the year. However these variations in composition did not affect the antimicrobial activity of most samples, and apparently the lack of one group of substances in one season was compensated by the presence of another group. This result corroborates with earlier studies of propolis from different geographical origins, which presented antimicrobial activity in spite of different chemical compositions [21].

Another pharmacologically important activity of propolis, antioxidant activity, although present in most samples analyzed was found to vary throughout the year. However, the results were directly influenced by the evaluation method used. Most samples contained different proportions of flavonoids and other phenolics, and specific assays correlated better with concentrations of one or the other class of compounds. It would seem that one class of antioxidant compounds, found in one season, is substituted by another class, in other seasons. However, no studies were found that evaluate how this variation affects the overall biological effect, in humans or animals.

## REFERENCES

[1] Pereira A. S. Própolis: 100 anos de Pesquisa e suas Perspectivas Futuras. *Química Nova,* 2002; 25(2):326.

[2] Sawaya A. C. H. F., Tomazela, D. M., Cunha I. B. S. et al. Electrospray ionization mass spectrometry fingerprint of propolis. *Analyst,* 2004; 129:739-744.

[3] Sawaya A. C. H. F., Cunha I. B. S., Marcucci M. C. et al. Electrospray ionization mass spectrometry fingerprinting of propolis of native Brazilian stingless bees. *Apidologie,* 2007; 38:93-103.

[4] Bankova V., Bourdounova-Krastev G., Popov S. et al. Seasonal variations of chemical composition of Brazilian propolis. *Apidologie,* 1998; 29:361-367.

[5] Cunha I. B. S., Sawaya A. C. H. F., Caetano F. M. et al, Factors that influence the yield and composition of Brazilian propolis extracts. *Journal Brazilian Chemical Society,* 2004; 15(6):964-970.

[6] Conti M. E., Botre F. Honeybees and their products as potential bioindicators of heavy metals contamination. *Environ. Monit. Assess. Netherlands.*, 2001-jul; 69(3):267-282.

[7] Campos R. C. de. Avaliação do Conteúdo de Metais em Plantas de Uso na Medicina Popular e em seus Extratos Aquosos. *Ciênc. Tecnol. Aliment.* 1996; 16(3):184-187.

[8] Carvalho A. A., Finger D., Machado C. S. et al. In vivo antitumoural activity and composition of an oil extract of Brazilian propolis. *Food Chemistry*, 2011; 126:1239-1245.

[9] Buriol L., Finger D., Schmidt E. M. et al. Composição química e atividade biológica de extrato oleoso de própolis: uma alternativa ao extrato etanólico. *Química Nova*, 2009; 32:296-302.

[10] Inoue H. T., De Sousa E. A., Orsi R. O., Funari S. R. C. et al. Produção de própolis por diferentes métodos de coleta, *Arch. Latinoam. Prod. Anim.*, 2007; 15(2):65-69.

[11] Schmidt E.,M., Santos C.,S., Stock D. et al. Effect of extraction solvent and collection time on propolis extracts quality: applications of multivariate analysis. *Food Research Internationa,*. 2011; Submitted.

[12] Bonvehi S. J., Collv F. Study on propolis quality from China and Uruguay. *Zeitschrift für Naturforschung*, 2000; 55(9-10):778-784.

[13] Funari C. S., Ferro V. O. Análise de Própolis. *Ciênc. Tecnol. Aliment.*, 2006 jan/mar; 26(1):171-178.

[14] Wosky R., Salatino A. J.Analysis of própolis: some parameters and procedures for chemical quality control. *Apicult. Res.*, 1998; 37(2):99-105.

[15] Sawaya A. C. H. F., Abdelnur P. V., Eberlin M. N. et al. Fingerprinting of propolis by easy ambient sonic-spray ionization mass spectrometry. *Talanta* (Oxford). 2010; 81(1-2):100-108. Acesso em in: PubMed; PMID 20188894.

[16] Sawaya A. C. H. F., Cunha I. B. S., Marcucci M. C. et al. Brazilian propolis of Apis mellifera and Tetragonisca angustula. *Apidologie,* 2006; 37:398-407.

[17] Sawaya A. C. H. F. Composition and antioxidant activity of propolis from three species of Scaptotrigona stingless bees. *Journal of ApiProduct and ApiMedical Science* 2009; 1(2):37-42.

[18] Nunes L. C. C., Deus A. S. O., Arcanjo D. D. et al. Variabilidade sazonal dos constituintes de própolis vermelha e bioatividade em Artemia salina. *Revista Brasileira de Farmacognosia,* 2009; 19:524-529.

[19] Silva B. B., Rosalen P. L., Cury J. Á. et al. Chemical Composition and Botanical Origin of Red Propolis, a New Type of Brazilian Propolis. *Evidence-Based Complementary and Alternative Medicine,* 2008; 5:313-316.

[20] Nunes L. C. C., Galindo A. B., Deus A. S. O. de et al. Variabilidade sazonal dos constituintes da própolis vermelha e bioatividade em Artermia salina. *Revista Brasileira de Farmacognosia*. 2009 abr-jun; 19(2B):524-529.

[21] Kujumgiev A., Tsvetkova I., Bankova V. et al. Antibacterial, antifungal and antiviral activity of propolis of different geographic origin. *Journal of Ethnopharmacology,* 1999; 64:235-240.

[22] Sforcin J. M., Fernandes A. Jr., Lopes C. A. M. et al. Seasonal effect on Brazilian propolis antibacterial activity. *Journal of Ethnopharmacology,* 2000; 73:243-249.

[23] Sforcin J. M., Fernandes A. Jr., Lopes C. A. M. et al. Seasonal effect on Brazilian propolis on Candida albicans and Candida tropicalis. *Journal of Venoms and Animal Toxins,* 2001; 7(1):63-69.

[24] Sforcin J. M., Kaneno R., Funari S. R. C. Absence of seasonal effect on the immunomodulatory action of Brazilian propolis on natural killer activity. *Journal of Venomous Animals and Toxins,* 2002; 8(1):19-29.

[25] Sforcin J. M., Novelli E. L. B., Funari S. R.C. Seasonal effect of Brazilian propolis on seric biochemical variables. *Journal of Venomous Animals and Toxins*, v. 8, n. 2, p. 244-254, 2002.

[26] Silva B. B. *Characterization of red propolis: its botanical origin and the seasonal effect on its chemical composition and biological activity.* Master Tesis, Universidade Estadual de Campinas, Faculdade de Odontologia de Piracicaba, 2008, 40pp.

[27] Da Silva J. F. M., Souza M. C. de, Matta S. R. et al. Correlation analysis between phenolic levels of Brazilian propolis extracts and their antimicrobial and antioxidant activities. *Food Chemistry*, 2006; 99(3):431–435.

[28] Prior R. L., Wu X., Schaich K. Standardized Methods for the Determination of Antioxidant Capacity and Phenolics in Foods and Dietary Supplements. *J. Agric. Food Chem.*, 2005; 53:4290-4302.

[29] Silici S., Kutluca S. Chemical composition and antibacterial activity of propolis collected by three different races of honeybees in the same region. *Journal of Ethnopharmacology,* 2005; 99(1):69-73.

[30] Leopoldini M., Russo N., Toscano M. The molecular basis of working mechanism of natural polyphenolic antioxidants. *Food Chemistry,* 2011; 125:288-306.

[31] Huang D., Ou B., Prior R. L. The Chemistry behind Antioxidant Capacity Assays. *J. Agric. Food Chem.* 2005; 53(6):1841-1856. DOI http:/ /pubs.acs.org/doi/abs/10.1021 /jf030723c.

[32] Simões-Ambrosio L. M. C., Gregório L. E., Sousa J. P. B. et al. The role of seasonality on the inhibitory effect of Brazilian green propolis on the oxidative metabolism of neutrophils. *Fitoterapia,* 2010; 81(8):1102-1108.

[33] Cottica S. M., Sawaya A. C. H. F., Eberlin M. N. et al. Antioxidant Activity and Composition of Propolis Obtained by Different Methods of Extraction. *J. Braz. Chem. Soc.* 2011; 22(5): 929-935.

[34] Miguel M. G., Nunes S., Dandlen S. A. et al. Phenols and antioxidant activity of hydro-alcoholic extracts of propolis from Algarve, South of Portugal. *Food and Chemical Toxicology*, 2010; 48(12):3418-3423

[35] Sawaya A. C. H. F., Calado J. C. P., Santos L. C. dos et al. Composition and antioxidant activity of propolis from three species of Scaptotrigona stingless bees. *Journal of ApiProduct and ApiMedical Science,* 2009; 1(2):37-42.

In: Beneficial Effects of Propolis on Human Health ... ISBN: 978-1- 62081-440-6
Editors: Tahira Farooqui and Akhlaq A. Farooqui 

*Chapter 4*

# Which Flavonoids Are Responsible for Anti-inflammatory and Anti-allergic Activities of Propolis?

***Salvatore Chirumbolo****
Department of Medicine, Section Geriatry, University of Verona, piazzale AL Scuro, Verona, Italy

## Abstract

In recent years, research on plant-derived phytochemicals has gained a significant role in medicine and attracted most of the scientific and medical community around this research topic. Traditional treatments such as propolis, commonly used against many infectious and inflammatory diseases, are currently expanding the scientific debate because of the discovery of many active ingredients in these natural compounds able to behave as promising new drugs. Many flavonoids with anti-inflammatory, anti-allergic and anti-cancer potential, known to be present in several edible plants and beverages, can also be found in propolis (chrysin, kaempferol, galangin, quercetin, etc.), although in various chemical proportions. Actually, an impressive amount of plant flavonoids has hampered a thorough comprehension of their role in human health and, *de facto*, difficulties have been shown in finding a straightforward answer to the question about which component represents the main active principle of some natural products such as propolis. One good perspective is to highlight the many complex mechanisms by which signals are read within cellular machinery and interpreted within the articulated network of intracellular components. The individual or concerted action of propolis flavonoids might strengthen the role of this natural product in human health, particularly in inflammation and allergy.

**Keywords:** Propolis, flavonoids, quercetin, chrysin, anti-inflammatory, anti-allergic, anti-microbial

---

* Correspondence concerning this article should be addressed to: dr. Salvatore Chirumbolo-Department of Medicine-Section Geriatry-Azienda Ospedaliera Universitaria Integrata (AOUI)-Ospedale Civile Maggiore-Geriatrico-c/o Studio prof. M. Zamboni, lato via Mameli, 37100 Verona.

## Introduction

Propolis is a honeybee product, a resinous substance probably produced by the first phase of pollen digestion in bees by small organs placed between the sac and the lower gut of these hymenoptera. Generally, propolis appears as a resinous mixture that honey bees collect from tree buds, sap flows, or other botanical sources (willow, birch, poplar, fir, horse, pine, chestnut). Bees use propolis as a sealant for unwanted open spaces in the hive: propolis mixture is therefore applied to small gaps (5-6 mm, approximately), while larger spaces are usually filled with beeswax. This might explain why propolis is sticky above room temperature (20° C) while at lower temperatures it becomes quite a hard and very brittle substance.

The use of propolis goes back to antiquity, principally to Egyptian people about 3,000 years ago but Greeks gave to this natural resinous substance its current name [1]. Propolis possesses many biological properties, including immuno-modulatory, anti-inflammatory, antioxidant, antibacterial, antiviral, antifungal and antiparasite ones [2-4]; furthermore, an anti-cancer activity of propolis components has been recently reported [5]. In recent years, *in vitro* and *in vivo* assays provided new information concerning its mechanisms of action, and new data from several laboratories, which focused on its chemical composition, botanical sources and biological properties, have recently been reported. Presence of flavonoids in propolis has been estimated in several occasions [6-9] but the extreme variability of raw propolis itself, as it comes from different geographical regions, has rendered this analytical task very difficult. Biodiversity is higher in tropical countries than in northern or European regions. For example, a spectrophotometer analysis of flavonoids, performed in twenty propolis samples collected from ten different geographic localities in northern Croatia and using two complementary methods, reported that the contents of flavones and flavonols were quite similar for most samples and ranged from 2% to 2.3%, except for one sample, which showed a concentration of 1.3% and one sample in which it was not possible to detect flavones and flavonols [6]. This extreme variability influences propolis composition and its role as an anti-allergic substance. In many propolis samples, flavones and flavonols were determined using aluminum chloride and expressed as quercetine equivalent while flavanones were determined using 2,4-dinitrophenylhydrazine and were expressed as naringenin. Furthermore, contents of flavanones in these propolis samples were quite variable, as 55% of samples contained flavanones between 15% and 24% and 45% of samples between 4% and 10%, while total levels of flavonoids in raw propolis samples ranged between 5% and 26%. For the majority of samples (75%), the total level of flavonoids ranged between 15% and 25.9% [6]. This composition shows wider variability when propolis coming from other geographical regions is considered, but some countries show variability in propolis biochemistry also when different internal regions are considered, depending on climate conditions, plants biodiversity (genetics and type of cultivation) and surface extension. Typical examples come from Brazil, from which two different types of propolis have been characterized, namely green propolis and red propolis. Due to the existence of a large amount of different propolis types and different compositions, research is hampered by several difficulties in tracing a possible chemical characterization of this bee-derived substance to justify its role in allergy prevention and therapy. However, most of the raw propolis extracts, which were analyzed worldwide, should contain a few group of well known flavonoids, whose activity is still under investigation and whose mode of action is becoming a promising research field to understand cell molecular biology and cell response to phytochemicals. The role and the activity of these flavonoids, listed in Table 1, are yet puzzling because of their huge possibility to combine as different molecules, as conjugates, metabolites and molecules acting in a synergistic way with other phenolics, such as phenolic acids, caffeic acid, CAPE, artepillin C. In this perspective, while we are considering the metabolic transformation of most known flavonoids contained in propolis by gut microflora, a real effectiveness of propolis *in vivo* has not yet been demonstrated, i.e. few data have been reported concerning whether the activity is caused by a particular flavonoid or another, although very interesting evidence is coming from *in vitro* experimentations with purified and synthetic molecules from propolis. Therefore, one possible scenario able to highlight the importance of this natural substance in medicine, arises from deepening the role of the main components contained in propolis towards cell function and survival.

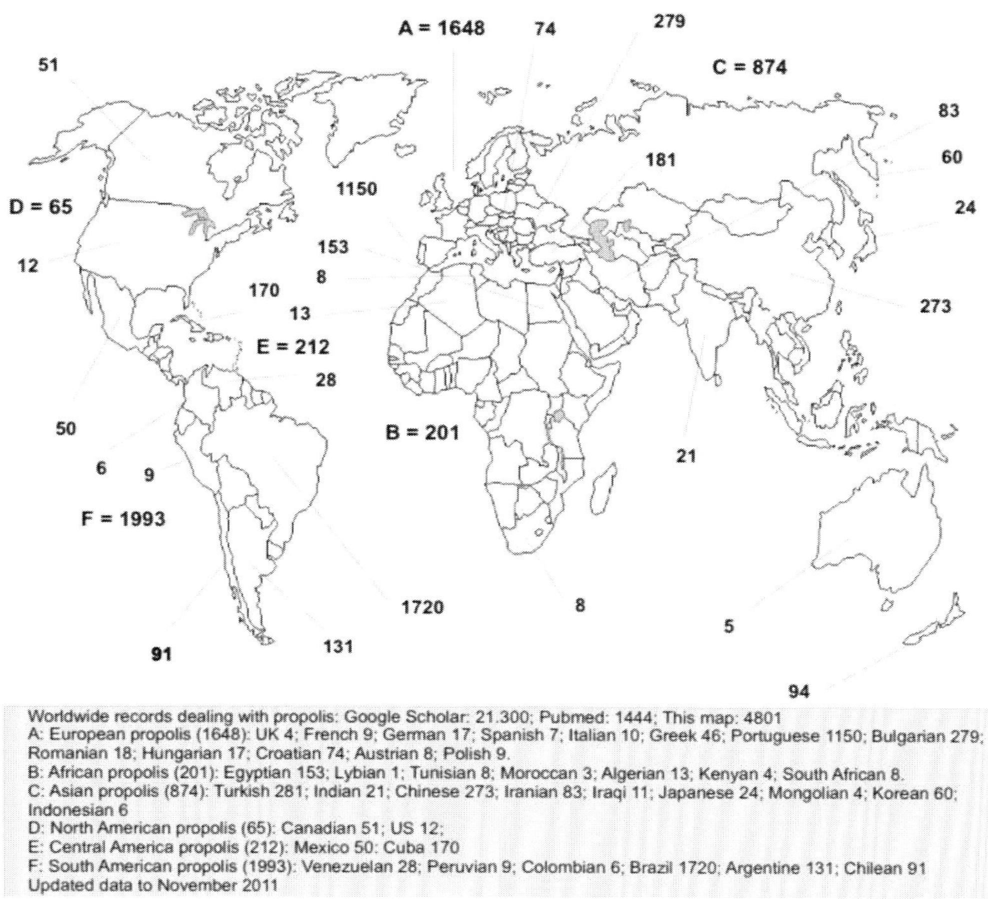


Figure 1. Distribution map of current reports dealing with propolis worldwide. Data refer to November 2011 and includes all scientific references in Scopus, PubMed, Science Direct and other search engines about medical publication.

**Table 1. Main flavonoids identified in propolis**

| Flavonoid | IUPAC name | Class |
|---|---|---|
| Acacetin | 5,7-dihydroxy-2-(4-methoxyphenyl)chromen-4-one | O-methylated-flavone |
| Apigenin | 5,7-Dihydroxy-2-(4-hydroxyphenyl)-4*H*-1-benzopyran-4-one | Flavone |
| Chrysin | 5,7-dihydroxy-2-phenyl-4H-chromen-4-one | Flavanone |
| Galangin | 3,5,7-trihydroxy-2-phenylchromen-4-one | Flavonol |
| Hesperetin | (S)-2,3-dihydro-5,7-dihydroxy-2-(3-hydroxy-4-methoxyphenyl)-4H-1-benzopyran-4-one | Flavanone |
| Kaempferol | 3,5,7-Trihydroxy-2-(4-hydroxyphenyl)-4*H*-chromen-4-one | Flavonol |
| Kaempferide | 3,5,7-trihydroxy-2-(4-methoxyphenyl)chromen-4-one | O-methylated-flavonol |
| Isalpinin | 7-O methyl-3,5,7-trihydroxy-2-phenylchromen-4-one | 7-O-methyl-flavanone |
| Luteolin | 2-(3,4-Dihydroxyphenyl)- 5,7-dihydroxy-4-chromenone | Flavone |
| Myricetin | 3,5,7-Trihydroxy-2-(3,4,5-trihydroxyphenyl)- 4-chromen-one | Flavonol |
| Morin | 2-(2,4-dihydroxyphenyl)-3,5,7-trihydroxychromen-4-one | Flavonol |
| Naringenin | 5,7-dihydroxy-2-(4-hydroxyphenyl)chroman-4-one | Flavanone |
| Pinocembrin | (2*R*,3*R*)-3,5,7-Trihydroxy-2-phenyl-chroman-4-one | Flavanone |
| Pinobanksin | (2S,3R)-3,5,7-Trihydroxy-2-phenyl-chroman-4-one | Dihydroflavonol |
| Pinobanksin-3-acetate | (2S,3R)-3,5,7-Trihydroxy-2-phenyl-chroman-4-one-3-acetate | Dihydroflavonol-3-acetate |
| Pinostrobin | (S)-2,3-Dihydro-5-hydroxy-7-methoxy-2-phenyl-4H-1-benzopyran-4-one | 5-hydroxy-7-methoxy-flavanone |
| Quercetin | 2-(3,4-dihydroxyphenyl)-3,5,7-trihydroxy-4*H*-chromen-4-one | Flavonol |
| Tectochrysin | 5-hydroxy-7-methoxy-2-phenyl-4H-1-benzopyran-4-one | 7-Methoxy-flavanone |
| Tricetin | 5,7-dihydroxy2-(3,4,5-trihydroxyphenyl)-4H-1-benzopyran-4-one | Flavone |

## A First Survey about those Reports Dealing with Propolis Worldwide

To understand the availability of nature-derived propolis for inflammation and allergy prevention, some consideration about propolis diffusion throughout the world has to be highlighted. Figure 1 describes an overall distribution of scientific reports about propolis composition and effects published in literature worldwide. What is striking is the huge number of studies in the Portuguese language areas, about 5-10 times as many as those in countries with the highest amount of publication concerning propolis. For example, the amount of evidence and reports concerning Brazilian propolis is slightly higher than manuscripts dealing with European countries as a whole. In this continent, Portuguese propolis has been extensively studied, as it has been used as an anti-inflammatory agent for many years [10-12]. Its composition has been investigated mainly as total phenols [13] and with different methods such as mass spectroscopy [14]. In a previously published study, flavonoids present in twenty samples of Portuguese heather honey were analyzed by reversed-phase HPLC and the flavonoid fraction purified by a combination of chromatography on Amberlite XAD-2 and Sephadex LH-20 columns. The total amount of flavonoids ranged between 60 μg/100g and 500 μg/100g honey, values which were much smaller than those previously found for Spanish rosemary honey samples (500-2000 μg/100 g honey). This study has assessed that the main flavonoids present in Portuguese heather honey and propolis were the flavanones pinocembrin and pinobanksin and the flavones chrysin and galangin: actually, these flavonoids are represented in propolis from different geographical areas with high frequency. The reported analyses showed that all the samples contained a similar flavonoid pattern composed of at least 22 compounds. Main substances were myricetin, myricetin 3-methyl ether, myricetin 3'-methyl ether and tricetin [15]. Portuguese propolis has been tested in many infectious and inflammatory models [16] and also as a neuro-protective promising sources of phenolics [17, 18]. Moreover, effectiveness of Portuguese propolis on hereditary spherocytosis was recently reported [19]. Maybe it is not only a mere coincidence that in Europe propolis is so extensively studied within that country historically related to Brazil. Brazilian propolis is perhaps the most diffused propolis in the world. The origin and the chemical variation of this propolis has been recently investigated [20-22] and attempts were made to characterize those phenolics involved in propolis anti-microbial and anti-inflammatory property [23-25]; in addition, many components derived from Brazilian propolis have been tested on tumors [26-28]. The high frequency in Brazilian propolis might affect propolis distribution as a purchasable product in the world. Therefore, industrialized and/or northern countries, frequently affected by allergic pathologies, might use mainly brazilian propolis to address their own health problem: this is interesting, because our cellular response to propolis from tropical countries should be quite different compared to local propolis and may affect its anti-inflammatory and anti-allergic potential. Most of this difference depends on intestinal flora composition and on human genetics. The distribution of interest regarding propolis throughout the world, as indicated in Figure 1, might suggest that propolis consideration in medicine in more frequent in those countries where people are used to referring to traditional and complementary medicine, although attention to folk medicine is also present among common people from Northern civilized nations [29] and propolis is becoming an intriguing topic in pharmacology and in the chemistry of plant products also in modern, industrialized countries [30, 31]. Furthermore, the highest number of reports dealing with propolis comes from countries with warm and temperate climate. In these regions, propolis composition shows a significant variability among different geographical places and environments, depending on the wider biodiversity concerning plants and hymenoptera species. Although the biological activity of propolis, especially its antimicrobial and anti-inflammatory activity, can always be demonstrated, in samples from different geographic and climatic zones this activity is due to different chemical constituents and to their proportion in the complete polyphenol mixture. Actually, chemical composition of propolis is a very complex issue and phenolics content depends on the plants present in the areas where propolis is collected. Therefore, it is very difficult to discover properly which flavonoid may cause an anti-inflammatory or anti-allergic effect. A detailed and reliable overview of comparative data on biological activities, combined with chemical evidence, in order to decide whether some specific areas of application of a particular propolis can be formulated as preferable, is a fundamental hallmark to comprehend propolis pharmacology. More than 200 compounds have been identified in propolis from different geographical origins including phenolic acids, flavonoids, terpenes, lignans, amino acids, fatty acids, vitamins, and minerals. In countries such as Europe, North America, and the non-tropical regions of Asia, the main source of propolis is the resinous exudates of the buds of poplar trees (*Populus* species). These samples of propolis are characterized by similar chemical composition – main compounds belonging to the phenolic class and include flavonoid aglycones, aromatic acids, and their esters. Propolis from warm regions, such as Brazilian green (Alecrim) propolis, which originates from *Baccharis dracunculifolia* (Asteraceae) is characterized by the presence of prenylated derivatives of *p*-coumaric acid and *o*-hydroxy-acetophenone. These substances are typical chemical constituents of Brazilian propolis, and they are not present in propolis from other regions. Flavonoids different from those in European propolis, as well as diterpenes and lignans, have also been found in samples of Brazilian propolis. Red propolis, which can be found also in Brazil, is a typical propolis of Cuba, where its plant source was identified as *Clusia nemorosa* (Clusiaceae), and of Venezuela, where bees collect it from *C. scrobiculata*. Typical components of Cuban propolis are polyprenylated benzophenones, and this makes Cuban propolis different from both European and Brazilian propolis. However, propolis, regardless of its plant source and chemical composition, always possesses antimicrobial and anti-oxidative activity. The antimicrobial activity of propolis is mainly attributed to the presence of flavonoids such as pinocembrin, galangin, pinobanksin, pinobanksin-3-acetate, chrysin, in addition to chlorogenic and cafeic acid phenetyl-ester (CAPE). Propolis with strong antioxidant activity contained compounds such as kaempherol, caffeic acid, and phenethyl caffeate. The concentration of bioactive principles in propolis may vary substantially according to the origin of the sample, and such differences may affect its biological activities. Therefore, the chemical constituents of propolis have to be identified and quantified using appropriate methods. Nevertheless, flavonoids described in propolis are very few and are listed in Table 1, while existing commercial propolis comes principally from tropical places: Brazilian propolis accounts for the largest diffusion of propolis worldwide and constitutes a significant component in the commercial raw substance: therefore, when this kind of propolis is considered for allergy or airway inflammatory ailments, phenolic acids may exert a dominant role compared to flavonoids. Attempts to describe a correlation between propolis composition and antimicrobial activity have been made [25] but a huge heterogeneity still exists. A chemical study on European propolis from Bulgaria, Italy and Switzerland showed that propolis from the Graubünden Alpine region, Switzerland, was rich in phenolic glycerides, while the one from Sicily contained only a limited number of phenolics and was rich in diterpenic acids [32]. Very few reports dealing with propolis composition and property can be found in cold and industrialized countries, such as Scandinavian, Russian, North American area, in addition to Australia, anyway. In Europe, interest in propolis pertains mainly to the Mediterranean region and to some Eastern countries, such as Bulgaria [33]. Geographical distribution of propolis has the utmost importance in propolis composition; phenolic content of propolis also depends on regional distribution of wider geographical areas [34, 35]. This issue is certainly interesting in tracing an overall perspective about propolis quality and composition based on its natural sources and geographical distribution. For example, following a rapid fingerprint method, which was developed to investigate and assess geographical origin of Chinese propolis by using high performance liquid chromatography–ultraviolet detection (HPLC–UV), eight major compounds were identified as flavonoids, including rutin, myricetin, quercetin, kaempferol, apigenin, pinocembrine, chrysin and galangin [36]. As an anti-inflammatory agent, a comparative investigation of the antibacterial activity of propolis from different geographical and climatic areas, has recently been attempted [37]. In the Asiatic continent, Chinese propolis represents the main component of the total amount of Asiatic propolis. Components of Chinese propolis have been analyzed by several Authors [38, 39] and preventive/protective effects, were described elsewhere [40, 41] but also propolis from other places in the Asiatic continent has been reported to be a potent anti-inflammatory and anti-microbial substance [42]. Actually, importance in the knowledge of plant sources has recently been suggested [43]. Bankova and colleagues have addressed a thorough investigation on propolis from different plant sources and geographical areas and showed that in tropical bee glue, flavonoids were important components of these samples, as in European ones, although their plant origin is different. In samples from the Sonoran Desert, Wollenweber and colleagues [44] identified flavonoid aglycones typical of leaf exudates from *Ambrosia deltoidea*; among them 5,7,4'-trihydroxy- 6,8-dimethoxyflavone and sideritiflavone, this being a novelty for propolis. Myricetin 3,7,4',5'-tetramethyl ether and quercetin 3,7,3'-trimethyl ether were isolated from Tunisian propolis, which originated from leaf exudates of *Cistus* species [45]. In Brazilian samples, kaempferid, 5,6,7-trihydroxy-3,4'-dihydroxyflavon, aromadendrine-4'methyl ether [46] and 3,5,7-trihydroxy-6,4'-dimethoxyflavon [47] were also identified. The activity of flavonoids from different geographical areas has already been analyzed and assessed the important role of these phytochemicals in human health prevention and protection. In a past study the antioxidant activities of propolis of various geographic origins, i.e., Argentina, Australia, Brazil, Bulgaria, Chile, China (Hebei, Hubei, and Zhejiang), Hungary, New Zealand, South Africa, Thailand, Ukraine, Uruguay, United States, and Uzbekistan were compared. Major constituents were identified in ethanol extracts of propolis by HPLC analysis with photo-diode array (PDA) and mass spectrometric (MS) detection, and quantitatively analyzed [48]. As mentioned above, the highest frequency in propolis from tropical areas, particularly from South America and Brazil, might suggest a concern about genetic response to different phenolic compounds by people living in different geographical areas who use propolis purchased from tropical sources. This may constitute an interesting topic for pharmacogenomics of different propolis extract in different populations worldwide.

## The Anti-inflammatory and Anti-allergic Property Depends on Propolis Biochemistry: Reports about Flavonoids Composition in Propolis

Many reports dealt with propolis composition. Propolis was analyzed with different analytical methods [12, 49-55], such as spectrophotometry [39, 56], capillary electrophoresis [57], reverse phase HPLC [58-62], HPLC-diode array detection [26, 28, 63, 64], HPLC-MS [65], HPLC-DAD and HPLC-ESI-MS/MS by comparing the performance of ion trap and triple quadrupole mass analyzers [66], gas chromatography coupled with mass spectrometry

(GC-MS) [32, 55, 67, 68], electrospray ionization mass spectrometry [60, 69], H-NMR [70, 71]. Studies about the chemical composition in flavonoids within propolis have been conducted for thirty years or more. Colorimetric methods with aluminum chloride reactions allowed to evaluate, as quercetin or naringenin equivalent, the content in flavonoids of most diffused raw propolis samples, namely Brazilian and Chinese propolis, leading to the assessment that Brazil propolis contained the lowest level of total flavonoids (10.38% ± 0.14), while samples obtained from Taiwan contained higher levels of total flavonoids (20.60%–24.91%), although, according to the Authors, due to the existence of a tremendous variation in total flavonoid contents of commercial propolis products, further verification of data has to be requested. Ethanolic extracts and essential oils from green propolis from South-East Brazil and leaf buds from its botanical origin *Baccharis dracunculifolia* were analyzed by reversed phase HPLC (RP-HPLC), by RP-HPLC and GC-MS and with thin layer chromatography (RP-HPTLC), leading to identification of thirteen major flavonoids and phenolic acids, namely artepillin C, chrysin, tectochrysin, quercetin, galangin, keamferide, kaempferol, apigenin, pinocembrin, rutin, pinobanksin, pinobanksin-3-acetate and quercetin, both in propolis and in its source plant, although for some of these compounds propolis presented a lower content in flavonoids than leaf buds, as mg/g [72]. This evidence would suggest that propolis composition in flavonoids may have a comparable pattern to its origin plant, at least for most of the analyzed flavone-derived polyphenols [7]. In Bulgarian propolis main flavonoids are represented by pinocembrin, galangin, chrysin, tectochrysin, isorhamnetin, quercetin and small amounts of kaemferol [73]. Conjugated forms of myricetin (myricetin 3, 7, 4‘, 5‘-tetramethyl ether) and quercetin (quercetin 3, 7, 3 - trimethyl ether), typical of *Cistus spp.*, were detected in Tunisian propolis [45]. Those flavonoids are represented also in Egyptian (Behera) and United Arabic Emirates (Dubai) propolis, with typical differences. The ethanolic extract of this propolis showed the presence of several polyphenolic substances, such as chrysin (5,7 - dihydroxyflavone), 5,7 - dihydroxydihydroflavone, physcion or emodin - 3 - methyl - ether (1, 7 - Dihydroxy - 3 - methoxy - 6 - methylanthraquinone), pinostrobin (5 - Hydroxy -7- methoxy-2 - phenyl - 4H - 1 - benzopyran - 4 - one), emodin (1,3,8-Trihydroxy - 6 - methylanthraquinone), 1 - (Dihydroxyphenyl) -3 - phenylpropenone [74]. A variability in the chemical nature of propolis coming from different origin and sources have been observed by many other Authors in the past [23, 43, 45, 76 - 88]. Said and colleagues have pointed out that even the two Egyptian samples of propolis investigated in previous studies (El-Saff and Ismailia) have been found to possess different chemical composition [82]. It is worthy to note that most of the compounds detected in the samples of Behera propolis are different from those present in the Egyptian propolis of other origin that has previously been investigated [82]: as well as other propolis sources, this may be due to the existence of differences in the source of poplar buds and other plants from which the propolis was collected. Furthermore, seasonality influences the chemical composition of the commercial classes of raw Brazilian green propolis [89]. Understanding the composition in flavonoids of propolis represents a real challenge for analysts because this might allow researchers to find possible active principles in this resinous beeswax: main significant information about the molecular nature of propolis reported effects, should come from further knowledge concerning purified components *in vitro.* Very few papers, which have shown the anti-inflammatory and anti-microbial effect of propolis, have focused onto the role of single determined compounds, such as flavonoids or phenolic acids, in elucidating the molecular mechanisms by which propolis exerted its preventive and health promoting effect [90, 91]; most of them were attracted by the consideration of water (WEP) or ethanol extracts (EEP) of propolis, whose composition has been highlighted, but without ascribing effect to any particular compound [92-97]. On the other hand, research on single components extracted from raw propolis, along with current discoveries of other natural flavonoids [98] and newly synthesized molecules, is becoming a very promising research field; therefore, most evidence about the role of flavonoids in propolis comes from those reports dealing with the activity of these single compounds on cell or animal models.

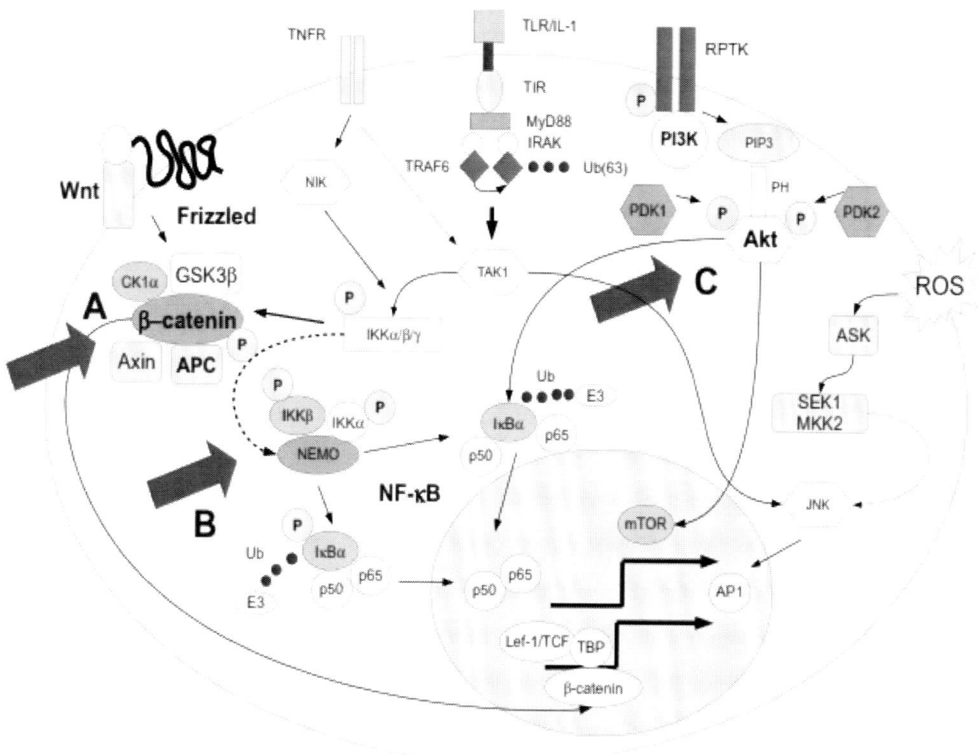


Figure 2. Carton describing the main signaling pathways (as arrows indicated by letters) affected by flavonoids contained in propolis. Flavonoids target many intracellular kinases and signaling proteins, such as phosphoinositide-3-kinse (PI3K) and downstream kinases such as Akt, JNK and others (ERK-1/2 or p38MAPK, non shown in the figure). Along with the Wnt/Frizzled-beta-catetin pathway, these systems can be related to NF-κB signaling, which can be considered the bottleneck of both intracellular function and gene expression/regulation. This model may explain the concurrent anti-inflammatory or cytoprotective effect with the anti-replicative (or also pro-apoptotic) action, which render flavonoids possible guns against tumors. See text for further explanations.

## THE ANTI-INFLAMMATORY AND ANTI-ALLERGIC ACTIVITY OF PROPOLIS-DERIVED FLAVONOIDS

The most diffused flavonoids in propolis are chrysin, galangin and pinocembrin. Other flavonoids, such as quercetin, kaempferol, kaempferide, morin, acacetin, pinostrobin or other molecules derived from the above flavonoids such as pinobanksin or tectochrysin, are less represented and their content in propolis varies widely from one geographical area to another. Their diffusion in plant-derived food and beverage makes it difficult to unveil if an anti-inflammatory effect following propolis assumption may derive also from ingested flavonoids from fruits or vegetables present in daily diet. Purified compounds showed interesting effects, anyway. Pinostrobin showed efficacy against herpes simplex virus-1 [99], evidence reported in the past also for propolis and for other propolis-derived flavonoids, such as galangin [100]. Pinocembrin and galangin were the most represented flavonoids in propolis extract exhibiting an *in vitro* activity against *Streptococcus pyogenes* [101]. Most propolis flavonoids are flavanones or flavones and their molecular targeting within cell is summarized in Figure 2. Three main pathways, described in the figure, illustrate possible targets of propolis flavonoids on intracellular signalling: a) the Wnt/β-catenin pathway; b) the NF-κB pathway; c) the PI3K-Akt pathway. NF-κB represents a possible cross-point of other signaling pathways and this may explain why most flavonoids affect NF-κB function and behave as anti-inflammatory agents [102, 103]. Another pathway regards the relationships between reactive oxygen species (ROS) and other free radicals with intracellular signaling, mitochondrial function, apoptosis and gene regulation. All of these signaling routes lead to intracellular function such as receptor-intracellular target communication, exocytosis of mediators-containing granules, protein trafficking and cytoskeleton re-organization but also to genetic expression of cytokines and inflammatory molecules, to cell cycle regulation and to apoptosis [102, 103]. This should suggest the complex role of many flavonoids in inflammation and their task in cancer onset and progression. For certain aspects, the anti-inflammatory role of most flavonoids is strictly related to their claimed effectiveness in chemoprevention. This does not mean immediately the possible effectiveness of propolis against cancer, of course, but purified molecules would promise a possible horizon in prevention or therapy. What has to be highlighted and further explained with new emerging insights, concerns the question why flavonoids are able to inhibit cancer cells almost selectively, by promoting in those cells apoptosis and cell cycle arrest. This is one of the most intriguing issues of the anti-inflammatory potential pertaining flavonoids. Probably, tumours have lost stress-response mechanisms that enable non tumour cells to suppress the genotoxic and cytotoxic action of plant derived polyphenols. Nevertheless, few reports exist dealing with the use of propolis against cancer [5, 65]. Propolis worldwide is a well known natural substance for upper respiratory tract infections (URTIs) [104] but its potential against many other chronic inflammatory pathologies, including tumours, lays on its chemical composition and on the evidence emerging from assaying its single phenolic components [31].

## Chrysin

Chrysin is probably the most represented flavonoid in propolis and it is used with galangin as a standard in chromatographic assays evaluating propolis composition. Its beneficial effects have been shown in several reports, even in reproductive physiology [105, 106], in hypotension [107] and as a hepatoprotective molecule [108]. Chrysin can also be found in some *Passiflora* plant genus, where it is discovered as an anxiolytic active principle [109]: furthermore, hyperalgesia induced by chrysin via $GABA_A$ receptor has also been reported [110]. Actually, chrysin tropism for neuronal cells allows this phenolic to play a role also as a neuro-protective compound. Neurodegenerative diseases are often caused by neuroinflammation mediated by microglia. In this perspective suppression of microglial activation might contribute to neuronal cell survival. Some evidence was reported showing that chrysin significantly inhibited the release of nitric oxide (NO) and pro-inflammatory cytokines such as TNF-α and interleukin-1β (IL-1β), the expression of inducible NO synthase (iNOS) and cyclooxygenase-2 (COX-2) [111]. At a molecular level, chrysin inhibited the activations of c-Jun N-terminal kinase (JNK) and nuclear factor-κB (NF-κB), which are signaling molecules involved in neuro-inflammation [111]. The neuroprotective effect of chrysin was also associated to a decrease in C/EBPδ protein level, mRNA expression, and DNA-binding activity, with no effect on C/EBPβ and p65 nuclear protein levels or DNA-binding activity, pointing out C/EBPδ as a possible mediator of chrysin effects [112].

Recently reported evidence has shown that chrysin, together with epicatechin, p-coumaric acid, morin, 3,4-dimethoxycinnamic acid, naringenin, ferulic acid, cinnamic acid and pinocembrin is the major functional phenolic compound in Chinese water extract of propolis [39]. As well as many other flavanones contained in this resinous substance, chrysin (5,7-dihydroxy-phenyl-4H-chromen-4-one) exerts an immuno-modulatory action that enables this polyphenolic compound to be a potential anti-microbial, anti-inflammatory (by modulating the activity of NK cells) and anti-tumoral substance [39, 113]. It exerts a pro-apoptotic action in tumors [114, 115], for example by enhancing apoptosis induced by TRAIL [117] and plays an anti-inflammatory role. In a pneumonia murine model, the flavanone is a potent inhibitor of α-haemolysin expression by *Staphylococcus aureus*, then conferring to animals a significant degree of protection against *S. aureus* pneumonia [117]. The anti-inflammatory property of chrysin, known also as galangin flavanone, encouraged many researchers to address synthetic approaches to chemically modified forms of chrysin [118, 119], for example 5,7-dihydroxy-8-(pyridine-4yl)-flavone, which showed higher efficacy than nature-derived chrysin as a potential anti-inflammatory agent [120, 121], or dimethoxyflavone (DMF), a methylated form of chrysin, which showed efficacy in the suppression of the development of pre-neoplastic lesions induced by N-nitrosodiethylamine (DEN) in rats [122]. A role against UV-induced damage in HaCaT keratinocytes has also been reported. Chrysin can attenuate apoptosis, reactive oxygen species (ROS) production, and cyclooxygenase 2 (COX-2) expression induced by UVB and UVA; furthermore, reversion of down-regulation of aquaporin 3 (AQP-3) induced by UVB and of JNK activation, as well as the mild inhibition of p38 activation triggered by UVA and UVB, has been reported [123]. A role for chrysin in melanogenesis has been recently addressed. Involvement of chrysin in alpha-MSH and forskolin-induced cAMP signaling within a cell based assay was examined and the results strongly suggested that chrysin directly inhibited the activity of adenylyl cyclase, downregulated forskolin-induced cAMP-production pathway and consequently inhibited melanogenesis, thus suggesting a possible therapeutic role in hyperpigmentation [124]. The role of chrysin in inflammation has spreading light on the action of this propolis-derived component also in tumors [125-127]: a possible explanation of this, which includes many other propolis-derived flavonoids, needs yet to be addressed. Chrysin promotes apoptosis, likewise other flavone-ring sharing phenolics from propolis [128] and actually chrysin inhibits cell growth, by inducing cell cycle arrest and/or apoptosis. Flavonoids are in fact well known substances that inhibit proliferation, angiogenesis, and/or metastasis; and exhibit anti-inflammatory and/or antioxidant effects. In turn, these effects involve multiple molecular and biochemical mechanisms of action, which are still not completely characterized. Thus, caution is mandatory when attempting to extrapolate the observations obtained in *in vitro* tumour cells to humans. Notwithstanding, a recent interesting evidence described the effect of topotecan and chrysin in breast cancer. ATP-driven efflux pumps such as phosphoglycoprotein-170 (P-gp), multidrug-resistance-associated protein-2 (MRP-2), or breast cancer resistance protein (BCRP) play altogether a crucial role in hampering the efficacy of tumor pharmacotherapy. Some flavonoids have proved to inhibit individual efflux-transporters and to act therefore as multidrug-resistance reversing agents. Chrysin acts as a potent inhibitor of P-gp, MRP-2, and BCRP in Caco-2 colon carcinoma cells [129]: this leads to a higher accumulation of the apoptosis-inducing chemotherapeutic topotecan in the presence of chrysin, although under these conditions the expression of the transporters can be markedly increased. However, in spite of raising the cellular concentrations of topotecan, chrysin potently inhibits the apoptosis-inducing activities of the anti-tumor drug, probably by suppressing caspase-activation of apoptosis, a mechanism caused by transport-independent functions of ABC-transporters [129]. A relationship can be outlined by focusing onto the role of intracellular signalling and of key factors, known to be targeted by flavonoids, such as several intracellular kinases and NF-κB. This scenario may explain also the inhibitory activity exerted by chrysin towards IL-6-mediated angiogenesis [130]. The IL-6-induced binding of STAT3 was significantly suppressed by chrysin. Chrysin suppresses IL-6-induced angiogenesis through modulation of the sIL-6R/gp130/JAK1/STAT3/VEGF signaling pathway [130]. Probably, conjugated or enzyme-modified forms of chrysin, enhance its efficacy in fighting tumors [131]. Dimethoxy flavone (DMF), a methylated flavone derived from chrysin, significantly suppressed the development of pre-neoplastic lesions induced by N-nitrosodiethylamine (DEN) in rats. Although the mechanism of action was not known; the study has been conducted on the effects of DMF administration on gene expression changes related to the inflammation-mediated NF-kB pathway, Wnt pathway and apoptotic mediators in DEN-induced pre-neoplastic nodules [115]. A significant increase in inflammatory markers like cyclooxygenase-2 (COX-2) and inducible nitric oxide synthase (iNOS) and a decrease in apoptotic mediators like p53, caspase-3 and bax in DEN-treated rats, when compared to the control group, was also reported [115]. In this context, activation of NF-κB was noticed by an elevated expression of nuclear protein expression of NF-kB and cytoplasmic phospho-IkBαSer(32/36) in the same animals; likewise, up-regulation of canonical Wnt pathway was observed by elevated expression of nuclear protein levels of phospho-β-cateninThr(393) and cytoplasmic casein kinase-2 (CK2), Dvl2 and cyclin D1 levels, along with a simultaneous decrease in expression of phospho-GSK3β (Ser9) [115]. DMF also reversed the activation of NF-κB and Wnt pathway, as shown by the decrease in protein expression of several proteins. This results provided evidence that attenuation of Wnt pathway and suppression of inflammatory response mediated by NF-κB could be implicated, in part, in the chemopreventive effects of methylated chrysin.

Much evidence about chrysin as a natural and biologically active flavonoid with anticancer effects has been recently reported, therefore, but cancer cells often perform an adaptive response to this flavanone. What it is recently acknowledged is that chrysin has proteasome inhibitor activity. As like as many other phenolics, chrysin too can inhibit enzyme function but also the role of proteasome in cell function [132]: this evidence supports the idea that many down-regulating effects ascribed to chrysin may arise because it counteracts a strategic function of some enzymatic pathway involving protein changes and turn over. The ubiquitin-proteasome pathway plays a fundamental role in regulating apoptosis and the cell cycle. The function of proteasomes is mediated by three main catalytic activities: a) chymotrypsin-like (CT-L), b) trypsin-like (T-L), and c) peptidylglutamyl peptide hydrolyzing (PGPH) activity. Some evidence recently reported has revealed that proteasome inhibitors possess an antitumor effect, having been used to treat cancers such as multiple myeloma. Chrysin inhibited CT-L and T-L catalytic activities in a dose-dependent manner, whereas its effect on PGPH catalytic activity appeared weaker [132].

Previous studies demonstrated that proteasome inhibitors might induce endoplasmic reticulum (ER) stress response. Chrysin inhibits hepatoma cells growth and induces apoptosis in a dose-dependent manner; in this pathogenic model, chrysin induces GRP78 overexpression, X-box binding protein-1 splicing and eukaryotic initiation factor 2α phosphorylation, hallmarks of the unfolded protein response [133]. In this scenario, GRP78 knockdown potentiates chrysin-induced caspase-7 cleavage in hepatoma cells and enhances chrysin-induced apoptosis. Catechins, such as EGCG, overcome chrysin-induced GRP78 expression and a combination of EGCG and chrysin potentiates chrysin-induced caspase-7 and poly (ADP-ribose) polymerase (PARP) cleavage and sensitizes hepatoma cells to chrysin through caspase-mediated apoptosis [133]. In allergy, where chrysin seems to be provided with a higher effectiveness than chromolyn, the flavanone is able to inhibit mast cell releasability and also to suppress gene expression of pro-inflammatory cytokines such as, TNF-α, IL (interleukin)-1β, IL-4, and IL-6 in mast cells; the inhibitory effect of chrysin on the pro-inflammatory cytokine was nuclear factor-κB and caspase-1 dependent [134]. Actually, the anti-inflammatory property of chrysin appears to be mainly related to the inhibition of NF-κB signalling: the flavanone inhibits the activations of c-Jun N-terminal kinase (JNK) and nuclear factor-κB (NF-κB), which are signaling molecules involved in neuro-inflammation [111]. In lipopolysaccharide (LPS)-treated BV-2 mouse microglial cell lines, 10 μmol/L chrysin inhibits phosphorylation of JNK, but does not influence phosphorylation of p38-MAPK and ERKs [111]. This neuro-inflammatory model appears interesting to comprehend the molecular mechanism by which chrysin exerts its anti-inflammatory action. As an anti-allergic substance, chrysin showed anti-asthmatic potential, probably due to the alteration of Th1/Th2 polarization via the suppression of inducible nitric oxide synthase, NF-κB, and activation protein involved in this mechanism [135]. The anti-oxidant property of chrysin has been shown in many pathogenic models, where chrysin was able to prevent organ toxicity from other drugs [136-140]. Chrysin may express a biphasic behaviour, as like as many other flavonoids; for example, a chrysin-copper complex is able to interact with cell membrane, thus modifying the electrical characteristics of planar lipid bilayers, a property that might be used to ameliorate both technical application of liposome vehicles suited to enhance bioavailability of several pharmacological compounds and erythrocyte osmotic membrane disruption induced by drugs. At relatively low concentrations (20 μM), a chrysin-copper complex exhibited twice the protection against hypotonic stress-induced membrane disruption when compared to chrysin but this stabilizing effect gradually decreased and became comparable to chrysin at higher concentrations, so performing a biphasic behavior, which needs to be further explored [141]. The anti-inflammatory effect of chrysin has been reported mainly in cancer research. In this field, chrysin, as many other flavonoids such as quercetin, may act synergistically with other effective compounds, such as doxorubricin in human lung epithelial cancer [142] or nitrofurantoin in breast cancer [143]. Current research is planning synthetic molecules in order to improve chrysin effectiveness against tumors and to solve possible problems about bioavailability; for example, 5-allyl-7-

gen-difluoromethoxychrysin (AFMC) is a novel synthetic analogue of chrysin that has been reported to inhibit proliferation in various cancer cell lines, namely it enhances TRAIL-mediated apoptosis in human non-small cell lung cancer [144], the novel chrysin analog 8-bromo-7-methoxychrysin (BrMC) has been reported to induce apoptosis of various cancer cell lines [145]. In human prostate cancer cell line PC-3, chrysin reduces cell proliferation and induces apoptosis [146]. The activity of this flavanone towards receptor-mediated intracellular signaling appears not so different from many other related flavonoids derived from plants. An inhibitory activity against mitogens, such as platelet derived growth factor (PDGF) has been reported: the action exerted by chrysin, on PDGF signaling and protein tyrosine phosphatase function, was reversed by depletion of intracellular glutathione (GSH), suggesting an involvement of chrysin on GSH/glutaredoxin system for PTP reactivation [147].

## Galangin

Galangin or norizalpinin is a 3,5,7-trihydroxyflavone. As like as many other flavonoids, galangin inhibits many biochemical proteins, mainly ezymes [148, 149], a possible reason for which galangin may express an anti-microbial effect [149-151]. Together with chrysin and caffeic acid phenetyl ester (CAPE), galangin is considered one of the main phenolic compound in propolis. Ethanolic extracts of propolis, deprived from CAPE and galangin, did not exhibit any anti-inflammatory effect in rat using a carrageenin foot oedema model [152, 153]. Its anti-oxidant property has been confirmed also recently. A recent study examined the effects of galangin on oxidative stress, inflammatory cytokine levels and NF-κB activation in fructose-fed rat liver [154], giving some suggestion as a possible therapeutic against insulin-resistance [155]. Compared to control diet-fed animals, fructose-fed animals developed hyperglycemia, hyperinsulinemia, hypertriglyceridemia and insulin resistance (IR) (all $p<0.01$). Galangin prevented the rise in plasma glucose, insulin and triglycerides and improved insulin sensitivity. Tumor necrosis factor-α (TNF-α) and interleukin-6 (IL-6) levels in plasma and the mRNA and protein levels of TNF-α and transforming growth factor-β1(TGF-$\beta_1$) in liver were significantly higher in fructose-fed rats than control rats. However, treatment with galangin down-regulated the expression of these cytokines. As an anti-inflammatory natural agent in cancer, galangin activates apoptosis in cancer cells [156] and possesses genotoxic-preventive potential, as it can counteract the genotoxicity of many chemicals in chemoprevention [157, 158]. Synergistic effects between galangin and other drugs have been also reported: galangin increases the cytotoxic activity of imatinib-mesylate in Bcr-abl expressing leukemia cells [159]. Galangin and pinocembrin are, together with chrysin, the most abundant flavonoids present in propolis [160]. Past reports showed that at a molecular level, galangin was able to inhibit cytochrome $P_{450}$1A1 (CYP1A1) activity and aryl-hydrocarbon receptor [161]: evidence showing that CYP1A1 can oxidize galangin was also reported [162]. Actually, galangin is metabolized to kaempferol by TCDD-inducible CYP1A1 in Caco-2 cells and in this configuration the flavonoid, which can inhibit CYP1A1 expression induced by 2,3,7,8-tetrachlorodibenzo-*p*-dioxin (TCDD), is less effective163. From a molecular point of view, intracellular targets affected by galangin are represented by the GSK-3β signaling pathway; structure-activity data indicated that the major structural requirements for galangin-mediated β-catenin degradation are hydroxyl groups at positions 3,

5, and 7164. In this model, inhibition of glycogen synthase kinase-3β (GSK-3β) activity or mutation of the GSK-3β-targeted sequence from β-catenin was unable to abrogate the galangin-mediated degradation of β-catenin. The flavonoid galangin actually down-regulated the intracellular β-catenin levels in cancer cells with inactivating mutations of adenomatous polyposis coli (APC) or axin, which are components of the β-catenin destruction complex. As a matter of fact, evidence was reported showing that galangin repressed the expression of β-catenin/T-cell factor-dependent genes, such as cyclin D1 and c-myc, and thus inhibited the proliferation of CRT-positive cancer cells [164].

## Pinocembrin

An anti-inflammatory potential of pinocembrin has been described in permanent cerebral ischemic rats [165-169]: the polyphenolic compound is able to reduce the expressions of TNF-α, IL-1β, ICAM-1, vascular cell adhesion molecule-1, inducible NO synthase and aquaporin-4, inhibit the activation of microglias and astrocytes; and downregulate the expression of matrix metalloproteinases (MMPs) in the ischemic brain [165]. This role in cerebral ischemia has been recently confirmed [166]: pinocembrin decreased the neurological scores, alleviated brain edema, reduced the permeability of blood brain-barrier (BBB) and mitigated the ultrastructural changes of 'neurovascular unit' in the global cerebral ischemia/reperfusion (GCI/R) rats. Pinocembrin also improved cerebral blood flow in the GCI/R rats and protected rat cerebral microvascular endothelial cells against oxygen-glucose deprivation/reoxygenation mediated injury [166]. These data, besides to evidence reported elsewhere also by others [167-171], suggests a role for pinocembrin as a neuroprotective natural substance. There are increasing evidence that pinocembrin has better neuroprotective effect than other flavonoids, for it acts on mitochondrial respiratory function in global brain ischemia/ reperfusion models and improve ATP content in brain mitochondria, both *in vitro* and in neuronal SH-SY5Y cell line [169]. This was confirmed also with Chinese propolis [172]. Some reports would suggest that the effect of pinocembrin may be considered comparable to that of borneol, a bicyclic organic compound and a terpene [173], although there is no apparent molecular likeness between borneol and the flavanone present in propolis. However, as like as borneol, this 5,7-dihydroxyflavanone seems to affect the intracellular NF-κB signalling pathway. Acute liver injury and fibrosis is characterized by an increased expression and cross-linking activity of tissue trans-glutaminase (tTG). Propolis components prevent both the tTG expression *in vitro* and fibrogenesis *in vivo*. In this model, both ERK1/2 and PI3K/Akt pathways can regulate the effects of ethanol on NF-κB-dependent transcription and these signaling pathways may be involved in activation of ethanol-mediated tTG expression; the administration of pinocembrin inhibited tTG activation and significantly prevented the development of thioacetamide (TAA)-induced liver cirrhosis. This participation of pinocembrin in preventing liver fibrosis may involve an effect on NF-κB. Although the exact causal relationship between activation of NF-κB and alcoholic liver injury remains speculative, an hypothetical mechanism for such a relationship has been previously addressed [174]. NF-κB is associated with the tTG expression in Hep 3B liver cells exposed to ethanol. One model suggests that NF-κB, acting as an intermediate, increases the expression of cytokines and fibrosis-related genes. The molecular activation of NF-κB occurs secondarily to the proteolytic degradation of IkBα, allowing free NF-κB to translocate to the nucleus and initiate gene transcription. In this perspective, the role of pinocembrin towards NF-κB would be argued by its ability in affecting that relationship between ROS and NF-κB, as many other flavone-derived substances [175]. In rats, following treatment with 10 and 100 mg/kg pinocembrin, heme oxygenase activity significantly increased ($p<0.05$), although the flavanone did not affect neither the activities of NADPH: cytochrome P450 reductase, NADPH: quinone reductase, UDP-glucuronosyltransferase and glutathione-S-transferase, not the expression of phase I metabolizing enzymes, including CYP1A1, CYP2B1, CYP2C11, CYP2E1, CYP3A2, and NADPH: cytochrome P450 reductase [176]. Furthermore, mithocondrial targeting is a typical hallmark of several anti-oxidant and pro-apoptotic flavonoids; pinocembrin, as for instance, exhibited proteasome inhibitory activities in a human 20S proteasome bioassay with $IC_{50}$ values of 3.45 ± 0.18 and 2.87 ± 0.26 μM, respectively, so showing that C-benzylated dihydroflavones have an apoptotic effect associated with disruption of the mitochondrial transmembrane potential [177]. Isolation of pinocembrin as a bacteriostatic substance goes back to more than 40 years ago [178], but the molecule proved to be effective also against fungi [179] and against *Neisseria gonorrhoeae* [180]. Pinocembrin from the leaves of *Cryptocarya sinensis* exhibited antituberculosis activity against *Mycobacterium tuberculosis in vitro* with MIC values of 3.5 and 25.0 μg/ml, respectively [181] but this property has not yet showed with pinocembrin from propolis. An anti-inflammatory effect showing a participation of pinocembrin was recently reported: seed ethanolic extract of *Alpinia katsumadai* H (var. Ayata) exerts anti-inflammatory effects for NO and $PGE_2$ production. This extract, which contains a significant amount of pinocembrin, significantly inhibited the LPS-induced production of IL-6 and TNF-α, as well as the expression of iNOS and moreover induced HO-1 expression in RAW264.7 cells (the extract may have anti-inflammatory activity via induction of HO-1 expression) and inhibited the nuclear translocation of NF-κB by preventing degradation of the inhibitor kappa B-alpha [182]. However this evidence, although confirming the activity of flavone-derived substances on HO-1 expression, has to be reappraised, as the extract contained cardamonin, a chalcone that exhibits an inhibitory effect on LPS-induced NO production more pronounced than pinocembrin [183]. Furthermore, the anti-inflammatory effect of pinocembrin, as well as other propolis derived flavonoids, has to be interpreted as a synergistic action between phenolic acids and flavonoids; for example, an anti-proliferative and cytotoxic effect of propolis on the HeLa cells may be not correlated with the concentration of particular components such as specific flavonoids but on establishing the possible synergistic anti-proliferative activity of individual phenolic acid and flavonoids altogether [58]. As like as many other polyphenols, pinocembrin inhibits several enzymatic activities [184, 185].

## FUTURE PERSPECTIVES

Propolis is a widespread natural substance that can be used, with very little side effects, to address inflammatory reactions caused by pathogen bacteria or other microbes. Normally, propolis is suggested for people suffering from URTIs but the analysis of its phenolic components and their testing on cells and animals in several inflammation models, has encouraged and promoted the biochemical and pharmacological investigation on propolis extracts, which merit to be considered as potential new guns against chronic pathologies such as neurodegenerative diseases and cancer. This claimed and assessed efficacy of propolis in different protocols, both *in vitro* and *in vivo*, should suggests for a more pronounced decision as a therapeutic agent, but before establishing a strategy using this bee product, it is necessary to obtain further insights on: (1) the chemical nature of the propolis sample and the activity of main flavonoids, including synergistic effects with CAPE and other phenolic acids; (2) propolis efficacy should be compared to well-established parameters, e.g. positive or negative controls in the experiments and with standardized procedures. Furthermore, possible interactions between propolis and other medicines should be investigated in humans as well; (3) clinical investigation is requested to evaluate propolis potential in patients or healthy individuals, to understand under which conditions propolis may promote human health and prevent inflammatory ailments. Many insights are still requested; since propolis-containing products have been marketed and humans have used propolis for different purposes, the goal of future research is to address and deepen the potential of propolis for the development of new drugs, by comparing data from the literature that suggest candidate areas for the establishment of drugs against cancer, microbial and viral infections, allergy, diabetes, ulcers, neurodegenerative disorders and with immuno-modulatory action.

## ACKNOWLEDGMENTS

A special thank to Katia Mazzau, from Verona (Italy) for her kind contribution in reviewing the text.

## REFERENCES

[1] Makashvili Z. A. From the history of propolis. In Remarkable hive product : Propolis. *Scientific data and suggessions concerning its composition, properties and possible use in therapeutics*.APIMONDIA standing Commission on Beekeeping technology and Equipment, Bucharest, 1978.

[2] Salatino A., Fernanes-Silva C. C., Righi A. A., Salatino M. L. F. Propolis research and the chemistry of plant products. *Nat Prod Rep* 2011; 28:925-936.

[3] Cherniack E. P. Bugs as drugs, Part 1: Insects: the new alternative medicine for the 21st century? *Altern Med Rev*. 2010 Jul;15(2):124-35.

[4] Boukraâ L., Sulaiman S. A. Rediscovering the antibiotics of the hive. *Recent Pat Antiinfect Drug Discov*. 2009 Nov;4(3):206-13.

[5] Watanabe M. A., Amarante M. K., Conti B. J., Sforcin J. M. Cytotoxic constituents of propolis inducing anticancer effects: a review. *J Pharm Pharmacol*. 2011 Nov;63(11):1378-86.

[6] Kosalec I., Bakmaz M., Pepeljnjak S., Vladimir-Knezevic S. Quantitative analysis of flavonoids in raw propolis from Northern Croatia 2004; *Acta Pharm* 54:65-72.

[7] Chang C. C., Yang M. H., Wen H. M., Chern J. C. Estimation of total flavonoid content in propolis by two complementary colorimetric methods, *J Food Drug Anal* 2002; 10(3):178-182.

[8] Lima B., Tapia A., Luna L., Fabani M. P., Schmeda-Hirschmann G,, Podio N. S, Wunderlin D. A., Feresin G. E. Main Flavonoids, DPPH Activity, and Metal Content Allow Determination of the Geographical Origin of Propolis from the Province of San Juan (Argentina). *J Agric Food Chem*, 2009; 57(7):2691-2698.

[9] Cvek J., Medic-Saric M., Jasprica. I, Mornar A. High-performance thin-layer chromatographic analysis of the phenolic acid and flavonoid content of Croatian propolis samples. *Anal Chem* 2007; 20(6):429-35.

[10] Valente M. J., Baltazar A. F., Henrique R., Estenìnho L, Carvalho M. Biological activities of Portuguese propolis: Protection against free radical-induced erythrocyte damage and inhibition of human renal cancer cell growth in vitro. *Food Chem Toxicol* 2011; 49:86-92.

[11] Falcao S. I., Vilas-Boas M., Estevinho L. M., Barros C., Domingues M. R. M., Cardoso SM. Phenolic characterization of Northeast Portuguese propolis: usual and unusual compounds. *Anal Bioanal Chem* 2010; 396:887-897.

[12] Miguel M. G., Nunes S., Dandlen S. A., Cavaco A. M., Antunes M. D. Phenols and antioxidant activity of hydro-alcoholic extracts of propolis from Algarve, South of Portugal. *Food Chem Toxicol.* 2010 Dec; 48(12):3418-23.

[13] Moreira L., Dias L. G., Pereira J. A., Estevinho L. Antioxidant properties, total phenols and pollen analysis of propolis samples from Portugal. *Food Chem Toxicol* 2008; 46:3482-3485.

[14] Falcao S., Vilas-Boas M., Freire C., Domingues M. R. M., Cardoso S. M. Characterization of new phenolic derivatives in Portuguese propolis by electrospray mass spectroscopy. *In EuroFoodChem XV - Food for the Future - Proceeding 2.* Copenhaghen p. 64-67, 2009.

[15] Ferreres F., Andrade P., Tomàs-Berbèras F.A. Flavonoids from Portuguese heather honey Z Lebensm Unters Forsch 1994; 1991:32-37.

[16] Fokt H., Pereira A., Ferreira A. M., Cunha A., Aguiar C. *How do bees prevent hive infections*? The antimicrobial properties of propolis in Current Research Technology and Education Topics in Applied Microbiology and Microbial Biotechnology A-Mendez-Vilas, Ed, Formatex, 2010.

[17] Cardoso S. M., Ribeiro M., Ferreira I. L., Falcao S., Vilas-Boas M., Rego A. C. *Northeast Portuguese propolis protects against neurotoxic events in cerebral cortical neurons, in Trends in Natural Products Research*, Ed Leicester, 2010.

[18] Cardoso S. M., Ribeiro M., Ferreira I. L., Rego A. C. Northeast Portuguese propolis protects against staurosporine and hydrogen peroxide-induced neurotoxicity in primary cortical neurons *Food Chem Toxicol* 2011; 49(11):2862-2868.

[19] Moreira L. L., Dias T., Dias L. G., Rogão M., Da Silva J. P., Estevinho L. M. Propolis influence on erythrocyte membrane disorder (hereditary spherocytosis): A first approach. *Food Chem Toxicol* 2011; 49:520-526.

[20] Salatino A., Teixeira E. W., Negri G., Message D. Origin and chemical variations of Brazilian propolis. *eCAM J* 2005; 2(1):33-38.

[21] Silva B. B., Rosalen P. L., Cury J. A., Ikegazi M., Souza V. C., Esteves A., Alencar S.M. Chemical Composition and Botanical Origin of Red Propolis, a New Type of Brazilian Propolis. *eCAM J* 2008; 5(3):313-318.

[22] Daugsch A., Moraes C. S., Fort P., Park Y.K. Brazilian red propolis-chemical composition and botanical origin. *eCAM J* 2008; 5(4):435-441.

[23] Bankova V., Christov R., Kujumgiev A., Marcucci M. C., Popov S. Chemical composition and antibacterial activity of Brazilian propolis Zeitschrift fur Naturforschung. *C. Journal of Biosciences* 1995; 50(3-4):167-72.

[24] Marcucci M. C., Ferreres F., Garcia-Viguera C., Bankova V. S., De Castro S. L., Dantas A. P., Valente P. H. M., Paulino N. Phenolic compounds from Brazilian propolis with pharmacological activities. *J Ethnopharmaco,*. 2001; 74(2):105-112.

[25] Salomao K., Pereira P. R. S., Campo L. C., Borba C. M., Cabello P. H., Marcucci M. C., De Castro S. L. Brazilian propolis. Correlation between chimica composition and antimicrobial activity. *eCAM J* 2008; 5(3):317-324.

[26] Szliszka E., Zydowicz G., Janoszka B., Dobosz C., Kowalczyk-Ziomek G., Krol W. Ethanolic extract of Brazilian green propolis sensitizes prostate cancer cells to TRAIL-induced apoptosis. *Int J Oncol,* 2011 Apr;38(4):941-53.

[27] Bufalo M. C., Candeias J. M. G., Sforcin J. M. In vitro Cytotoxic Effect of Brazilian Green Propolis on Human Laryngeal Epidermoid Carcinoma (HEp-2) Cells. *eCAM J* 2009: 6(4):483-487.

[28] Ahn M. R., Shigenori Kumazawa S., Usui Y., Nakamura J., Matsuka M., Zhu F, Nakayama T. Antioxidant activity and constituents of propolis collected in various areas of China. *Food Chem* 2007; 101(4):1383-1392.

[29] Baumann L. S. Less-known botanical cosmeceuticals. *Dermatol Ther.* 2007 Sep-Oct;20(5):330-42.

[30] Salatino A., Fernanes-Silva C. C., Righi A. A., Salatino M. L. F. Propolis research and the chemistry of plant products, *Nat Prod Rep* 2011; 28:925-936.

[31] Sforcin J. M., Bankova V. Propolis: is there a potential for the development of new drugs? *J Ethnopharmacol* 2011; 133(2):253-60.

[32] Bankova V., Popova M., Bogdanov S., Sabatini A. G. Chemical composition of European propolis: expected and unexpected results. *Z Naturforsch C,* 2002 May-Jun;57(5-6):530-3.

[33] Prytzyk E., Dantas A. P., Salomão K., Pereira A. S., Bankova V. S., De Castro S. L. Aquino Neto FR Flavonoids and trypanocidal activity of Bulgarian propolis, *J Ethnopharmacol* 2003;88:189-193.

[34] Moţ A. C., Soponar F., Sârbu C. Multivariate analysis of reflectance spectra from propolis: geographical variation in Romanian samples. *Talanta.* 2010 May 15;81(3):1010-5.

[35] Marcucci M. C., Ferreres F., Custódio A. R., Ferreira M. M., Bankova V. S., García-Viguera C., Bretz W.A. Evaluation of phenolic compounds in Brazilian propolis from different geographic regions. *Z Naturforsch C.* 2000 Jan-Feb;55(1-2):76-81.

[36] Zhou J., Li Y., Zhao J., Xue X., Wu L., Chen F. Geographical traceability of propolis by high-performance liquid chromatography fingerprints. *Food Chem* 2008; 108:749-59.

[37] Seidel V., Peyfoon E., Watson D. G., Fearnley J. Comparative study of the anti-bacterial activity of propolis from different geographical and climatic zones. *Phytother Res* 2008; 22:1256-1263.

[38] Usia T., Banskota A. H., Tezuka Y., Midorikawa K., Matsushige K., Kadota S. Constituents of Chinese Propolis and Their Antiproliferative Activities. *J Nat Prod* 2002; 65(5):673-676.

[39] Guo X. L., Chen B., Liping L., Zhang X., Dai X. M., Gong S. J. Chemical compositions andantioxidant activities of water extract of Chinese propolis. *J Agric Food Chem.* 2011 Oct 25, in press DOI: 10.1021/jf202818p.
[40] Zhu W., Li Y. H., Chen M. L., Hu F. L. Protective effects of Chinese and Brazilian propolis treatment against hepatorenal lesion in diabetic rats. *Hum Exp Toxicol,* 2011 Sep;30(9):1246-55.
[41] Nakamura R., Nakamura R., Watanabe K., Oka K., Ohta S., Mishima S., Teshima R. Effects of propolis from different areas on mast cell degranulation and identification of the effective components in propolis. *Int Immunopharmacol.* 2010 Sep;10(9):1107-12.
[42] Kim M. J., Kim C. S., Kim B. H., Ro S. B., Lim Y. K., Park S. N., Cho E., Ko J. H., Kwon S. S., Ko Y. M., Kook J. K. Antimicrobial effect of Korean propolis against the mutans streptococci isolated from Korean. *J Microbiol,* 2011 Feb;49(1):161-4.
[43] Bankova V. S., De Castro S. L., Marcucci M. C. Propolis: recent advances in chemistry and plant origin, *Apidologie* 2000; 31:3-15.
[44] Wollenweber E., Buchmann S. L., Feral honey bees in the Sonoran Desert: propolis sources other than poplar (*Populus* spp.), *Z. Naturforsch* 52c (1997) 530–535.
[45] Martos I., Cossentini M., Ferreres M., Barberan-Thomas F. A. Flavonoid composition of Tunisian honeys and propolis. *J agric Food Chem,* 1997; 45(8):2824-2829.
[46] Boudourova-Krasteva G., Bankova V., Sforcin J. M., Nikolova N., Popov S., Phenolics from Brazilian propolis, *Z. Naturforsch,* 52c (1997) 676–679.
[47] Banskota A. H., Tezuka Y., Prasain J. K., Matsushige K., Saiki I., Kadota S. H. Chemical constituents of Brazilian propolis and their cytotoxic activities. *J. Nat. Prod,* 61 (1998) 896–900.
[48] Kumazawa S., Hamasaka T., Nakayama T. Antioxidant activity of propolis of various geographic origins. *Food Chem,* 2004; 84:329-339.
[49] Dudonné S., Poupard P., Coutière P., Woillez M., Richard T., Mérillon J. M., Vitrac X. Phenolic composition and antioxidant properties of poplar bud (Populus nigra) extract: individual antioxidant contribution of phenolics and transcriptional effect on skin aging. *J Agric Food Chem,* 2011 May 11;59(9):4527-36.
[50] Kalogeropoulos N., Konteles S. J., Troullidou E., Mourtzinos I., Karathanos V. T. Chemical composition, anti-oxidant activity and antimicrobial properties of propolis extracts from Greece and Cyprus. *Food Chem* 2009; 116(2):452-461.
[51] Trusheva B., Popova M., Koendhori E. B., Tsvetkova I., Naydenski C., Bankova V. Indonesian propolis: chemical composition, biological activity and botanical origin. *Nat Prod Res,* 2011 Mar;25(6):606-13.
[52] Sawaya A. C., Barbosa da Silva Cunha I., Marcucci M. C. Analytical methods applied to diverse types of Brazilian propolis. *Chem Cent J.* 2011 Jun 1;5(1):27.
[53] Koshechkina A. S., Vlasov A. M., Eller K. I., Kovalenko D. N. [The estimation of biological value and quality of propolis and propolis based food products and food dietary supplements]. *Vopr Pitan.* 2007;76(2):53-6.
[54] Koru O., Toksoy F., Acikel C. H., Tunca Y. M., Baysallar M., Uskudar Guclu A., Akca E., Ozkok Tuylu A., Sorkun K., Tanyuksel M., Salih B. In vitro antimicrobial activity of propolis samples from different geographical origins against certain oral pathogens. *Anaerobe,* 2007 Jun-Aug;13(3-4):140-5.

[55] Uzel A., Sorkun K., Onçağ O., Cogŭlu D., Gençay O., Salih B. Chemical compositions and antimicrobial activities of four different Anatolian propolis samples. *Microbiol Res,* 2005;160(2):189-95.

[56] Popova M., Chen C. N., Chen P. Y., Huang C. Y., Bankova V. A validated spectrophotometric method for quantification of prenylated flavanones in pacific propolis from Taiwan. *Phytochem Anal,* 2010 Mar;21(2):186-91.

[57] Fu S. H., Yang M. H., Wen H. M., Chern J. C. Analysis of Flavonoids in Propolis by Capillary Electrophoresis. *J Food Drug Anal,* 2005; 13(1):43-50.

[58] Barbarić M., Mińković K., Bojić M., Lončar M. B., Smolčić-Bubalo A., Debeljak Z., Medić-Ńarić M. Chemical composition of the ethanolic propolis extracts and its effect on HeLa cells. *J Ethnopharmacol,* 2011 Jun 1;135(3):772-8.

[59] Silva V., Genta G., Möller M. N., Masner M., Thomson L., Romero N., Radi R., Fernandes D. C., Laurindo F. R., Heinzen H., Fierro W., Denicola A. Antioxidant activity of uruguayan propolis. In vitro and cellular assays. *J Agric Food Chem,* 2011 Jun 22;59(12):6430-7.

[60] Piccinelli A. L., Lotti C., Campone L., Cuesta-Rubio O., Campo Fernandez M., Rastrelli L. *Cuban and Brazilian red propolis: botanical origin and comparative analysis by high-performance liquid chromatography-photodiode array etection/electrospray ionization tandem mass spectrometry.*, 2011 Jun 22;59 (12): 6484-91.

[61] Ramanauskiene K., Savickas A., Inkeniene A., Vitkevicius K., Kasparaviciene G., Briedis V., Amsiejus A. Analysis of content of phenolic acids in Lithuanian propolis using high-performance liquid chromatography technique. *Medicina* (Kaunas). 2009;45(9):712-7.

[62] Koo H., Rosalen P. L., Cury J. A., Park Y. K., Ikegaki M., Sattler A. Effect of Apis mellifera propolis from two Brazilian regions on caries development in desalivated rats. *Caries Res,* 1999 Sep-Oct;33(5):393-400.

[63] Kumazawa S., Ahn M. R., Fujimoto T., Kato M. Radical-scavenging activity and phenolic constituents of propolis from different regions of Argentina. *Nat Prod Res,* 2010 May;24(9):804-12.

[64] Ahn M. R., Kumazawa S., Hamasaka T., Bang K. S., Nakayama T. Antioxidant Activity and Constituents of Propolis Collected in Various Areas of Korea, *J agric Food Chem,* 2004; 52(24):7286-7292.

[65] Hernandez J., Goycoolea F. M., Quintero J,. Acosta A., Castañeda M., Dominguez Z., Robles R., Vazquez-Moreno L., Velazquez E.F., Astiazaran H., Lugo E., Velazquez C. Sonoran propolis: chemical composition and antiproliferative activity on cancer cell lines. *Planta Med,* 2007 Nov;73(14):1469-74.

[66] Pellati F., Orlandini G., Pinetti D., Benvenuti S. HPLC-DAD and HPLC-ESI-MS/MS methods for metabolite profiling of propolis extracts. *J Pharm Biomed Anal,* 2011 Jul 15;55(5):934-48.

[67] Duran N., Muz M., Culha G., Duran G., Ozer B. GC-MS analysis and antileishmanial activities of two Turkish propolis types. *Parasitol Res,* 2011 Jan;108(1):95-105.

[68] Popova M. P., Graikou K., Chinou I., Bankova V. S. GC-MS profiling of diterpene compounds in Mediterranean propolis from Greece. J Agric *Food Chem,* 2010 Mar 10;58(5):3167-76.

[69] Sawaya A. C., Tomazela D. M., Cunha I. B., Bankova V. S., Marcucci M. C., Custodio A.R., EberlinMN. Electrospray ionization mass spectrometry fingerprinting of propolis. *Analys*, 2004 Aug;129(8):739-44.

[70] Bertelli D., Papotti G., Bortolotti L., Marcazzan G. L., Plessi M. (1) H-NMR Simultaneous Identification of Health-Relevant Compounds in Propolis Extracts. *Phytochem Anal,* 2011, *in press* Aug 18. DOI: 10.1002/pca.1352.

[71] Vera N., Solorzano E., Ordoñez R., Maldonado L., Bedascarrasbure E., Isla M.I. Chemical composition of Argentinean propolis collected in extreme regions and its relation with antimicrobial and antioxidant activities. *Nat Prod Commun*, 2011 Jun;6(6):823-7.

[72] Maróstica Junior M. R., Daugsch A., Silveira Moraes C. S., Queiroga C.L., Pastore G.M., Parki Y.K. Comparison of volatile and polyphenolic compounds in Brazilian green propolis and its botanical origin *Baccharis dracunculifolia,Ciênc Tecnol Aliment* 2008; 28(1):178-181.

[73] Bankova V. S., Popov S. S., Marekov N. L. A study of flavonoids of propolis, *J Nat Prod* 1983; 46(4):471-474.

[74] Said S. A., Khan S. A., Ahmad I., Ali H. S. Chemical composition of Egyptian and UAE propolis. *Pak J Pharm Sci* 2006; 19(1):58-61.

[75] Abd El Hady F. K. and Hegazi A. G. Egyptian propolis: 2. Chemical composition, antiviral and antimicrobial activities of East Nile Delta propolis, *Z. Naturforsch.*, 2002; 57c: 386-394.

[76] Pápay V., Soltész M., Csizmadia B., Tóth L. [Chemical and pharmacological study of propolis samples from various locations]. *Acta Pharm Hung.,* 1987 Jul;57(3-4):143-51.

[77] Abd El Hady F. K. and Hegazi A. G. Egyptian propolis: 2. Chemical composition, antiviral and antimicrobial activities of East Nile Delta propolis, *Z. Naturforsch.*, 2002; 57c: 386-394.

[78] Pereira A. S., Norsell M., Cardoso J. N., Aquino Neto F. R., Ramos M. F. Rapid screening of polar compounds in Brazilian propolis by high-temperature high-resolution gas chromatography-mass spectrometry. *J Agric Food Chem.* 2000 Nov;48(11):5226-30.

[79] Hegazi A. G., Abd El Hady F. K., Abd Allah F. A. Chemical composition and antimicrobial activity of European propolis. *Z Naturforsch C.* 2000 Jan-Feb;55(1-2):70-5.

[80] Velikova M., Bankova V., Sorkun K., Houcine S., Tsvetkova I., Kujumgiev A. Propolis from the Mediterranean region: chemical composition and antimicrobial activity. *Z Naturforsch C.* 2000 Sep-Oct;55(9-10):790-3.

[81] Hegazi A. G., Abd El Hady F. K., Abd Allah F. A. Chemical composition and antimicrobial activity of European propolis. *Z Naturforsch C.* 2000 Jan-Feb;55(1-2):70-5.

[82] Hegazi A. G., Abd El Hady F. K. Egyptian propolis: 3. Antioxidant, antimicrobial activities and chemical composition of propolis from reclaimed lands. *Z Naturforsch C.* 2002 Mar-Apr;57(3-4):395-402.

[83] Keskin N., Hazir S., Baser K. H., Kürkçüoglu M. Antibacterial activity and chemical composition of Turkish propolis. *Z Naturforsch C.* 2001 Nov-Dec;56(11-12):1112-5.

[84] Rhajaoui M., Oumzil H., Faid M., Lyagoubi M., Elyachioui M. Antibacterial activity of a moroccan propolis extracts. *Science Letters* 2001; 3(3): 201-207.

[85] Sorkun K., Süer B., Salih B. Determination of chemical composition of Turkish propolis. *Z Naturforsch C.* 2001 Jul-Aug;56(7-8):666-8. 514.

[86] Melliou E., Chinou I. Chemical analysis and antimicrobial activity of Greek propolis. *Planta Med.* 2004 Jun;70(6):515-9.

[87] Salomão K., Dantas A. P., Borba C. M., Campos L. C., Machado D. G., Aquino Neto F. R., de Castro S. L. Chemical composition and microbicidal activity of extracts from Brazilian and Bulgarian propolis. *Lett Appl Microbiol.* 2004;38(2):87-92.

[88] Popova M., Silici S., Kaftanoglu O., Bankova V. Antibacterial activity of Turkish propolis and its qualitative and quantitative chemical composition. *Phytomedicine.* 2005 Mar;12(3):221-8.

[89] Nunes C. A., Guerreiro M. C. Characterization of Brazilian green propolis throughout the seasons by headspace GC/MS and ESI-MS. *J Sci Food Agric.*, 2011, *in press* DOI:: 10.1002/jsfa.4596.

[90] Otoguro K., Iwatsuki M., Ishiyama A., Namatame M., Nishihara-Tsukashima A., Kiyohara H., Hashimoto T., Asakawa Y., Omura S., Yamada H. In vitro antitrypanosomal activity of some phenolic compounds from propolis and lactones from Fijian Kawa (Piper methysticum). *J Nat Med.* 2011, *in press* DOI: 10.1007/s11418-011-0613-z.

[91] Cheung K. W., Sze D. M., Chan W. K., Deng R. X., Tu W., Chan G. C. Brazilian green propolis and its constituent, Artepillin C inhibits allogeneic activated human CD4 T cells expansion and activation. *J Ethnopharmacol.* 2011 Nov 18;138(2):463-71.

[92] Inouye S., Takahashi M., Abe S. Composition, antifungal and radical scavenging activities of 4 propolis. *Med Mycol J.* 2011;52(4):305-13.

[93] Montoro A., Soriano J. M., Barquinero J. F., Almonacid M., Montoro A., Verdú G., Sahuquillo V., Villaescusa J.I., Sebastià N. Assessment in vitro of cytogenetic and genotoxic effects of propolis on human lymphocytes. *Food Chem Toxicol.* 2011, *in press* DOI: 10.1016/j.fct.2011.10.053.

[94] Aliyazicioglu Y., Demir S., Turan I., Cakiroglu T.N., Akalin I., Deger O., Bedir A. Preventive and protective effects of turkish propolis on H2O2-induced DNA damage in foreskin fibroblast cell lines. *Acta Biol Hung*, 2011 Dec;62(4):388-96.

[95] Gjertsen A. W., Stothz K. A., Neiva K. G, Pileggi R. Effect of propolis on proliferation and apoptosis of periodontal ligament fibroblasts. Oral *Surg Oral Med Oral Pathol Oral Radiol Endod.*, 2011 Dec;112(6):843-8.

[96] Motallebnejad M., Ghassemi L., Zabihi E., Moslemi D., Seyedmajidi M., Moghadamnia A. A. Dose-dependent profile of ethanolic extracts of Iranian propolis on radiation-induced mucositis in rats. *Saudi Med J.* 2011 Nov;32(11):1196-8.

[97] Cigut T., Polak T., Gašperlin L., Raspor P., Jamnik P. Antioxidative activity of propolis extract in yeast cells. *J Agric Food Chem,* 2011 Nov 9;59(21):11449-55.

[98] Li F., He Y. M., Awale S., Kadota S., Tezuka Y. Two new cytotoxic phenylallylflavanones from Mexican propolis. *Chem Pharm Bull* (Tokyo). 2011;59(9):1194-6.

[99] Wu N., Kong Y., Zu Y., Fu Y., Liu Z., Meng R., Liu X., Efferth T. Activity investigation of pinostrobin towards herpes simplex virus-1 as determined by atomic force microscopy. *Phytomedicine* 2011; 18(2-3):110-118.

[100] Amoros M., Simões C. M., Girre L., Sauvager F., Cormier M. Synergistic effect of flavones and flavonols against herpes simplex virus type 1 in cell culture. Comparison with the antiviral activity of propolis. *J Nat Prod.* 1992 Dec;55(12):1732-40.

[101] Bosio K., Avanzini C., D'Avolio A., Ozino O., Savoia D. In vitro activity of propolis against Streptococcus piogene, *Lett Appl Microbiol* 2000; 31:174-177.

[102] Shin E. K., Kwon H. S., Kim Y. H., Shin H. K., Kim J. K. Chrysin, a natural flavone, improves murine inflammatory bowel diseases. *Biochem Biophys Res Commun,* 2009 Apr 17;381(4):502-7.

[103] Nam N. H. Naturally occurring NF-kappaB inhibitors. *Mini Rev Med Chem,* 2006 Aug;6(8):945-51.

[104] Sforcin J. M. Propolis and the immune system: a review. *J Ethnopharmacol.* 2007 Aug 15;113(1):1-14.

[105] Ciftci O., Ozdemir I., Aydin M., Beytur A. Beneficial effects of chrysin on the reproductive system of adult male rats. *Andrologia,* 2011, *in press.* DOI: 10.1111/j.1439-0272.2010.01127.x.

[106] Jana K., Yin X., Schiffer R. B., Chen J. J., Pandey A. K., Stocco D. M., Grammas P., Wang X. Chrysin, a natural flavonoid enhances steroidogenesis and steroidogenic acute regulatory protein gene expression in mouse Leydig cells. *J Endocrinol.,* 2008 May;197(2):315-23.

[107] Cherkaoui-Tangi K., Lachkar M., Wibo M., Morel N., Gilani A. H., Lyoussi B. Pharmacological studies on hypotensive, diuretic and vasodilator activities of chrysin glucoside from Calycotome villosa in rats. *Phytother Res.,* 2008 Mar; 22(3):356-61.

[108] Sathiavelu J., Senapathy G. J., Devaraj R., Namasivayam N. Hepatoprotective effect of chrysin on prooxidant-antioxidant status during ethanol-induced toxicity in female albino rats. *J Pharm Pharmacol,* 2009 Jun;61(6):809-17.

[109] Brown E., Hurd N. S., McCall S., Ceremuga T. E. Evaluation of the anxiolytic effects of chrysin, a Passiflora incarnata extract, in the laboratory rat. *AANA J.* 2007 Oct;75(5):333-7.

[110] Zhai K., Hu L., Chen J., Fu C. Y., Chen Q. Chrysin induces hyperalgesia via the GABAA receptor in mice. *Planta Med,* 2008 Aug;74(10):1229-34.

[111] Ha S. K., Moon E., Kim S. Y. Chrysin suppresses LPS-stimulated proinflammatory responses by blocking NF-κB and JNK activations in microglia cells. *Neurosci Lett.* 2010 Nov 26;485(3):143-7.

[112] Gresa-Arribas N., Serratosa J., Saura J., Solà C. Inhibition of CCAAT/enhancer binding protein δ expression by chrysin in microglial cells results in anti-inflammatory and neuroprotective effects. *J Neurochem.,* 2010 Oct;115(2):526-36.

[113] Beaumont D. M., Mark T. M. Jr, Hills R., Dixon P., Veit B., Garrett N. The effects of chrysin, a Passiflora incarnata extract, on natural killer cell activity in male Sprague-Dawley rats undergoing abdominal surgery. *AANA J.* 2008 Apr;76(2):113-7.

[114] Pichichero E., Cicconi R., Mattei M., Muzi M. G., Canini A. Acacia honey and chrysin reduce proliferation of melanoma cells through alterations in cell cycle progression. *Int J Oncol.,* 2010 Oct;37(4):973-81.

[115] Khan M. S., Halagowder D., Devaraj S. N. Methylated chrysin induces co-ordinated attenuation of the canonical Wnt and NF-kB signaling pathway and upregulates apoptotic gene expression in the early hepatocarcinogenesis rat model. *Chem Biol Interact.* 2011 Aug 15;193(1):12-21.

[116] Li X., Wang J. N., Huang J. M., Xiong X. K., Chen M. F., Ong C. N., Shen H. M, Yang X. F. Chrysin promotes tumor necrosis factor (TNF)-related apoptosis-inducing ligand (TRAIL) induced apoptosis in human cancer cell lines. *Toxicol In Vitro,* 2011 Apr;25(3):630-5.

[117] Wang J., Qiu J., Dong J., Li H., Luo M., Dai X., Zhang Y., Leng B., Niu X., Zhao S., Deng X. Chrysin protects mice from Staphylococcus aureus pneumonia. *J Appl Microbiol.*, 2011 Oct 4, *in press*, DOI: 10.1111/j.1365-2672.2011.05170.x.

[118] Lv P. C., Cai T. T., Qian Y., Sun J., Zhu H. L. Synthesis, biological evaluation of chrysin derivatives as potential immunosuppressive agents. *Eur J Med Chem.* 2011 Jan;46(1):393-8.

[119] Zou X. Q., Peng S. M., Hu C. P., Tan L. F., Yuan Q., Deng H. W., Li Y. J. Synthesis, characterization and vasculoprotective effects of nitric oxide-donating derivatives of chrysin. *Bioorg Med Chem.* 2010 May 1;18(9):3020-5.

[120] Lim H., Jin J. H., Park H., Kim H. P. New synthetic anti-inflammatory chrysin analog, 5,7-dihydroxy-8-(pyridine-4yl)flavone. *Eur J Pharmacol.* 2011 Sep 21, *in press* DOI: 10.1016/j.ejphar.2011.09.010.

[121] Che H., Lim H., Kim H. P., Park H. A chrysin analog exhibited strong inhibitory activities against both PGE2 and NO production. *Eur J Med Chem.* 2011 Sep;46(9):4657-60.

[122] Khan M. S., Devaraj H., Devaraj N. Chrysin abrogates early hepatocarcinogenesis and induces apoptosis in N-nitrosodiethylamine-induced preneoplastic nodules in rats. *Toxicol Appl Pharmacol.* 2011 Feb 15;251(1):85-94.

[123] Wu N. L., Fang J. Y., Chen M., Wu C. J., Huang C. C., Hung C. F. Chrysin protects epidermal keratinocytes from UVA- and UVB-induced damage. *J Agric Food Chem.* 2011 Aug 10;59(15):8391-400.

[124] Kim D. C., Rho S. H., Shin J. C., Park H. H., Kim D. Inhibition of melanogenesis by 5,7-dihydroxyflavone (chrysin) via blocking adenylyl cyclase activity. *Biochem Biophys Res Commun.* 2011 Jul 22;411(1):121-5.

[125] Phan T., Yu X. M., Kunnimalaiyaan M., Chen H. Antiproliferative effect of chrysin on anaplastic thyroid cancer. *J Surg Res.* 2011 Sep;170(1):84-8. Epub 2011 Apr 20.

[126] Pichichero E., Cicconi R., Mattei M., Canini A. Chrysin-induced apoptosis is mediated through p38 and Bax activation in B16-F1 and A375 melanoma cells. *Int J Oncol.* 2011 Feb;38(2):473-83.

[127] Hong T. B., Rahumatullah A., Yogarajah T., Ahmad M., Yin K. B. Potential effects of chrysin on MDA-MB-231 cells. *Int J Mol Sci.* 2010 Mar 11;11(3):1057-69.

[128] Khoo B. Y., Chua S. L., Balaram P. Apoptotic effects of chrysin in human cancer cell lines. *Int J Mol Sci.* 2010 May 19;11(5):2188-99.

[129] Schumacher M., Hautzinger A., Rossmann A., Holzhauser S., Popovic D., Hertrampf A., Kuntz S., Boll M., Wenzel U. Chrysin blocks topotecan-induced apoptosis in Caco-2 cells in spite of inhibition of ABC-transporters. *Biochem Pharmacol.* 2010 Aug 15;80(4):471-9.

[130] Lin C. M., Shyu K. G., Wang B. W., Chang H., Chen Y. H., Chiu J. H. Chrysin suppresses IL-6-induced angiogenesis via down-regulation of JAK1/STAT3 and VEGF: an in vitro and in ovo approach. *J Agric Food Chem.* 2010 Jun 9;58(11):7082-7.

[131] Zheng X., Zhao F. F., Liu Y. M., Yao X., Zheng Z. T., Luo X., Liao D. F. Synthesis and preliminary biological evaluation of chrysin derivatives as potential anticancer drugs. *Med Chem.* 2010 Jan;6(1):6-8.

[132] Wu Y. X., Fang X. Apigenin, chrysin, and luteolin selectively inhibit chymotrypsin-like and trypsin-like proteasome catalytic activities in tumor cells. *Planta Med.* 2010 Feb;76(2):128-32.

[133] Sun X., Huo X., Luo T., Li M., Yin Y., Jiang Y. The anticancer flavonoid chrysin induces the unfolded protein response in hepatoma cells. *J Cell Mol Med.* 2011 Nov;15(11):2389-98.

[134] Bae Y., Lee S., Kim S. H. Chrysin suppresses mast cell-mediated allergic inflammation: involvement of calcium, caspase-1 and nuclear factor-κB. *Toxicol Appl Pharmacol.* 2011 Jul 1;254(1):56-64.

[135] Wadibhasme P. G., Ghaisas M. M., Thakurdesai P. A. Anti-asthmatic potential of chrysin on ovalbumin-induced bronchoalveolar hyperresponsiveness in rats. *Pharm Biol.* 2011 May;49(5):508-15.

[136] Tahir M., Sultana S. Chrysin modulates ethanol metabolism in Wistar rats: a promising role against organ toxicities. *Alcohol.* 2011 Jul-Aug;46(4):383-92.

[137] Ciftci O., Vardi N., Ozdemir I. Effects of quercetin and chrysin on 2,3,7,8-tetrachlorodibenzo-p-dioxin induced hepatotoxicity in rats. *Environ Toxicol.* 2011, in press DOI: 10.1002/tox.20707.

[138] Ciftci O., Ozdemir I. Protective effects of quercetin and chrysin against 2,3,7,8-tetrachlorodibenzo-p-dioxin (TCDD) induced oxidative stress, body wasting and altered cytokine productions in rats. *Immunopharmacol Immunotoxicol.* 2011 Sep;33(3):504-8.

[139] Anand K. V., Anandhi R., Pakkiyaraj M., Geraldine P. Protective effect of chrysin on carbon tetrachloride (CCl4)--induced tissue injury in male Wistar rats. *Toxicol Ind Health.* 2011 Nov;27(10):923-33.

[140] Pushpavalli G., Veeramani C., Pugalendi K. V. Influence of chrysin on hepatic marker enzymes and lipid profile against D-galactosamine-induced hepatotoxicity rats. *Food Chem Toxicol.* 2010 Jun;48(6):1654-9.

[141] Selvaraj S., Krishnaswamy S., Devashya V., Sethuraman S., Krishnan U.M. Investigations on membrane perturbation by chrysin and its copper complex using self-assembled lipid bilayers. *Langmuir.* 2011 Nov 1;27(21):13374-82.

[142] Brechbuhl H. M., Kachadourian R., Min E., Chan D., Day B.J. *Chrysin enhances doxorubicin-induced cytotoxicity in human lung epithelial cancer cell lines: The role of glutathione.* Toxicol Appl Pharmacol. 2011, in press.

[143] Kawase A., Matsumoto Y., Hadano M., Ishii Y., Iwaki M. Differential effects of chrysin on nitrofurantoin pharmacokinetics mediated by intestinal breast cancer resistance protein in rats and mice. *J Pharm Pharm Sci.* 2009;12(2):150-63.

[144] Xie Z. H., Quan M. F., Liu F., Cao J. G., Zhang J. S. 5-allyl-7-gen-difluoromethoxychrysin enhances TRAIL-induced apoptosis in human lung carcinoma A549 cells. *BMC Cancer.* 2011 Jul 29;11:322.

[145] Xiao G., Tang X., Yao C., Wang C. Potentiation of arsenic trioxide-induced apoptosis by 8-bromo-7-methoxychrysin in human leukemia cells involves depletion of intracellular reduced glutathione. *Acta Biochim Biophys Sin* (Shanghai). 2011 Sep;43(9):712-21.

[146] Samarghandian S., Afshari J. T., Davoodi S. Chrysin reduces proliferation and induces apoptosis in the human prostate cancer cell line pc-3. *Clinics* (Sao Paulo). 2011;66(6):1073-9.

[147] Lo H. M., Wu M. W., Pan S. L., Peng C. Y., Wu P. H., Wu W. B. Chrysin restores PDGF-induced inhibition on protein tyrosine phosphatase and reduces PDGF signaling in cultured VSMCs. *J Nutr Biochem.* 2011, *in press.*

[148] Guo A. J. Y., Xie H. Q., Roy C. Y., Zheng K. Y. Z., Bi C. W. C., Xu S. L., Dong T. T. X., Tsim K. W. K. Galangin, a flavonol derived fromRhizoma Alpiniae Officinarum, inhibits acetylcholinesterase activity *in vitro Chem-Biol Interact* 2010: 187(1-3):246-248.

[149] Chen C. C., Huang C. Y. Inhibition of Klebsiella pneumoniae DnaB helicase by the flavonol galangin. *Protein J.* 2011 Jan;30(1):59-65.

[150] Eumkeb G., Sakdarat S., Siriwong S. Reversing β-lactam antibiotic resistance of Staphylococcus aureus with galangin from Alpinia officinarum Hance and synergism with ceftazidime. *Phytomedicine.* 2010 Dec 15;18(1):40-5.

[151] Campana R., Patrone V., Franzini I. T., Diamantini G., Vittoria E., Baffone W. Antimicrobial activity of two propolis samples against human Campylobacter jejuni. *J Med Food.* 2009 Oct;12(5):1050-6.

[152] Borrelli F., Maffia P., Pinto L., Ianaro A., Russo A., Capasso F., Ialenti A. Phytochemical compounds involved in the antiinflammatory effect of propolis extract. *Fitoterapia* 2002; 73(1):S53-S63.

[153] Russo A., Longo R., Vanella A. Anti-oxidant activity of propolis: role of caffeic acid phenetyl ester and galangin. *Fitoterapia* 2002; 73(1):S21-S29.

[154] Sivakumar A.S., Anuradha C. V. *Effect of galangin supplementation on oxidative damage and inflammatory changes in fructose-fed rat liver.* Chem Biol Interact. 2011, in press DOI: 10.1016/j.cbi.2011.06.003.

[155] Sivakumar A. S., Viswanathan P., Anuradha C. V. Dose-dependent effect of galangin on fructose-mediated insulin resistance and oxidative events in rat kidney. *Redox Rep.* 2010;15(5):224-32.

[156] Zhang H. T., Luo H., Wu J., Lan L. B., Fan D. H., Zhu K. D., Chen X. Y., Wen M., Liu H.M. Galangin induces apoptosis of hepatocellular carcinoma cells via the mitochondrial pathway. *World J Gastroenterol.* 2010 Jul 21;16(27):3377-84.

[157] Kanazawa K., Kawasaki H., Samejima K., Ashida H., Danno G. Specific Desmutagens (Antimutagens) in Oregano against a Dietary Carcinogen, Trp-P-2, Are Galangin and Quercetin. *J. Agric. Food Chem* 1995;43 (2): 404–409.

[158] Heo M. Y., Sohn S. J., Au W. W. Anti-genotoxicity of galangin as a cancer chemopreventive agent candidate. *Mut Res Rev* 2001:488(2):135-150.

[159] Tolomeo M., Grimaudo S., Di Cristina A., Pipitone R. M., Dusonchet L., Meli M., Crosta L., Gebbia N., Invidiata F. P., Titone L., Simoni D. Galangin increases the cytotoxic activity of imatinib-mesylate in imatinib-sensitive and imatinib-resistant Bxr-Abl expressing leukemia cells, *Can Lett* 2008; 265(2):289-297.

[160] Pietta P. G., Gardana C., Pietta A. M. Analytical methods for quality control of propolis. *Fitoterapia* 2002; 73(1):S7-S20.

[161] Ciolino H. P., Ye G. C. The flavonoid galangin is an inhibitor of CYP1A1 activity and an agonist/antagonist of the aryl hydrocarbon receptor, *Br J Cancer* 1999; 79(9-10):1340-46.

[162] Otake Y. and Walle T. Oxidation of the flavonoid galangin and kaempferide by human liver microsomes and CYP1A1, CYP1A2 and CYP2C9. *Drug Metabolism Dispos* 2002; 30(2):103-105.

[163] Hamada M., Satsu H., Ashida H., Konishi Y. S., Shimizu M. Metabolites of Galangin by 2,3,7,8-Tetrachlorodibenzo-*p*-dioxin-Inducible Cytochrome P450 1A1 in Human Intestinal Epithelial Caco-2 Cells and Their Antagonistic Activity toward Aryl Hydrocarbon Receptor. *J Agric Food Chem* 2010; 58(13):8111-8118.

[164] Gwak J., Oh J., Cho M., Bae S. K., Song I. S., Liu K. H., Jeong Y., Kim D. E., Chung Y. H. and Oh S. Galangin Suppresses the Proliferation of β-Catenin Response Transcription-Positive Cancer Cells by Promoting Adenomatous Polyposis Coli/Axin/Glycogen Synthase Kinase-3β-Independent β-Catenin Degradation, *Mol Pharmacol* 2011; 79(6):1014-1022.

[165] Gao M., Zhu S. Y., Tan C. B., Xu B., Zhang W. C., Du G. H. Pinocembrin protects the neurovascular unit by reducing inflammation and extracellular proteolysis in MCAO rats. *J Asian Nat Prod Res* 2010; 12(5):407-418.

[166] Meng F., Liu R., Gao M., Wang Y., Yu X., Xuan Z., Sun J., Yang F., Wu C., Du G. Pinocembrin attenuates blood–brain barrier injury induced by global cerebral ischemia–reperfusion in rats. *Brain Res* 2011; 1391:93-101.

[167] Guang H. M., Du G. H. Protection of pinocembrin on brain mithocondria contribute to cognitive improvement in chronic cerebral hypoperfused rats, *Eur J Pharmacol* 2006; 542(1-3):77-83.

[168] Gao M., Liu R., Zhu S. Y., Du G. H. Acute neurovascular unit protective action of pinocembrin against permanent cerebral ischemia in rats. *Journal of Asian Natural Products Research* 2008; 10(6): 551-558.

[169] Shi L. L., Chen B. N., Gao M., Zhang H. A., Li Y. J., Wang L., Du G. H. The characteristics of therapeutic effect of pinocembrin in transient global brain ischemia/reperfusion rats. *Life Sci.* 2011 Mar 14;88(11-12):521-8.

[170] Gao M., Zhang W. C., Liu Q. S., Hu J. J., Liu G. T., Du G. H. Pinocembrin prevents glutamate-induced apoptosis in SH-SY5Y neuronal cells via decrease of bax/bcl-2 ratio. *Eur J Pharmacol.* 2008 Sep 4;591(1-3):73-9.

[171] Liu R., Gao M., Yang Z. H., Du G. H. Pinocembrin protects rat brain against oxidation and apoptosis induced by ischemia-reperfusion both in vivo and in vitro. *Brain Res.* 2008 Jun 24;1216:104-15.

[172] Izuta H., Shimazawa M., Tazawa S., Araki Y., Mishima S., Hara H. Protective effects of Chinese propolis and its component, chrysin, against neuronal cell death via inhibition of mitochondrial apoptosis pathway in SH-SY5Y cells. *J Agric Food Chem.* 2008 Oct 8;56(19):8944-53.

[173] Liu R., Zhang L., Lan X., Li L., Zhang T. T., Sun J. H., Du G. H. Protection by borneol on cortical neurons against oxygen-glucose deprivation/reperfusion: involvement of anti-oxidation and anti-inflammation through nuclear transcription factor kappa-B signaling pathway. *Neuroscience* 2011; 176:408-411.

[174] Chen C. S., Wu C. H., Lai Y. C., Lee W. S., Chene H. M, Chene R. J., Chend L. C., Hoc Y.S., Ying-Jan Wang Y.J. NF-κB-activated tissue transglutaminase is involved in ethanol-induced hepatic injury and the possible role of propolis in preventing fibrogenesis. *Toxicology* 2008;246:148-157.

[175] Farooqui T., Farooqui A. A. Beneficial effects of propolis on human health and neurological diseases, *Front Biosci* 2012, E4.779-793.

[176] Punvittayagul C., Wongpoomchai R., Taya S., Pompimon W. Effect of pinocembrin isolated from Boesenbergia pandurata on xenobiotic-metabolizing enzymes in rat liver. *Drug Metab Lett.* 2011 Jan;5(1):1-5.

[177] Pan L., Matthew S., Lantvit D. D., Zhang X., Ninh T. N., Chai H., Carcache de Blanco E. J., Soejarto D. D., Swanson S. M., Kinghorn A. D. Bioassay-Guided Isolation of Constituents of Piper sarmentosum Using a Mitochondrial Transmembrane Potential Assay. *J Nat Prod.* 2011 Oct 28;74(10):2193-9.

[178] Villanueva V. R., Barbier M., Gonnet M., Lavie P. [The flavonoid of propolis, isolation of a new bacteriostatic substance: pinocembrin (dihydroxy-5,7-flavanone)] *Ann Inst Past* (Paris) 1970; 118(1):84-7.

[179] Castaldo S., Capasso F. Propolis, an old remedy used in modern medicine. *Fitoterapia.*, 2002 Nov;73 Suppl 1:S1-6.

[180] Ruddock P. S., Charland M., Ramirez S., López A., Neil Towers G. H., Arnason J. T., Liao M., Dillon J. A. Antimicrobial activity of flavonoids from Piper lanceaefolium and other Colombian medicinal plants against antibiotic susceptible and resistant strains of Neisseria gonorrhoeae. *Sex Transm Dis.* 2011 Feb;38(2):82-8.

[181] Chou T. H., Chen J. J., Peng C. F., Cheng M. J., Chen I. S. New Flavanones from the Leaves of Cryptocarya chinensis and Their Antituberculosis Activity. *Chem Biodivers.* 2011 Nov;8(11):2015-24.

[182] Lee M. Y., Seo C. S., Lee J. A., Shin I. S., Kim S. J., Ha H., Shin H. K. Alpinia katsumadai H(AYATA) *Seed Extract Inhibit LPS-Induced Inflammation by Induction of Heme Oxygenase*-1 in RAW264.7 Cells. Inflammation. 2011, in press.

[183] Takahashi A., Yamamoto N., Murakami A. Cardamonin suppresses nitric oxide production via blocking the IFN-γ/STAT pathway in endotoxin-challenged peritoneal macrophages of ICR mice. *Life Sci.* 2011 Aug 29;89(9-10):337-42.

[184] Bajgai S. P., Prachyawarakorn V., Mahidol C., Ruchirawat S., Kittakoop P. Hybrid flavan-chalcones, aromatase and lipoxygenase inhibitors, from Desmos cochinchinensis. *Phytochemistry,* 2011 Nov;72(16):2062-7. Epub 2011 Jul 28.

[185] Mapunya M. B., Hussein A. A., Rodriguez B., Lall N. Tyrosinase activity of Greyia flanaganii (Bolus) constituents. *Phytomedicine,* 2011 Aug 15;18(11):1006-12.

In: Beneficial Effects of Propolis on Human Health ... ISBN: 978-1- 62081-440-6
Editors: Tahira Farooqui and Akhlaq A. Farooqui 

*Chapter 5*

# CAN PROPOLIS AFFECT IMMUNITY?

***José Maurício Sforcin[*] and Bruno José Conti***
Biosciences Institute, UNESP, Botucatu, SP, Brazil

## ABSTRACT

Authors from different parts of the world have demonstrated the therapeutic properties of propolis. Our group has focused on the immunomodulatory action of propolis, and different approaches have been carried out *in vitro* and *in vivo* in order to understand its mechanism of action. Results from our laboratory and from others researchers have pointed the potential of propolis for the development of immunomodulators, but there is still a lack of clinical research on the effects of propolis. Articles should include propolis chemical composition in order to compare the results from different authors, and biological assays should include well-established positive or negative controls. Since propolis modulates the immune response, we pose a question in this chapter: can propolis affect immunity in humans and animals so that the pharmaceutical industry may create new immunomodulators? Herein we discussed propolis influence on the immune system, the problem of propolis standardization, concentration, intake period, its pro- or anti-inflammatory activity, its association with vaccines and new insights in this research field.

**Keywords:** Propolis, immune system

## HISTORICAL PERSPECTIVE

People most commonly think of plants when talking about natural products, but bee products are also included in “natural products”, providing excellent sources of material as the basis of new therapeutic agents.

---

[*] Correspondence concerning this article should be addressed to: José Maurício Sforcin, PhD, Department of Microbiology and Immunology, Biosciences Institute, UNESP, 18618-000, Botucatu, SP, Brazil. sforcin@ibb.unesp.br; Telephone: +55 14 3811-6058; Fax: +55 14 3811-6058236.

Bees produce propolis from secretions of trees, flowers, leaves and pollen, adding wax and substances secreted by their glands [1]. Propolis has been used for medicinal purposes since antiquity, due its remarkable therapeutic qualities [2]. In some countries, propolis is used for the treatment of a wide range of human ailments, such as cardiovascular and blood systems disorder (anemia), respiratory apparatus (for various infections), dental care [3], dermatology (tissue regeneration, ulcers, healing of burn wounds, mycosis, mucous membrane infections and lesions), cancer treatment [4-6], immune system support and improvement [7], digestive tract disorders (ulcers and infections), liver protection, and many others. The large number of chemical components in propolis may justify its several biological activities.

In temperate zones all over the world, poplar bud exudates (mainly *Populus nigra* L.) have been shown to be the main source of propolis. On the other hand, propolis primarily contains pollen from *Clusia* species in Cuba [8], while *Baccharis dracunculifolia* DC. was found to be the main source of propolis in Brazil [9, 10].

A significant number of papers dealing with propolis chemistry have been published and researchers realized that its chemical composition is highly variable, depending on the local flora [11, 12]. Some studies have revealed the chemical variability among propolis samples and the existence of different chemical types of propolis according to plant sources.

Pharmacological variability among propolis samples is expected, and although propolis composition is determined mainly by the phytogeographic characteristics, it is not possible to systematically compare the studies with propolis sample. Thus, propolis biological properties should be linked to its chemical composition and botanical sources, and a universal standardization still remains impossible [13, 14].

*Baccharis dracunculifolia* DC. is the main vegetal source of our propolis sample in Botucatu, São Paulo State, Brazil, followed by *Eucalyptus citriodora* Hook and *Araucaria angustifolia* (Bert.) O. Kuntze [15]. Our propolis sample, collected in the Beekeeping Section of the University, was analyzed by gas-chromatography, gas-chromatography-mass spectrometry and thin layer chromatography, revealing that its main components are phenolic compounds (flavonoids, aromatic acids, benzopyranes), di- and triterpenes, essential oils, among others.

The main constituents of our propolis sample were isolated and identified: flavonoids are present in small quantities in Brazilian propolis (kaempferid, 5,6,7-trihydroxy-3,4'-dimethoxyflavone, aromadendrine-4'-methyl ether); a prenylated *p*-coumaric acid and two benzopyranes: *E* and *Z* 2,2-dimethyl-6-carboxyethenyl-8-prenyl-2H-benzopyranes); essential oils (spathulenol, (2Z,6E)-farnesol, benzyl benzoate and prenylated acetophenones); aromatic acids (dihydrocinnamic acid, *p*-coumaric acid, ferulic acid, caffeic acid, which are common for poplar propolis, 3,5-diprenyl-*p*-coumaric acid, 2,2-dimethyl-6-carboxy-ethenyl-8-prenyl-2H-1-benzo-pyran); di- and triterpenes, among others. Seasonal variations in propolis composition are not significant and are predominantly quantitative [16-18].

Although there are few works dealing with propolis consumption for a long-term, it is possible to hypothesize that its complex composition may lead to damage in the organism [19]. Nevertheless, propolis seems to be safe to humans [1], and no side effects were related after propolis administration to rats [19-21].

Our group has focused on the immunomodulatory action of propolis, and different approaches have been carried out *in vitro* and *in vivo* in order to understand its mechanism of action. However, before the problem of propolis standardization, the greatest problem to carry out the immunological assays was to design the experimental protocols, since researchers have used different concentrations of propolis *in vivo* and *in vitro*, as well as different extracts, intake period and routes of administration [22]. Moreover, biological assays should include well-established positive or negative controls, in order to compare propolis efficiency with stimulatory or inhibitory parameters, respectively.

## PROPOLIS EFFECTS ON INNATE IMMUNITY

Immunity comprises different mechanisms aiming to protect the body from all sorts of diseases. The immune system comprises a network of cells, lymphoid organs and tissues, as well as chemicals that fight against antigens. Immunity can be didactically divided into innate or nonspecific immunity and adaptive or specific immunity. The innate immunity is a primary defense mechanism against invading pathogens, whereas the adaptive or acquired immunity acts as a second line of defense and is specific to the pathogen, taking several days to build up. The acquired immune response also involves the development of immunological memory, a state in which the immune system can quickly mount a response to an infectious agent that was faced before.

Innate immune response is not specific to the pathogen to which the system is responding, and it happens almost immediately when an infectious agent invades the body. Innate immunity includes physical and chemical barriers and phagocytic cells.

Some cells are collectively called “antigen presenting cells” (APC), since they are able to present different sets of antigens to activate T cells. APCs are specialized white blood cells that help fight off foreign antigens that enter the body such as different bacteria, virus or toxins. First, the APC engulfs the antigen quickly during a process called phagocytosis and then enzymes inside the APC break down the antigen into smaller particles. The processed antigens are transported to the surface of the APC, bound with either an MHC (major histocompatibility complex) class I or class II molecule, which the T-cell receptor (TCR) recognizes and binds to. Once the T-cell recognizes and binds to the MHC molecule complex, the APC sends out an additional co-stimulatory signal to activate the T cells.

There are three types of APC: dendritic cells, B cells and macrophages. Macrophages have been extensively studied in assays with propolis. These cells express a broad range of membrane receptors that mediate their interactions with natural and altered-self components of the host as well as with a range of microorganisms. Toll-like receptors (TLRs) are crucial for innate immunity response, since they recognize microbial products known as pathogen-associated molecular patterns. TLRs activation induces downstream signaling cascades that activate the nuclear factor κB (NF-κB) resulting in the transcription of pro-inflammatory genes. TLR-2 and TLR-4 have been widely studied due to their importance against microorganisms: TLR-2 recognizes, for example, components from Gram-positive bacteria and fungi zymozan, while TLR-4 recognizes Gram-negative bacteria lipopolysaccharide (LPS).

Recent articles have provided information of propolis influence on the immune system [14, 22].

In order to verify whether propolis could affect the initial events of the immune response, TLR-2 and TLR-4 expression and the production of pro-inflammatory cytokines (IL-1β and

IL-6) were evaluated after the treatment of male BALB/c with propolis (200 mg/kg) for three consecutive days [23]. TLR-2 and TLR-4 expression as well as IL-1β and IL-6 production were assessed in peritoneal macrophages and spleen cells. Basal IL-1β production and TLR-2 and TLR-4 expression were increased in peritoneal macrophages of propolis-treated mice. TLR-2 and TLR-4 expression and IL-1β and IL-6 production were also upregulated in the spleen cells of propolis-treated mice. It has been observed previously that propolis (0.2 – 1.0 mg/ml) stimulated cytokines production, such as IL-1β and TNF-α by peritoneal macrophages of mice [24].

The process of phagocytosis is complex and involves the binding of the target to the surface of macrophages and ingestion, which usually triggers the so-called oxidative burst. Propolis (2.5 and 5 mg/kg) also increased hydrogen peroxide ($H_2O_2$) generation by peritoneal macrophages, favoring the microorganisms killing [25].

Thus, propolis could exert its function by increasing directly the liberation of fungicidal substances by macrophages, such as oxygen and nitrogen metabolites, as well as inducing the production of some pro-inflammatory cytokines.

After incubation of macrophages with Brazilian or Bulgarian propolis (5, 10 and 20 μg/100μl) *in vitro*, these cells were subsequently challenged with *Paracoccidioides brasiliensis*. Propolis increased the fungicidal activity of macrophages, and no differences were seen between the samples. Since propolis was able to activate macrophages and enhance its fungicidal action, an indirect effect might be postulated [26].

Brazilian and Bulgarian propolis effects on the bactericidal activity of macrophages *in vitro* against *Salmonella* Typhimurium – causative agent of typhoid fever in humans, were also analyzed. Both Brazilian and Bulgarian samples increased the bactericidal activity of macrophages against *S.* Typhimurium, depending on its concentration (3, 10, 30 and 100 μg/100μl). No differences were seen between these samples, although they were produced in different geographic regions. Data also showed that the bactericidal activity of macrophages, using different ratios macrophage/bacteria and different propolis concentrations, might have occurred through oxygen and nitrogen intermediates [27]. However, a possible role of other microbicidal mechanisms should be investigated further. It is important to mention that no ethanol effects (propolis solvent) were seen in all immunological assays of our group.

In models of immunosupression, the administration of a water-soluble derivative (WSD) of propolis (50 mg/Kg) to mice prevented the cyclophosphamide effects and enhanced the survival rate of the animals [28]. These authors suggest that propolis modulates the non-specific immunity, via macrophage activation *in vivo*.

Propolis capsules (500 mg) were administered to humans for 2 weeks, and a significant increase of both spontaneous and LPS-induced cytokine (TNF-α, IL-1β, IL-6 and IL-8) secretion capacity of peripheral blood leukocytes [29].

One may conclude that propolis activates the initial steps of the immune response by upregulating TLRs expression, the production of pro-inflammatory cytokines and the respiratory burst in mice, modulating the mechanisms of the innate immunity and contributing to the recognition of microorganism by lymphocytes.

## PROPOLIS EFFECTS ON ACQUIRED IMMUNITY

Adaptive immunity is important to the recognition of "non-self" antigens, in order to eliminate specific pathogens or pathogen infected cells, followed by the development of immunological memory, so that each pathogen is "remembered" after the first exposure to the immune system and is eliminated quickly before an infection occurs. When a T helper cell (Th) interacts with an APC, some events are necessary to its activation: 1) TCR-CD3 complex binds to the antigen-MHC on the APC surface, and 2) CD28 on Th cell binds to CD80 (B7.1) or CD86 (B7.2) on APC. After these two signals, Th cells produce IL-2, which acts in an autocrine way to induce their proliferation. Afterwards, Th cells develop into effector cells and differentiate into two subtypes: Th1 and Th2 cells. Th1 cells produce IFN-γ and IL-2, among others, and active cell-mediated immunity, favoring the defense against intracellular pathogens, by activating macrophages, CD8+ T cells and natural killer cells. On the other hand, Th2 cells produce predominantly IL-4, IL-5, IL-6, IL-10 and IL-13, which promote humoral immunity, inducing antibody production against extracellular microorganisms.

Propolis' immunomodulatoty action was thought to be limited mainly to macrophages, with no influence on lymphocyte proliferation [28]. However, it has been demonstrated that splenocytes from mice treated with cinnamic acid – a propolis constituent, possessed an enhanced ability to incorporate thymidine, in the presence of mitogens such LPS, phytohemagglutinin (PHA) or concanavalin A (Con A), suggesting a proliferative tendency of these cell culture in the absence of mitogens [30]. Serum IL-1β of these animals was elevated, suggesting that cinnamic acid could activate macrophages, affecting the initial events of the immune response.

On the other hand, an inhibitory effect of propolis (5-100 μg/ml) on splenocyte proliferation was observed *in vitro* [31]. This immunosuppressor effect on the lymphoproliferative response may be attributed to flavonoids [32]. Propolis suppresses DNA synthesis of human peripheral blood mononuclear cells (PBMC) and purified T cells, and these effects were at least in part mediated by caffeic acid phenethyl ester (CAPE) and by the flavonoids quercetin and hesperidin [33].

CAPE (1, 5 and 10 μM) had inhibitory effects on transcription factors NF-κB and NFAT [34], and, as a consequence, CAPE inhibited IL-2 gene transcription, IL-2R (CD25) expression, and proliferation of human T cells, providing new insights into the molecular mechanisms involved in the anti-inflammatory and immunomodulatory activities of this natural compound.

The anti-inflammatory action of propolis has been reported by several researchers, using different experimental models [35-38]. Propolis administration (200 mg/kg) over a short-term (3 days) to mice inhibited IFN-γ production in splenocyte cultures [39]. Moreover, C57BL/6 mice treated with propolis (200 mg/kg) for 14 days showed an inhibition of IL-1β, IL-6, IFN-γ, IL-2 and IL-10 production by spleen cells, suggesting its anti-inflammatory activity once it is well established that cytokines orchestrate and perpetuate the chronic inflammatory features of several diseases [40, 41].

Thus, one may verify that propolis possesses both pro- and anti-inflammatory action, depending on concentration, intake period and experimental model.

With regards to the humoral immune response, treatment of rats with propolis 10% stimulated antibody production [42]. CAPE administration (5, 10 and 20 mg/kg) to BALB/c mice increased antibody production as well [43], but besides the effect of individual constituents, synergistic effects of several compounds may be responsible for the different pharmacological activities to propolis.

The biological properties of propolis are due to a natural mixture of its components, and a single constituent of propolis would not have an activity greater than that of the total extract [44]. These data strongly suggest the adjuvant capacity of propolis in association with vaccines. As an example, propolis (5 mg/dose) was associated to inactivated Suid herpesvirus type 1 (SuHV-1) vaccine, verifying that mice inoculated with SuHV-1 vaccine plus aluminium hydroxide and propolis showed higher antibodies titers [45]. Propolis was also efficient as an adjuvant to the inactivated vaccine against *Aeromonas hydrophila* in carps, since the phagocytic activity of these fishes and their serum antibodies against *A. hydrophila* were higher comparing to non-adjuvant vaccinated fishes [46].

The effects of propolis on immobilization stress-challenged animals were also investigated. In acutely stressed mice, propolis (200 mg/kg for 3 days) restored TLR-2 and TLR-4 expression [47], contributing to the recognition of microorganisms during stressful conditions, and increased IL-4 production, favoring humoral immune response [48]. In chronically stressed mice, propolis treatment (200 mg/kg for 7 days) potentiated $H_2O_2$ generation by macrophages and counteracted the alterations found in the spleen [49]. Propolis (200 mg/kg for 14 days) also exerted an immunomodulatory activity in melanoma-bearing mice submitted to chronic stress [40, 41].

In humans, CAPE (1, 2 and 4 μg/ml) showed protective effect against hyperthermal stress in athletes, enhancing the hyperthermal tolerance in immune mononuclear cells of competitive cyclists [50]. Since the modern life comprises a wide range of stressful conditions, these results point out the importance of further research in order to understand propolis usefulness during stress and for the development of new medicaments, affecting both innate and adaptive immunity.

## PROPOLIS EFFECTS ON TUMOR CELLS

Several authors have been investigating propolis' antitumor activity [22]. In fact, propolis has been always mentioned as an antitumoral and immunomodulatory agent. In recent years, *in vitro* and *in vivo* assays provided new information concerning its mechanisms of action.

*In vitro* assays have shown a cytotoxic action of propolis and its isolated compounds on various tumor cells [51, 52], and the main mechanisms of action of propolis involve apoptosis, cell cycle arrest and interference in metabolic pathways.

Although propolis may exert a direct effect on different tumor cells *in vitro*, the administration of propolis to animals or humans is followed by its solubility and systemic bioavailability. Thus, propolis action *in vivo* may occur mainly due to its immunomodulatory action, exerting either chemopreventive or therapeutic effects. Propolis and its isolated constituents exerted antitumoral effects *in vivo* as well, due to an immunomodulatory action [53], affecting the non-specific antitumor immunity via macrophages activation, which in turn could produce soluble factors and interfere directly in the tumor cells or in the functions of other immune cells [54].

The administration of 10% propolis to rats for 3 days increased the cytotoxic activity of natural killer cells against murine lymphoma [55]. Propolis (50 and 150 mg/kg) and some isolated polyphenolic compounds (caffeic acid, CAPE and quercetin) decreased the number of tumor nodules in the lung; however, the antimetastatic effectiveness of propolis was higher than that presented by its constituents [56]. Propolis, caffeic acid and CAPE (50 mg/kg) could be useful tools in the control of tumor growth. Orsolic et al. [53] reported that propolis antitumor action could be the consequence of synergistic activities of its polyphenolic compounds. Moreover, propolis action should be compared to antitumor drugs or even be tested in association with them, in order to investigate a possible synergistic action.

Cellular immune responses mediated primarily by activated T lymphocytes play an important role in eliminating malignant tumor cells. Different strategies to stimulate antitumor immunity have been extensively studied in humans, but an effective immunotherapy has not yet been developed for any type of malignancy. Thus, the role of propolis associated or not to immunotherapy against tumors may be a new perspective of investigation.

## Comments and Implications

Propolis biological properties have been intensely investigated in the last years, attracting a great interest of consumers in propolis-containing products marketed by health-food.

With respect to the immune system, propolis may modulate both innate and adaptive responses, showing pro- and anti-inflammatory activities, depending on concentration, intake period and experimental conditions. Thus, it all should be taken into consideration to obtain the expected results, since inhibitory or stimulatory activities may be expected.

Little is known concerning propolis efficiency clinically, although there have been a great number of publications lately considering the immunomodulatory and antitumor action of propolis and its constituents, what indicates their potential for the development of new pharmaceutical agents.

## References

[1] Burdock G. A. Review of the biological properties and toxicity of bee propolis (propolis). *Food and Chemical Toxicology*. 1998;36:347-363.

[2] Ghisalberti E. L. Propolis: a review. *Bee World*. 1979;60:59-84.

[3] Ikeno K., Ikeno T., Miyazawa C. Effects of propolis on dental caries in rats. *Caries Research*. 1991;25:347–351.

[4] Grunberger D., Banerjee R., Eisinger K., Oltz E. M., Efros L., Caldwell M., Estevez V., Nakanishi K. Preferential cytotoxicity on tumor cells by caffeic acid phenethyl ester isolated from propolis. *Experientia*. 1988;44:230–232.

[5] Scheller S., Krol W., Swiacik J., Owczarek S., Gabrys J., Shani J. Antitumoral property of ethanolic extract of propolis in mice-bearing Ehrlich carcinoma, as compared to bleomycin. *Zeitschrift für Naturforschung*. 1989;44:1063–1065.
[6] Hausen B. M., Evers P., Stuwe H. T., Konig W. A., Wollenweber E. Propolis allergy (IV). Studies with further sensitizers from propolis and constituents common to propolis, poplar buds and balsam of Peru. *Contact Dermatitis*. 1992;26:34–44.
[7] Scheller S., Gazda G., Krol W., Czuba Z., Zajusz A., Gabrys J., Shani J. The ability of ethanolic extract of propolis (EEP) to protect mice against gamma irradiation. *Zeitschrift für Naturforschung*. 1989;44:1049–1052.
[8] Cuesta Rubio O., Cuellar A., Rojas N, Velez Castro H, Rastrelli L, Aquino R. A polyisoprenylated benzophenone from Cuban Propolis. *Journal of Natural Products*. 1999;62:1013-1015.
[9] Bankova V. Chemical diversity of propolis and the problem of standardization. *Journal of Ethnopharmacology*. 2005;100:114-117.
[10] Montenegro G, Avila G, Peña R. C. 2001. Botanical origin and seasonal production of propolis in hives of Central Chile. *Boletim de Botânica da Universidade de São Paulo*. 2001;19:1-6.
[11] Marcucci M. C. Propolis: chemical composition, biological properties and therapeutic activity. *Apidologie*. 1995;26:83–99.
[12] Bankova V., de Castro S. L., Marcucci M. C. Propolis: recent advances in chemistry and plant origin. *Apidologie*. 2000;31:3–15.
[13] Bankova V. Recent trends and important developments in propolis research. *Evidence-based Complementary and Alternative Medicine*. 2005;2:29-32.
[14] Sforcin J. M., Bankova V. Propolis: is there a potential for the development of new drugs? *Journal of Ethnopharmacology*. 2011;133:253-260.
[15] Bankova V., Boudourova-Krasteva G., Sforcin J. M., Frete X., Kujumgiev A., Maimoni-Rodella R., Popov S. Phytochemical evidence for the plant origin of Brazilian propolis from São Paulo State. *Zeitschrift für Naturforschung*. 1999;54c:401-405.
[16] Boudourova-Krasteva G., Bankova V., Sforcin J.M., Nikolova N., Popov S. Phenolics from Brazilian propolis. *Zeitschrift für Naturforschung*. 1997;52c:676-679.
[17] Bankova V., Boudourova-Krasteva G., Popov S., Sforcin J. M., Funari S. R. C. Seasonal variations of the chemical composition of Brazilian propolis. *Apidologie*. 1998;29:361-367.
[18] Bankova V., Boudourova-Krasteva G., Popov S., Sforcin J. M., Funari S. R. C. Seasonal variations in essential oil from Brazilian propolis. *Journal of Essential Oil Research*. 1998;10:693-696.
[19] Sforcin J. M., Novelli E. L. B., Funari S. R. C. Seasonal effect of Brazilian propolis on seric biochemical variables. *The Journal of Venomous Animals and Toxins*. 2002;8:244–254.
[20] Mani F., Damasceno H. C. R., Novelli E. L. B., Martins E. A. M., Sforcin J.M. Propolis: effect of different concentrations, extracts and intake period on seric biochemical variables. *Journal of Ethnopharmacology*. 2006;105:95-98.
[21] Mani F., Damasceno H. C. R., Novelli E. L. B., Sforcin JM. Biochemical determinations of propolis-treated rats: effect of different concentrations, extracts and intake period. *Biosaúde*. 2008;10:3-16.

[22] Sforcin J. M. Propolis and the immune system: a review. *Journal of Ethnopharmacology*. 2007;113:1-14.

[23] Orsatti C. L., Missima F., Pagliarone A. C., Bachiega T. F., Búfalo M. C., Araújo Jr. J.P., Sforcin J.M. Propolis immunomodulatory action *in vivo* on Toll-like receptors 2 and 4 expression and on pro-inflammatory cytokines production in mice. *Phytotherapy Research*. 2010;24:1141-1146.

[24] Moriyasu J., Arai S., Motoda R., Kurimoto M. *In vitro* activation of mouse macrophage by propolis extract powder. *Biotherapy*. 1994;8:364-365.

[25] Orsi R. O., Funari S. R. C., Soares A. M. V. C., Calvi S.A., Oliveira S.L., Sforcin JM, Bankova V. Immunomodulatory action of propolis on macrophage activation. *The Journal of Venomous Animals and Toxins*. 2000;6:205-219.

[26] Murad J. M., Calvi S. A., Soares A. M. V. C., Bankova V., Sforcin J. M. Effects of propolis from Brazil and Bulgaria on fungicidal activity of macrophages against Paracoccidioides brasiliensis. *Journal of Ethnopharmacology*. 2002;79:331-334.

[27] Orsi R. O., Sforcin J. M., Funari S. R., Bankova V. Effects of Brazilian and Bulgarian propolis on bactericidal activity of macrophages against Salmonella Typhimurium. *International Immunopharmacology*. 2005;5:359–368.

[28] Dimov V., Ivanovska N., Manolova N., Bankova V., Nikolov N., Popov S. Immunomodulatory action of propolis. Influence on anti-infections protection and macrophage function. *Apidologie*. 1991;22:155-162.

[29] Bratter C., Tregel M., Liebenthal C., Volk H. D. Prophylaktische wirkungen von propolis zur immunstimulation: eine klinische pilotstudie. *Forschende Komplementarmedizin*. 1999;6:256-260.

[30] Ivanovska N., Neychev H., Stefanova Z., Bankova V., Popov S. Influence of cinnamic acid on lymphocyte proliferation, cytokines release and *Klebsiella* infection in mice. *Apidologie*. 1995;26:73-81.

[31] Sá-Nunes A., Faccioli L. H., Sforcin J. M. Propolis: lymphocyte proliferation and IFN-γ production. *Journal of Ethnopharmacology*. 2003;87,93-97.

[32] You K. M., Son K. H., Chang H. W., Kang S. S., Kim H. P. Vitexicarpin, a flavonoid from the fruits of *Vitex rotundifolia*, inhibits mouse lymphocyte proliferation and growth of cell lines *in vitro*. *Planta Medica*. 1998;64: 546-550.

[33] Ansorge S., Reinhold D., Lendeckel U. Propolis and some of its constituents down-regulate DNA synthesis and inflammatory cytokine production but induce TGF-β1 production of human immune cells. *Zeitschrift für Naturforschung*. 2003;58c:580-589.

[34] Márquez N., Sancho R., Macho A., Calzado M. A., Fiebich B. L., Muñoz E. Caffeic acid phenethyl ester inhibits T-cell activation by targeting both nuclear factor of activated T-cells and NF-κB transcription factors. *The Journal of Pharmacology and Experimental Therapeutics*. 2004;308:993-1001.

[35] Khayyal M. T., El-Ghazaly M. A., El-Khatib A. S. Mechanisms involved in the antiinflammatory effect of propolis extract. *Drugs under Experimental and Clinical Research*. 1993;19:192-203.

[36] Miyataka H., Nishiki M., Matsumoto H., Fujimoto T., Matsuka M., Satoh T. Evaluation of propolis. I. Evaluation of Brazilian and Chinese propolis by enzymatic and physic-chemical methods. *Biological & Pharmaceutical Bulletin*. 1997;20:496-501.

[37] Hu F., Hepburn H. R., Li Y., Chen M., Radloff S. E., Daya S. Effects of ethanol and water extracts of propolis (bee glue) on acute inflammatory animal models. *Journal of Ethnopharmacology*. 2005;100:276-283.

[38] Paulino N., Teixeira C., Martins R., Scremin A., Dirsch V. M., Vollmar A. M., Abreu S. R., De Castro S. L., Marcucci M. C. Evaluation of the analgesic and anti-inflammatory effects of a Brazilian green propolis. *Planta Medica*. 2006;72:899-906.

[39] Orsatti C. L., Missima F., Pagliarone A. C., Sforcin J. M. Th1/Th2 cytokines' expression and production by propolis-treated mice. *Journal of Ethnopharmacology*. 2010;129:314-318.

[40] Missima F., Pagliarone A. C., Orsatti C. L., Sforcin J. M. The effect of propolis on pro-inflammatory cytokines produced by melanoma-bearing mice submitted to chronic stress. *Journal of ApiProduct & ApiMedical Science*. 2009;1:11-15.

[41] Missima F., Pagliarone A. C., Orsatti C. L., Araújo Jr. J. P., Sforcin J. M. Propolis effect on Th1/Th2 cytokines' expression and production by melanoma-bearing mice submitted to stress. *Phytotherapy Research*. 2010;24:1501-1507.

[42] Sforcin J. M., Orsi R. O., Bankova V. Effects of propolis, some isolated compounds and its source plant on antibody production. *Journal of Ethnopharmacology*. 2005;98:301-305.

[43] Park J. H., Lee J. K., Kim H. S., Chung S. T., Eom J. H., Kim K. A., Chung S. J., Paik S. Y., Oh H. Y. Immunomodulatory effect of caffeic acid phenethyl ester in BALB/c mice. *International Immunopharmacology*. 2004;4:429-436.

[44] Kujumgiev A., Tsvetkova I., Serkedjieva Y., Bankova V., Christov R., Popov S. Antibacterial, antifungal and antiviral activity of propolis of different geographic origin. *Journal of Ethnopharmacology*. 1999;64:235-240.

[45] Fischer G., Conceição F. R., Leite F. P. L., Dummer L.A., Vargas G.D., Hübner S.O., Dellagostin O. A., Paulino N., Paulino A. S., Vidor T. Immunomodulation produced by a green propolis extract on humoral and cellular responses of mice immunized with SuHV-1. *Vaccine*. 2007;25:1250-1256.

[46] Chu W. H. Adjuvant effect of propolis on immunization by inactivated *Aeromonas hydrophila* in carp (*Carassius auratus gibelio*). *Fish & Shelfish Immunology*. 2006;21:113-117.

[47] Pagliarone A. C., Orsatti C. L., Búfalo M. C., Missima F., Bachiega T. F., Araújo Jr. J. P., Sforcin J. M. Propolis effects on pro-inflammatory cytokine production and Toll-like receptor 2 and 4 expression in stressed mice. *International Immunopharmacology*. 2009;9:1352-1356.

[48] Pagliarone A. C., Missima F., Orsatti C. L., Bachiega T. F., Sforcin J. M. Propolis effect on Th1/Th2 cytokines production by acutely stressed mice. *Journal of Ethnopharmacology*. 2009;125:230-233.

[49] Missima F., Sforcin J. M. Green Brazilian propolis action on macrophages and lymphoid organs of chronically stressed mice. *Evidence-based Complementary and Alternative Medicine*. 2008;5:71-75.

[50] Chen Y. J., Huang A. C., Chang H. H., Liao H. F., Jiang C. M., Lai L. Y., Chan J. T., Chen Y.Y., Chiang J. Caffeic acid phenethyl ester, an antioxidant from propolis, protects peripheral blood mononuclear cells of competitive cyclists against hyperthermal stress. *Journal of Food Science*. 2009;74:H162-167.

[51] Bassani-Silva S., Sforcin J.M., Amaral A. S., Gaspar L. F. J., Rocha N. S. Propolis effect *in vitro* on canine transmissible venereal tumor cells. *Revista Portuguesa de Ciências Veterinárias*. 2007;102:261-265.

[52] Búfalo M. C., Candeias, J. M. G., Sousa J. P. B., Bastos J. K., Sforcin J. M. *In vitro* cytotoxic activity of *Baccharis dracunculifolia* and propolis against HEp-2 cells. *Natural Product Research*. 2010;24:1710-1718.

[53] Orsolic N., Sver L., Terzic S., Basic I. Peroral application of water-soluble derivative of propolis (WSDP) and its related polyphenolic compounds and their influence on immunological and antitumor activity. *Veterinary Research Communications*. 2005;29:575-593.

[54] Orsolic N., Saranovic A. B., Basic I. Direct and indirect mechanism(s) of antitumour activity of propolis and its polyphenolic compounds. *Planta Medica*. 2006;72:20–27.

[55] Sforcin J. M., Kaneno R., Funari S. R. C. Absence of seasonal effect on the immunomodulatory action of Brazilian propolis on natural killer activity. *Journal of Venomous Animals and Toxins*. 2002;8:19-29.

[56] Orsolic N., Knezevic A. H., Sver L., Terzic S., Basic I. Immunomodulatory and antimetastatic action of propolis and related polyphenolic compounds. *Journal of Ethnopharmacology*. 2004;94:307-315.

In: Beneficial Effects of Propolis on Human Health ... ISBN: 978-1- 62081-440-6
Editors: Tahira Farooqui and Akhlaq A. Farooqui 

*Chapter 6*

# CHEMICAL COMPOSITION, ANTIVIRAL AND ANTIMICROBIAL ACTIVITIES OF EGYPTIAN PROPOLIS

***Faten K. Abd El-Hady****
Dept. Natural Product Chemistry, Nation-al Research Center, Egypt

## ABSTRACT

*Background:* Propolis (bee glue) is a resinous hive product collected by honeybees from various plant sources. Propolis chemical composition is variable, depending on the geographical differences. Propolis samples from Europe and Asia have different chemical compositions. Recently, propolis has attracted the interest of many investigators because of its antibacterial, antiviral, antiinflammatory, and immunestimulatory effects.

*Materials and Methods:* In this chapter, 11 Egypt propolis samples were collected from, Upper Egypt, Nile Delta, reclaimed lands, beach and oasis, evaluated for their antiviral and antimicrobial activities, their chemical composition was investigated by GC/MS and HPLC analysis.

*Results: Upper Egypt propolis* was characterized by the presence of : 7 caffeate esters and 4 triterpenoids in (B) sample; High amount of lactic acid and presence of 3 chalcones in (F); 4 prenylated coumarates in (As) and 5 aliphatic dicarboxylic acids in (So). (B) showed the highest antimicrobial activity against *Staph. aureus*; *E.coli* and *C. albicans,* while, (F) had moderate activity against all tested pathogen. (As) and (So) had the lowest antimicrobial activity.

*Nile Delta Propolis* was characterized by the presence of: New triterpenic acid methyl esters in (IS); Caffeate esters, some di- and triterpenoids in (Sh). (D) was a typical poplar propolis but it contained two new caffeate esters and two new triterpenoids. (D) showed the highest antiviral activity against (IBDV) and antimicrobial activity against *E. coli* and *C. albicans.* (Is) had the highest antiviral activity against Reo virus. (Sh) showed the highest antibacterial activity against *Staph. aureus.*

*Reclaimed lands:* The (Is-R) propolis was characterized by the presence of a highly significant amount of aromatic acid esters and triterpenoids, while (El) contained new

* Address correspondence to: Faten K. Abd El-Hady, Ph.D. Dept. Natural Product Chemistry, National Research Center, Egypt. Email: fatenkamal@hotmail.com. Mobile: +2 0100 613 88 30, fax: +202 333 70 931.

esters belonged to 4-methoxyhydrocinnamic, hydroferulic and ferulic acids. It had a very high significant amount of 2,6-bis-(pentanyloxy)- 4-pentanylphenethanol. (El) showed the highest antimicrobiall activity against *Staph. aureus* and *C. albicans*, while (Is-R) had the highest activity against *E. coli*.

*Matrooh beach and Siwa oasis were* characterized by the presence of : Diprenyl-dihydrocoumaric acids, coumarate esters, benzofuran lignans and valeric acids derivatives in (S); new ferulate esters, hydroxy acetophenones, furanon derivatives, furofuran lignans and pregnane sterol in (M).They showed antibacterial activity against *Clostridium oedematiens (Clostridium novyi)* type B associated to fascioliasis.

*HPLC analysis:* 42 Polyphenolic compounds quantitatively were identified in 10 samples. The major flavones identified are: Galangin-7-methylether, Acacetin, Quercetin-3,3'-dimethylether, Myricetin, Luteolin, while the flavanones are : Pinostrobin, Biochanin A, Pinocembrin, Naringenin and one major isoflavone: Formonontin. The samples showed variations in their *antiviral activity*; sample (D) induced the highest antiviral activity against *NDV and IBDV.*

*Conclusion:* Although, the chemical composition is qualitatively and quantitatively variable, most of the Egyptian propolis samples had high antiviral activity against NDV, Reo and IBDV and antimicrobial activity against *Staph. aureus, E. coli. C. albicans* and *Clostridium oedematiens.*[1]

**Keywords:** Egyptian Propolis, GC/MS, HPLC, Antiviral, Antimicrobial

# 1. INTRODUCTION

Propolis is a resinous substance with varying colors and consistencies, collected by *Apis mellifera* bees from several vegetal sources. The word propolis comes from the Greek *pro* meaning 'in defense of' and *polis* 'city', i.e. defense of beehives [1]. In fact, bees use propolis to protect themselves from insects and microorganisms, employing it as a cement to seal cracks or open spaces in the hive, to sterilize the queen-bee posture site, and to mummify insect invaders. Commonly, small animals or parts of them are found wrapped within propolis in perfect states of conservation [2].

Propolis is a honeybee product with a very complex chemical composition, made by gummy and balsamic material collected by bees from sprouts, flower-buds, trees and other vegetal-tissue resinous exudates. During propolis collection, bees mix the beeswax and the collected propolis with the 13-glicosidase enzyme found in their saliva, hydrolyzing flavonoids glycosides into flavonoid aglycones [3]. Afterwards, the collected material is augmented with enzymatic and salivary secretions.

Along with other honeybee products (honey, royal jelly, pollen), propolis has outstanding therapeutic properties [4], being used since 300 years B.C. in popular medicine in various parts of the world. However, interest in the correlation of propolis chemical composition with its pharmacological activities started only forty years ago [2]. Propolis is one of the few "natural drugs" being used for a long time by different civilizations [5]. Currently, several propolis products are being commercialized worldwide, including candies, chocolate bars,

[1] B, Banisweif; F, Fayoum; As, Assiut; So, Souhag; D, Dakahlia; Sh, Sharkia; Is, Ismailia; El, El-Saff and IsR, Ismailia; S, Siwa oasis; M, Matrooh beach. *Staph. aureus= Staphylococcus aureus; E. coli = Escherichia coli, C. albicans = Candida albicans,* IBDV=Infectious Bursal Disease Virus and NDV=Newcastle Disease Virus; GC/MS = gas chromatography /mass spectrometry; HPLC = high performance liquid chromatography.

shampoos, skin lotions, antiseptic mixtures, and toothpastes [6]. The Persians, Greeks, Romans and Incas also used propolis with therapeutic purposes. In ancient Egypt, it was employed to embalm the dead, while in the Balkans States propolis is widely used. In France, the term propolis is found in the general literature since the sixteenth century. In South Africa, during the Anglo-Boer War, more than 90 years ago, it was used with Vaseline for ointment preparation to heal war wounds. This helped save the lives of many soldiers, since antibiotics were not yet available [7]. In the Second World War, Soviet medical clinics studied propolis with excellent results.

The color of propolis depends on its origin. It varies from dark-brown to reddish-brown, with a greenish tone. It has a typical odor, which can vary from sample to sample, with some being odorless. Propolis obtained from beehives, also known as crude propolis, is composed of around 50% balsam resin, 30% wax, 10% essential and aromatic oils, 5% pollen, and 5% other substances, including wood fragments [8]. The resin found in propolis is collected in vegetation nearby beehives, where bees also collect pollen and nectar for feeding. Propolis composition is mainly determined by the phyto-geographic characteristics of beehive surroundings [9]. However, seasonal variation may occur within the same place [10]. Also, variation was observed among samples collected in the same place, but by different *A. mellifera* subspecies [11]. Several contaminants close by beehives can be collected and unexpectedly added to propolis, such as asphalt powder, pesticide, iron excess, copper, magnesium, [12] and even lead [13]. The nature of aromatic and terpene compounds found in propolis has a biological importance, allowing bees to determine which vegetal species to visit [2]. The pharmacological activities of propolis are more numerous in tropical regions than in temperate climates, reproducing the richer vegetal diversity observed in the former [14, 15]. More than 300 different compounds have been identified so far in propolis, including aliphatic acids, esters, aromatic acids, fatty acids, carbohydrates, aldehydes, amino acids, ketones, chalcones, dihydrochalcones, terpenoids, vitamins, and inorganic substances [2]. Of all, flavonoids are the ones which draw greater research interest [16]. Propolis has several therapeutic properties, such as antibacterial, anti-inflammatory, healing, anesthetic [17], anticariogenic [3], antifungal, antiprotozoan and antiviral activities.

## 2. Chemical Composition of Egyptian Propolis

This chapter demonstrated the chemical composition of Egypt propolis collected from eleven governorates belong to Upper Egypt (B, F, AS and SO samples), Nile Delta (D, IS and Sh samples), reclaimed lands (EL and Is-R samples), beach (M sample) and oasis(S sample).

246 individual compounds were identified by GC/MS and HPLC analysis [18-22]. The data obtained are presented in (Tables 1-9) and (Figures 1-).

The chemical composition of eleven Egyptian propolis samples was investigated by GC-MS after silylation. As expected, most samples not displayed the typical pattern of "poplar" propolis: they contained pinocembrin, pinobanksin and its 3-O-acetate, chrysin, galangin, prenyl esters of caffeic and ferulic acids, etc. The ratio between the main compound classes corresponded to that in *P. nigra* bud exudates. Some samples, however, differed significantly from the others.

## 2.a. Chemical Composition Assessment with GC/MS Analysis

In Tables (1-8), the composition of "poplar propolis"(B and D samples) is compared to the composition of the other nine propolis samples with unusual propolis composition (F, AS, SO IS, Sh, EL, Is-R, M and S samples).

### *Upper Egypt Propolis*

Propolis samples were collected from different governorates of Upper Egypt, each of them characterized by some types of predominant trees or shrubs. According to the difference in plant source, each propolis sample was characterized by certain specific compounds [18].

*Sample (B)* is the only sample contained benzoic acid, trans-p-coumaric acid, ferulic acid, dimethylallyl caffeate, benzyl caffeate and caffeate esters with long chain fatty alcohols and typical flavonoids from poplar origin (*Populus nigra* ).

It also contained high amounts of triterpenic alcohols including β-amyrin, unidentified triterpene of β-amyrin type, lanosterol and cycloartenol (Tables 1-3).Sample (F) was characterized by the presence of the following new compounds to propolis: 2,3,4,5 tetrahydroxypentanoic acid-1,4-lactone, 2-propenoic acid-3-methoxy-3-hydroxy methyl ester, monoethyl succinate and benzylmethylketone, the last compound present with high significant amount (Tables 2,4,5). *Sample (AS)* was characterized by the presence of 4 prenylated coumarate esters, 4-methoxycinnamic acid, 3-methyl-2-butenylcaffeate and benzyl-2-methylpropyl which is new to propolis (Tables 1, 2, 5). Sample (**F**) and (**AS**) did not contain any triterpenic alcohols.*Sample (SO)* was characterized by the presence of 15 aliphatic acids, from which 2-hydroxy-cyclohexane-1-caboxylic acid, 3-methyl-3-hydroxy-pentanedioic acid and 2,3-dihydroxy pentanedioic acid are new to propolis, and also other new compounds like: 1,2-dihydroxy cyclohexene, 1,2,3-trihydroxy butane, 1,2,4-trihydroxy butanal, 2,4-bis(dimethylbenzyl)-6-t-butylphenol and 1,8- dihydroxy-3-methyl anthraquinone (Tables 4, 5). Sample (SO) did not contain any aromatic acid esters.

On the basis of the data obtained, a conclusion could be drawn concerning the plant origin of the investigated samples. One of the plant sources appeared to be common for the first 3 samples is poplar, but with different species. Sample (B) appeared to be from the origin of *Populus nigra*. The high concentration of esters of phenolic acids, the presence of pentenyl caffeates (Table 2) and typical flavanones indicate this (Table 8). Samples (F) and (AS) appeared to be from other poplar species as sample (F) was rich in flavanones and flavones (Table 8), while sample (AS) was characterized by the presence of prenylated coumarates (Table 2). The primary source of the plant exudate incorporated into propolis samples( B, F and AS) is bud exudate of poplar trees. The composition of propolis is therefore directly related to the composition of the poplar bud exudate collected by the bees [23- 26]. Bud extracts of *P. balsamifera* and P. *candicans* are very high in dihydrochalcones and rich in cinnamic and coumaric acids plus their esters, *P. balsamifera* appeared to be higher in flavones. *P.nigra* and *P. x euramericana* bud exudates are very low in dihydrochalcones and low in cinnamic and coumaric acids plus their esters [27]. Also each poplar species has its own characteristic mixture of compounds in its bud exudates [28, 29] and there can be considerable difference in bud exudates composition between different poplar species [29, 30].

**Table 1. Phenolic acids assessed by GC- MS analysis of propolis samples**

| No | Phenolic acids | B | F | AS | SO | D | IS | SH | EL | Is | S | M |
|---|---|---|---|---|---|---|---|---|---|---|---|---|
| | | [a] TIC % | | | | | | | | | | |
| 1 | Benzoic acid | 0.20 | | | | 2.70 | | 0.01 | | | | |
| 2 | 2-Phenyl- 2-hydroxy acrylic acid | | | | | 0.40 | | | | | | |
| 3 | 4-Hydroxy benzoic acid | | | | 0.10 | 0.60 | | 0.02 | 0.01 | | | |
| 4 | 2,4- Dihydroxybenzoic acid | | | | | | | | | | | 0.03 |
| 5 | 2,6- Dihydroxybenzoic acid | | | | | | | | | | | 0.03 |
| 6 | 2,3,4- Trihydroxybenzoic acid | | | | | | | | | | | 0.08 |
| 7 | 2,4,6- Trihydroxybenzoic acid | | | | | | | | | | | 0.13 |
| 8 | 3,4,5- Trihydroxybenzoic acid | | | | | | | | | | | 0.03 |
| 9 | Dihydrocinnamic acid | | | | | 0.30 | | | | | | |
| 10 | Cinnamic acid | | | | | 2.80 | | | | | | |
| 11 | 4- Methoxy-cinnamic acid | | | | | 0.80 | | | | | | |
| 12 | cis-p-Coumaric acid | | | | | 0.40 | | | | | | |
| 13 | trans- p-Coumaric acid | 0.50 | | | | 2.30 | | | | | | |
| 14 | 3,4-Dimethoxy-cinnamic acid | | | | | 2.90 | | 0.05 | | | | |
| 15 | 4- Methoxy-cinnamic acid | | | 1.81 | | | | | | | | |
| 16 | 3,4-di-Methoxy-cinnamic acid | 0.40 | 0.13 | 1.57 | 0.01 | | | | 0.04 | | | |
| 17 | Isoferulic acid | | | 0.70 | | 1.10 | | | | | | |
| 18 | Ferulic acid | 0.20 | | | | 2.40 | | | | | | |
| 19 | Caffeic acid | 0.30 | 0.29 | 0.86 | 0.05 | 4.40 | | 0.30 | 0.15 | | | |
| 20 | 3,5-dimethoxy-4-pentanyl cinnam acid | | | | | | | | | | 0.5 | |
| 21 | 3,5-diprenyldihydrocoumaric acid | | | | | | | | | | 2.9 | |
| 22 | 3,5-diprenyldihydrocoumaric acid isomer | | | | | | | | | | 1.3 | |

[a] TIC = The ion current generated depends on the characteristics of the compound concerned and it is not a true quantitation.

**Table 2. Esters assessed by GC- MS analysis of propolis samples**

| *No* | *ESTERS* | B | F | AS | SO | D | IS | SH | El | Is-R | S | M |
|---|---|---|---|---|---|---|---|---|---|---|---|---|
| | | *TIC%* | | | | | | | | | | |
| 1 | 2-propenoic acid-3-MeO-3-OH- methyl ester | | 0.73 | | | | | | | | | |
| 2 | Monoethyl succinate | | 0.43 | | | | | | | | | |
| 3 | Methyl palmitate | | | | | 0.27 | | | | | | |
| 4 | Ethyl palmitate | 0.5 | | | 0.01 | 0.13 | | | | | | |
| 5 | Ethyl oleate | 1.2 | | | 0.40 | | | | | 0.02 | | 0.17 |
| 6 | Stearic acid methyl ester | | | | | 0.20 | | | | | | |
| 7 | Octadecenoic acid pentyl ester | | | | | | | | 0.05 | 0.04 | | |
| 8 | Octadecenoic acid methyl ester | | | | | | | | | | | 0.22 |

**Table 2. (Continued)**

| *No* | *ESTERS* | B | F | AS | SO | D | IS | SH | El | Is-R | S | M |
|---|---|---|---|---|---|---|---|---|---|---|---|---|
| | | *TIC%* | | | | | | | | | | |
| 9 | Hydroxyl-pentacosatrienoic acid methyl ester | | | | | | | | | | | 0.88 |
| 10 | 2- Hydroxy-hexandioic acid monodecenyl ester | | | | | | | | | | - | 0.17 |
| 11 | Tetradecyl -4-methoxyhydrocinnamate | | | | | | | | | 0.05 | | |
| 12 | Tetradecenyl -4-methoxyhydrocinnamate | | | | | | | | | 0.29 | | |
| 13 | Hexadecyl -4-methoxyhydrocinnamate | | | | | | | | | 1.12 | | |
| 14 | Hexadecenyl -4-methoxyhydrocinnamate [bc] | | | | | | | | | 0.61 | | |
| 15 | Octadecyl -4-methoxyhydro-cinnamate [bc] | | | | | | | | | *11.3* | | |
| 16 | *trans*-3-Penteny-*trans*-4-coumarate | | | | | | | | 0.09 | | | |
| *17* | 3-methyl 2-butenyl –cis-4- coumarate | | | 0.68 | | | | | | | | |
| 18 | 3-methyl 3-butenyl –trans-4- coumarate | | | 0.35 | | | | | 0.04 | | | |
| 19 | 2-methyl 2-butenyl –trans-4- coumarate | | | 0.13 | | | | | | | | |
| 20 | 3-methyl 2-butenyl –trans-4- coumarate | | | 0.35 | | | | | | | | |
| 21 | Tetradecanyl –*trans*-4-coumarate | | | | | | | | 0.04 | | | |
| 22 | Hexadecanyl –*trans*-4-coumarate | | | | | | | | 0.09 | | | |
| 23 | Benzyl benzoate | | | | | 0.40 | | | | | | |
| 24 | Benzyl –trans-4-coumarate | | | | | 0.03 | | | | | | |
| 25 | Cinnamyl –trans-4-coumarate | | | | | 0.09 | | | | | | |
| 26 | 3,5-diisopropoxy-nonanyl coumarate | | | | | | | | | | 4.4 | |
| 27 | 3,5-diisopropoxy-nonanyl coumarate isomer | | | | | | | | | | 3.1 | |
| 28 | 3,5-diisopropoxy-nonanyl coumarate isomer | | | | | | | | | | 2.6 | |
| 29 | 3,5-dimethoxy-tetradecenyl coumarate | | | | | | | | | | 0.9 | |
| 30 | 3,5-dimethoxy-tridecenyl dihydrocoumarate | | | | | | | | | | | 0.6 |
| 31 | Heindecenyl hydroferulate | | | | | | | | | 0.8 | | |

| *No* | *ESTERS* | B | F | AS | SO | D | IS | SH | El | Is-R | S | M |
|---|---|---|---|---|---|---|---|---|---|---|---|---|
| | | *TIC%* | | | | | | | | | | |
| 32 | Tridecatrienyl hydroferulate | | | | | | | | | 0.3 | | |
| 33 | Tridecatrienyl hydroferulate (isomer) | | | | | | | | | *6.0* | | |
| 34 | Tridecyl hydroferulate | | | | | | | | | 0.4 | | |
| 35 | Tridecyl hydroferulate (isomer) | | | | | | | | | 0.8 | | |
| *36* | *Tridecyl hydroferulate (isomer)* | | | | | | | | | *11.2* | | |
| 37 | Tridecenyl hydroferulate | | | | | | | | | 0.30 | | |
| 38 | Pentadecyl hydroferulate | | | | | | | | | 3.14 | | |
| *39* | *Pentadecyl hydroferulate (isomer)* | | | | | | | | | *10.4* | | |
| 40 | Pentadecenyl hydroferulate | | | | | | | | | 0.50 | | |
| 41 | 3-Pentanyl-octyldihydroferulate | | | | | | | | | | | 1.2 |
| 42 | 3-Hexanyl-octyldihydroferulate | | | | | | | | | | | 0.38 |
| 43 | 3-Hexanyl-octyldihydroferulate isomer | | | | | | | | | | | 0.71 |
| 44 | 3-Methyl-3-butenyl isoferulate | | | | | 0.07 | | | | | | |
| 45 | 3-Methyl-2-butenyl isoferulate | | | | | 0.14 | | | | | | |
| 46 | Octenyl ferulate | | | | | | | | 0.4 | | | |
| 47 | Octadecatrienyl ferulate | | | | | | | | 1.1 | | | |
| 48 | Isopentenyl caffeate | 0.9 | 0.5 | 0.8 | | | | | 0.2 | | | |
| 49 | Dimethyl allyl caffeate | 1.3 | | | | | | | | | | |
| 50 | 2-Methyl-2-buteny caffeate | | 1.0 | 0.8 | | 0.18 | | 0.1 | 0.3 | | | |
| 51 | 3-Methyl-2-butenyl caffeate | | | 1.4 | | 0.90 | | 0.8 | | | | |
| 52 | 3-Methyl-3-butenyl caffeate | | | | | 0.64 | | 0.5 | | | | |
| 53 | Benzyl caffeate | 0.6 | | | | 0.32 | | | | | | |
| 54 | Dodecyl caffeate | 1.1 | | | | | | | | | | |
| 55 | Tetradecyl caffeate | 3.1 | | | | 0.18 | | 0.8 | | | | |
| 56 | Tetradecenyl caffeate | 0.3 | | | | 0.05 | | 0.1 | | | | |
| 57 | Tetradecenyl caffeate (isomer) | | | | | 0.13 | | 1.3 | | | | |
| 58 | Tetradecanyl caffeate | | | | | 0.05 | | 0.7 | | | | |
| 59 | Hexadecyl caffeate | 4.7 | | | | 0.2 | | 0.4 | | | | |
| 60 | Phenylethyl caffeate | | | | | 0.3 | | | | | | |
| 61 | Cinnamyl caffeate | | | | | 0.1 | | | | | | |

So, the original source of sample (F) and (AS) needs more investigation to know the other poplar species. The presence of substances unusual for poplar buds such as sterol precursors in sample (B) and amyrins in samples (B) and (SO) rather than F and (AS) is an indication that there could be another plant source for propolis which.

### *Nile Delta Propolis*

Propolis samples were collected from three governorates in East area of Nile Delta region, each of them characterized by some types of predominant trees or shrubs [19].

*Sample D* showed the presence of the characteristic groups of poplar propolis. These groups are aromatic acids, aromatic acid esters, aliphatic acids and flavonoids (Tables 1, 2, 4, 8) and it was also characterized by the presence of some triterpenoids (Table 3).

**Table 3. Di- and triterpenes assessed by GC- MS analysis of propolis samples**

| No | *Diterpenes* | B | F | AS | SO | D | IS | SH | El | Is-R | S | M |
|---|---|---|---|---|---|---|---|---|---|---|---|---|
| | | [a]TIC % | | | | | | | | | | |
| 1 | Pimaric acid | | | | | | | 0.5 | | | | |
| 2 | Dehydroabietic acid | | | | 0.40 | 0.14 | | 1.1 | 0.08 | 0.24 | | |
| 3 | Abietic acid | | | | | | | 1.0 | | | | |
| 4 | Diterpene,$[M]^+$ = 274 | | | | | | | | 0.08 | | | |
| 5 | Diterpene,$[M]^+$= 274 | | | | | | | | 0.15 | | | |
| | *Triterpenes* | | | | | | | | | | | |
| 1 | Cycloartinol | 7.1 | | | | 0.58 | | 0.8 | | 2.05 | | |
| 2 | Cycloartinol isomer | | | | | | | | | 0.17 | | |
| 3 | Cycloartinol isomer | | | | | | | | | 2.12 | | |
| 4 | Cycloartinol with another double bond | | | | | | | | | 0.83 | | |
| 5 | Cycloartinol with another double bond | | | | | | | | | 1.73 | | |
| 6 | Lanosterol | 1.2 | | | | | | 0.3 | | | | |
| 7 | Lanosterol with another double bond | | | | | | | 0.2 | | | | |
| 8 | Lanosterol acetate | | | | | | | | 0.06 | | | |
| 9 | α -Amyrin | | | | | 0.30 | | 0.2 | 0.14 | 2.53 | | |
| 10 | β-Amyrin | 4.7 | | | 0.17 | 0.21 | | 0.8 | 0.44 | 2.24 | | |
| 11 | Triterpene of β-amyrin type | 4.8 | | | 0.08 | | | | | | | |
| 12 | Lupeol | | | | | 0.42 | | | | | | |
| 13 | Triterpene of β-amyrin type [M+] m/z = 498 | | | | | 0.44 | 0.73 | | | | | |
| 14 | 3- Oxo-triterpenic acid methyl ester (oleanane type) $[M^+]$ m/z = 468 | | | | | | 0.14 | | | | | |
| 15 | 3- Oxo-triterpenic acid methyl ester (oleanane type) $[M^+]$ m/z = 468 | | | | | | 0.21 | | | | | |
| 16 | 3- Oxo-triterpenic acid methyl ester (ursane type) $[M^+]$ m/z = 468 | | | | | | 0.46 | | | | | |

| No | *Diterpenes* | B | F | AS | SO | D | IS | SH | El | Is-R | S | M |
|---|---|---|---|---|---|---|---|---|---|---|---|---|
| | | [a]TIC % | | | | | | | | | | |
| 17 | 3- Oxo-triterpenic acid methyl ester (ursane type) [$M^+$] m/z = 468 | | | | | | 1.16 | | | | | |
| 18 | Triterpene of β-amyrin type [M+] m/z = 498 | | | | | | 0.13 | | | | | |
| 19 | Triterpene (lupane type) | | | | | | | | 0.44 | | | |
| 20 | Triterpene of β-amyrin type | | | | | | | | 0.15 | 3.61 | | |
| 21 | Triterpene of β-amyrin type | | | | | | | | 0.05 | 2.00 | | |
| 22 | Triterpenic acid methyl ester (oleanane type) | | | | | | | | 0.08 | | | |
| 23 | Triterpenic acid methyl ester (ursane type) | | | | | | | | 0.50 | | | |
| 24 | Triterpenic acid methyl ester (ursane type) | | | | | | | | 0.05 | | | |

[a] TIC = The ion current generated depends on the characteristics of the compound concerned and it is not a true quantitation.

From the aliphatic acids, it contained a significant concentration of palmitic, oleic, stearic, tetracosanoic and hexacosanoic acids. Sample D showed high concentrations of the following aromatic acids: benzoic, cinnamic, trans-p-coumaric, 3,4-dimethoxycinnamic, ferulic and caffeic acids. Sample D was characterized also by the presence of 11 caffeate esters, from which two are new to propolis: tetradecenyl caffeate (isomer) and tetradecanyl caffeate.

It also contained some triterpenoids, from which two are new to propolis : lupeol and α - amyrin. In contrary to Dakahlia (*D*) sample, the Ismailia (*IS*) sample did not contain any aromatic acids and aromatic esters. It contained 6 aliphatic acids from which three are new to propolis: pentonic acid- 2-deoxy-3,5-dihydroxy-γ-lactone and its isomer and 2,3,4,5-tetrahydroxypentanoic acid-1,4-lactone (isomer).

Also it was characterized by the presence of 5 new triterpenoids to propolis: four 3-oxo-triterpenic acid methyl esters belonging to oleanane and ursane types and one triterpene from the β-amyrin type (Table 3). Also 1,2,3-trihydroxy butanal (isomer), 1-methoxy-1,3-dihydroxypropane and dihydroxyacetone dimer were identified for the first time to propolis (Table 5).

Sharkia propolis (*Sh*) is extremely different from the (IS) sample. It shared with D sample in 6 aliphatic acids, 4 aromatic acids. It was characterized by the presence of caffeate esters only (8 esters) as well as 3 diterpenes, 5 triterpenes. It was also characterized by the presence of three isomers of myristicin (Tables 1-5).

From the above mentioned data it is clear that Dakahlia sample is a typical poplar propolis [31,32]. In this investigation 65 compounds were identified in the Dakahlia sample while in Christove's study there were 39 compounds. The study of Christove *et al.* (1998) was done on poplar sample collected from Banisiewief province (Upper Egypt), while Dakahlia is located in the East area of Nile Delta region. There were some differences in the chemical composition of these two poplar propolis samples, these variations are species specific.

**Table 4. Aliphatic Acids assessed by GC / MS of propolis samples**

| *No* | *Aliphatic Acids* | B | F | AS | SO | D | IS | SH | El | Is-R | S | M |
|---|---|---|---|---|---|---|---|---|---|---|---|---|
| | | % TIC [a] | | | | | | | | | | |
| 1 | Lactic acid | 1.3 | 18.5 | 4.54 | 0.31 | 0.25 | | 0.55 | 0.41 | | | |
| 2 | Hydroxyacetic acid | | 4.3 | 1.86 | 0.05 | 0.06 | | 0.02 | 0.10 | | 0.17 | |
| 3 | 3-Hydroxypropanoic acid | | | | 0.01 | | | | 0.10 | | 0.51 | |
| 4 | 2,3-Dihydroxypropanoic acid | | 0.29 | | 0.06 | | | 0.06 | 0.04 | | | |
| 5 | 5-Hydroxy-n-valeric acid | | | | | 0.28 | | | | | | |
| 6 | Propanoic acid-3-hydroxyl-2-oxo | | | | | | | | | | 0.17 | |
| 7 | Pentonic acid- 2-deoxy-3,5-dihydroxy-γ-lactone | | | | | | 0.02 | | | | | |
| 8 | Octanoic acid | | | | | | | | | | 0.08 | |
| 9 | Methyl-propanedioic a | | | | | | | | | | 0.12 | |
| 10 | 2,3-Dihydroxypropano acid | | | | | | | | | | 0.15 | |
| 11 | 2,3,4-Trihydroxybutyri acid | | | | | | | | | | 0.14 | |
| 12 | Malic acid | | 0.68 | | 0.32 | 0.70 | | 0.13 | 0.13 | | | |
| 13 | Succinic acid | 0.30 | 8.00 | | 0.16 | | | 0.14 | 0.18 | | | |
| 14 | 2-butenedioic acid (E) | | 0.11 | | 0.01 | | | | | | | |
| 15 | 2-hydroxy-cyclohexane-1-carboxylic acid | | | | 0.10 | | | | | | | |
| 16 | Pentanedioic acid- 3-methyl-3-hydroxy | | | | 0.02 | | | | | | | |
| 17 | 2-hydroxy-cyclohexane-1-carboxylic acid | | | | 0.10 | | | | | | | |
| 18 | 2,3 dihydroxypentanedioic acid | | | | 0.05 | | | | | | | |
| 19 | 2,3,4,5- tetrahydroxy-pentanoic acid-1,4-lactone | | 0.16 | | | | 0.12 | | 0.01 | | 0.21 | |
| 20 | Nonanoic acid | | 0.01 | | | 0.20 | | | | | | |
| 21 | Decanoic acid | | | | | 0.20 | | | | | | |
| 22 | Dodecanoic acid | | | | | 0.50 | | | | | | |
| 23 | Tetradecanoic acid | 0.50 | | | | | | | | | | |
| 24 | Palmitic acid | 3.00 | | 0.36 | 2.31 | 13.3 | 0.06 | 1.40 | 0.58 | 0.05 | 11.5 | 0.10 |
| 25 | 8-Methoxy hexadecanoic acid | | | | | | | | | | | 0.21 |
| 26 | Heptadecanoic acid | | | | 0.02 | | | 0.05 | | 0.01 | | |
| 27 | Linoleic acid | | | | 0.10 | 1.50 | | | | | | |
| 28 | Oleic acid | 4.00 | | | 2.13 | 2.30 | 0.02 | 3.20 | 0.31 | 0.03 | | 0.3 |
| 29 | Stearic acid | 0.90 | | | 0.44 | 6.40 | | 1.90 | 0.12 | | | |
| 30 | Tetracosanoic acid | 1.6 | | | | | | | | | | |

| *No* | *Aliphatic Acids* | B | F | AS | SO | D | IS | SH | El | Is-R | S | M |
|---|---|---|---|---|---|---|---|---|---|---|---|---|
| | | % TIC [a] | | | | | | | | | | |
| 31 | Octadecenoic acid | | | | | | | | | 0.04 | | |
| *32* | *Eicosanoic acid* | | | | | | | 0.30 | | | | |
| *33* | *Tetracosanoic acid* | | | | | 8.00 | | | | | | |
| 34 | Hexacosanoic acid | | | | | 2.00 | | | | | | |
| 35 | 2- Hydroxy hexacosanoic acid | | | | | | | 0.40 | | | | |
| 36 | Hydroxyl-octadecenoic acid | | | | | | | | | | | 0.08 |
| 37 | 3,5-Dihydroxy-3-heptenylvaleric acid | | | | | | | | | | 1.8 | 1.12 |
| 38 | 3,5-dihydroxy-3-octenyl valeric acid | | | | | | | | | | 2.0 | |
| 39 | 3,5-dihydroxy-3-octenyl valeric acid isomer | | | | | | | | | | 1.32 | |
| 40 | 3,5-dihydroxy-3-octenyl valeric acid isomer | | | | | | | | | | 6.3 | |
| 41 | Eintriacontenoic acid | | | | | | | | | | 4.62 | 0.03 |

[a] TIC = The ion current generated depends on the characteristics of the compound concerned and it is not a true quantitation.

Four triterpenic acid methyl esters belonging to ursane and oleanane types were identified for the first time in propolis. Ismailia governorate is rich with *Eucalyptus* trees, so these triterpenoids could originate from this plant. Younes *et al.*, isolated some ursonic acid derivatives from the leaves of Egyptian *Eucalyptus rostrata* [33]. Contrary to the propolis sample collected from an *Eucalyptus* forest in Sao Paulo, Brazil investigated by Marcucci *et al.*, which contained aromatic acids and esters and did not contain any triterpenoids [34]. Ismailia (IS) sample contained new triterpenoids to propolis and did not contain any aromatic acids and esters [19].

### *Reclaimed Lands Propolis*

*Is-R* propolis was characterized by high significant amounts of aromatic acid esters (47.3 %) and triterpenoids (17.5%) (Tables 2,3), while (*El*) propolis contained 2.16 % and 2.22%, respectively.

*Is-R* propolis contained five esters for the 4-methoxyhydrocinnamic acid (13.3 %) and 10 esters for hydroferulic acid (33.8 %). These esters appeared to be new compounds, they were tentatively identified from there mass spectra as esters with long chain alcohols: heindecenyl, tridecyl, tridecenyl, tetradecyl, tetradecenyl, pentadecyl, pentadecenyl, hexadecyl and hexadecenyl for the 4-methoxyhydrocinnamic or hydroferulic acids. *El* propolis appeared to have 2.16 % aromatic acid esters, from them two coumarate and two ferulate esters with long chain alcohols.

The *Is-R* propolis was characterized by the presence of a highly significant amount (17.5 %) of the triterpenoids: cycloartinol, cycloartinol isomers, cycloartinol with another double bond and its isomers, α -amyrin, β-amyrin and triterpenes of β-amyrin type.

Although the *El* propolis contained 2.22 % triterpenoids included the presence of new compound to propolis: lanosterol acetate and triterpene of lupane type.

It also contained a triterpene methyl ester (ursane type) and triterpenes of β-amyrin type (Table 3). (*El*) propolis contained a very high significant amount (27.0 %) of the compound; 2,6-bis-(pentanyloxy)- 4-pentanylphenethanol (Table 5).

It also contained the compounds; 2-pentanyloxy- 4-pentenyl phenethanol and tropine alkaloid which are new to propolis. *Is-R* propolis showed the presence of 2,6-bis(t-butyl)-4-(dimethylbenzyl) phenol and 2,4,6-tri(dimethylbenzyl) phenol (Table 5).

Concerning to the presence of aromatic and aliphatic acids in Reclaimed land propolis, it was clear that the (*Is-R*) propolis had no aromatic acids. While the (*El*) propolis contained 3 aromatic acids: 4- hydroxybenzoic acid, 3,4-dimethoxycinnamic acid and caffeic acid [20].

From the above mentioned data it is clear that reclaimed land propolis samples (*Is*-R) *and* (*E*l) possess different chemical composition. The specificity of the two propolis could be explained by the different geographic locations (it has been show earlier that in Egypt the chemical composition of propolis is changed very much with the location site [18,19,31].

As the chemical composition differs according to the geographic location or the type of trees and shrub in the same province (Ismailia) as mentioned above the Ismalia propolis (IS) contained no aromatic acids and esters [19], while in (*Is-R)* (Ismalia propolis; reclaimed land) collected from the same province showed the presence of 15 new aromatic acid esters (47.3 %) and had no aromatic acids. These esters belonged to 4- methoxyhydrocinnamic acid and hydroferulic acid. 4- methoxyhydrocinnamic acid was identified before in European propolis [32,35]. Hydroferulic acid was identified in the Brazilian propolis [36,37], No esters of long chain alcohols for these two acids have been identified before in propolis. So, that is the first time to identify these new esters.

*Is-R* Isamlia propolis (reclaimed land) contained 17.5 % of triterpenoids; mainly cycloartane type, while *(IS)* Isamlia propolis from old valley contained 2.8 % ; mainly triterpenic acid methyl esters of oleanane and ursane types [19]. Phenethyl alcohol was identified in European propolis [38], but that is the first time to identify derivatives from this compound from *El* propolis: 2-pentanyloxy-4-pentenylphenethanol (0.20 %) and 2,6-bis-(pentanyloxy)- 4-pentanylphenethanol (27.0 %).

### *Matrooh Beach and Siwa Oasis Propolis*

*(M)* propolis was characterized by the presence of the following new compounds: 3,5-Dihydroxy-3-heptenyl- valeric acid (Table 4), 3,5-diprenylcoumaric acid (Table 1), three new dihydroferulate esters; 3-pentanyl-octyldihydroferulate, two isomers of 3-hexanyl- octyl-dihydroferulate (Table 2) and two benzofuran lignans (Table 6). It was characterized by the presence of five steroids (pregnane-type, Table 6) and three hydroxy acetophenones (acetophenone-4′-hydroxy, acetophenone-2′-hydroxy and acetophenone-3′-hydroxy, Table 5), all these compounds were identified for the first time in propolis. It was also characterized by the presence of five hydroxy-benzoic acids: 2,4- dihydroxybenzoic acid, 2,6-dihydroxybenzoic acid, 2,3,4- trihydroxybenzoic acid, 2,4,6- trihydroxybenzoic acid and 3,4,5- trihydroxybenzoic acid (Table 1). *(M)* propolis was characterized by the presence of three furanon derivatives (Table 6).

Furofuran lignans (sesamin and isosesamin) were identified in *(M)* sample (first time in Egyptian propolis). Both **(S)** and *(M)* contained no di- and triterpenoids [21].

GC/MS analysis revealed that propolis samples from Siwa oases and Matrooh beach were completely different from that of Dakahlia province (D), where it was of poplar origin.

**Table 5. Other compounds assessed by GC / MS of propolis samples**

| No | Others | B | F | AS | SO | D | IS | SH | EL | Is-R | S | M |
|---|---|---|---|---|---|---|---|---|---|---|---|---|
| | | [a] TIC % | | | | | | | | | | |
| 1 | 2,3- Butanediol | | | | | | | | 0.02 | | | |
| 2 | 2(3H)-Furanone-5-butyl-dihydroxy | | | | | | | | | | | 0.02 |
| 3 | 2(3H)-Furanone-5-hexyl-dihydroxy | | | | | | | | | | | 0.04 |
| 4 | 2(3H)-Furanone-5-heptyldihydroxy | | | | | | | | | | | 0.02 |
| 5 | Glycerol | | 22 | 11.6 | 4.50 | 1.41 | 7.50 | 2.03 | 1.66 | 0.71 | 0.36 | |
| 6 | Phosphoric acid | 2.7 | 0.3 | 1.67 | 0.06 | 0.04 | | 0.07 | 0.06 | | 0.73 | |
| 7 | 2,3-dihydroxy butane | | 0.7 | | | | | | | | | |
| 8 | 1,2,4-trihydroxy butane | | | | 0.02 | | | 0.01 | | | | |
| 9 | 1,2,3-trihydroxy butanal | | 0.6 | 1.41 | 0.36 | | 0.60 | 0.07 | 0.09 | 0.11 | 0.74 | |
| 10 | 1,2,3-trihydroxy butanal (Isomer) | | | | | | 0.01 | | | | | |
| 11 | Eugenol | | | | 0.03 | | | | | | | |
| 12 | Vanillin | | | | | 0.50 | | | | | | |
| 13 | Benzyl-methyl ketone (Insect repellent) | | 11 | | | | | | | | | |
| 14 | Benzyl-2-methyl propyl | | | 0.98 | | | | | | | | |
| 15 | 1,4-Dihydroxy benzene | | | | | 0.06 | | | | | | |
| 16 | 4 –Hydroxy-benzaldehyde | | | | | 0.04 | | | | | | |
| 17 | 4 –Hydroxy-acetophenone | | | | | 0.10 | | | | | | |
| 18 | 3- hydroxy pyridine | | 0.2 | 1.87 | 0.01 | | | | | | | |
| 19 | 1,2-dihydroxy cyclohexene | | | | 0.01 | | | | | | | |
| 20 | 2,4-bis(dimethyl benzyl)-6-t- buty phenol | | | | 0.10 | | 0.04 | | 0.05 | 0.14 | | |
| 21 | 1,8-dihydroxy-3-methy l anthraquinone | | | | 0.10 | | | 1.43 | | | | |
| 22 | *Myristicin* | | | | | | | 0.27 | | | | |
| 23 | Myristicin (isomer) | | | | | | | 0.09 | | | | |
| 24 | Myristicin (isomer) | | | | | | | 0.04 | | | | |
| 25 | 1-Methoxy-1, 3-dihydroxypropane | | | | | | 1.63 | | | | | |
| 26 | Dihydroxyacetone dimer | | | | | | 0.17 | | | | | |
| 27 | 2-Pentanyloxy- 4-pentenyl phen-ethanol | | | | | | | | 0.20 | | | |
| *28* | *2,6-bis-(Pentanyloxy)-4-pentanyl-phenethanol* | | | | | | | | *27.0* | | | |
| 29 | 2,6-bis(t-Butyl)-4-(dimethyl benzyl) phenol | | | | | | | | | 0.04 | | |
| 30 | 2- Ethyl-1,3-dihydroxy-propane | | | | | | | | | 0.01 | | |
| 31 | 2,4,6-Tri(dimethylbenzyl) phenol | | | | | | | | | 0.17 | | |
| *32* | Tropine (alkaloide) | | | | | | | | 0.03 | | | |
| *33* | Acetophenone-4'-hydroxy | | | | | | | | | | | 0.03 |
| 34 | Acetophenone-2'-hydroxy | | | | | | | | | | | 0.02 |
| 35 | Acetophenone-3'-hydroxy | | | | | | | | | | | 0.09 |

[a] TIC = The ion current generated depends on the characteristics of the compound concerned and it is not a true quantitation.

**Table 6. Lignans and Sterols assessed by GC / MS of propolis samples**

| | lignans | B | F | AS | SO | D | IS | Sh | EL | Is-R | S | M |
|---|---|---|---|---|---|---|---|---|---|---|---|---|
| | | [a]TIC % | | | | | | | | | | |
| | ***furofuran lignan*** | | | | | | | | | | | |
| 1 | Sesamin | | | | | | | | | | | 0.13 |
| 2 | Iso sesamin | | | | | | | | | | | 0.01 |
| 3 | Dihydroxy-trimethoxy furofuran lignan | | | | | | | | | | 0.40 | 0.20 |
| | ***Benzofuran lignans:*** | | | | | | | | | | | |
| 4 | Benzofuran dodecenyl dihydrocaffeate | | | | | | | | | | 0.76 | 0.10 |
| 5 | Benzofuran dodecenyl dihydrocaffeate isomer | | | | | | | | | | 4.11 | - |
| 6 | Benzofuran dodecenyl dihydrocaffeate isomer | | | | | | | | | | 3.17 | - |
| 7 | Benzofuran-propyl ferulate | | | | | | | | | | 0.81 | - |
| 8 | Benzofuran –diprenyl dihydrocoumaric acid | | | | | | | | | | 4.62 | 0.03 |
| | ***Sterol*** | | | | | | | | | | | |
| 1 | Sterol ( pregnane type)[M+] m/z = 372 | | | | | | | | | | | 0.45 |
| 2 | Sterol ( pregnane type) [M+] m/z = 460 | | | | | | | | | | | 0.15 |
| 3 | Sterol ( pregnane type) [M+] m/z = 372 | | | | | | | | | | | 0.20 |
| 4 | Sterol ( pregnane type) [M+] m/z = 386 | | | | | | | | | | | 0.60 |
| 5 | Sterol ( pregnane type) [M+] m/z = 386 | | | | | | | | | | | 0.70 |
| 6 | Sterol (cholest- type) [M+] m/z = 458 | | | | | | | | | | | 0.17 |

[a] TIC = The ion current generated depends on the characteristics of the compound concerned and it is not a true quantitation.

Siwa *(S)* sample contained new compounds some of them were tentatively identified by mass fragmentation. Prenylated cinnamic acids, their esters and benzofurans turned out to be a salient chemical feature of Siwa Oasis propolis; diprenyl dihydro-coumaric acids, 3,5-diisopropoxy-nonanyl coumarates, benzofuran lignans and 3,5-dihydroxy-3-octenyl valeric acids which represented about 39.44% as new compounds. It was the first time to identify new prenylated dihydrocoumaric acids and benzofuran lignans from propolis. It was the first time to identify lignan from the furofuran type in Egyptian propolis; it was identified before by GC/MS analysis in Canary Islands propolis [37] and isolated as sasamin [39]. Three lignans from the furofuran type were identified in **(S)** sample, while in Canary Islands propolis 13 furofuran lignans were identified, the plant sources of Egyptian and Canary Islands propolis is still remain unknown. Three hydroxyacetophenones (acetophenone-4′-hydroxy, acetophenone-2′-hydroxy and acetophenone-3′-hydroxy) were identified in Matrooh beach propolis *(M),* other acetophenone derivatives were isolated from Barazilian propolis [40] and benzophenones from Venezuelan propolis [41,42] and from Cuban propolis [43]. Diprenyl coumaric acid, 3-prenyl coumaric acid and other isoprenylated compounds were isolated before from Brazilian Propolis [44-46]. Prenylated cinnamic acids turned out to be a salient chemical feature of green propolis, among them artipillin C had attracted great attention not only for its antimicrobial [47], but also for its cytotoxic activity [48]. Prenylated cinnamic acids might also present as esters [49]. Dihydrobenzofurans were isolated from Chilean propolis had moderate growth inhibitory activity against Mycobacterium avium, M. Tuberculosis and two strains of Staph. aureus [50,51]. Benzofuran derivatives had mild cytotoxic activity against liver-metastatic murine colon 26-L5 carcinoma and human HT-1080 fibrosarcoma cells were isolated from Brazilian propolis [44].

## 2.b. Chemical Composition Assessment with HPLC Analysis

Quantitative comparison of polyphenolic profile of propolis collected from 10 Egyptian governorates was assessed by HPLC analysis. 42 polyphenolic compounds which are characteristics of propolis were identified by comparison with authentic markers (Table 7, concentration mg/g propolis). 13 aromatic acids, esters, alcohols and 29 flavonoids were identified. Six flavonoids were identified for the first time in propolis: Liquiriteginin, 5,7,4'-trihydroxyisoflavone, formonontin, 5,4'-dihydroxy-7- methoxyisoflavone, 7-hydroxy-4'-methoxyflavone and Biochanin A [21,22].

***Upper Egypt Propolis***

*(As)* sample was characterized by the presence of highly significant concentrations of ; caffeic and cinnamic acids (10.16 and 6.14 mg/g propolis), myricetin and luteolin (34.29 and 38.74 mg/ g propolis). Quercetin-3,3'-dimethylether and pinocembrin were highly present in *(As)* sample (10.31 and 22.83 mg/ g propolis respectively). Luteolin-3'-methylether, and acacetin were present with the highly significant concentrations in sample (As) (12.22 and 24.52 mg/ g propolis respectively). Also it has the highest concentrations of quercetin-3-methylether, apigenin quercetin-7-methylether and chrysin (9.35, 7.50, 6.30 and 7.56 mg/g propolis respectively). Hydrocinnamic acid, biochanin A were highly present in *(F)* propolis (4.86, 3.1 mg/g propolis respectively), while quercetin, formonontin, prunetin, galangin were present only in *(F)* propolis. Vanillic acid, kaempferol and quercetin-7,3'-dimethylether were present only in (SO) propolis.

***Nile Delta Propolis***

Hydrocinnamic acid and hydrocaffeic acid were present with highly significant concentrations in samples *(Is)* and *(Sh)* (42.50 and 18.05 and 22.86 and 15.70 mg/g propolis respectively). Naringenin was present with large amount in *(Sh)* sample (14.46 mg/g propolis). Quercetin-3,3'-dimethylether, pinocembrin, formonontin and biochanin A were highly present in *(Sh)* sample (47.05, 39.36, 10.14 and 10.16 mg /g propolis respectively) [22]. Propolis (D) was characterized by the presence of two caffeate estres (dimethylallylcaffeate and phenylethylcaffeate) and 15 flavonoids from which pinobankasin, quercetin-3-methylether, pinocembri, chrysin, pinobankasin-3-acetate, 7-hydroxy-4'-methoxyflavone, galangin, biochanin A and pinostrobin [21,22].

***Reclaimed Lands Propolis***

Sample (El) showed the highest concentration of dimethylallylcaffeate and galangin-7-methylether (31.09 and 10.64 mg / g. propolis respectively). Most of the flavonoids present in (El) and (Is-R) propolis existed in minor quantities [22].

**Table 7. Polyphenolic compounds assessed by HPLC of Egyptian propolis (mg/g propolis)**

| No | Name | F | As | So | D | Sh | Is | El | Is-R | S | M |
|---|---|---|---|---|---|---|---|---|---|---|---|
| *1* | *Hydrocinnamic acid* | *4.86* | *2.38* | *1.27* | *1.72* | *18.1* | *42.6* | *8.88* | *1.00* | | |
| *2* | *Hydrocaffeic acid* | *0.35* | *6.14* | *0.27* | *0.87* | *15.7* | *22.9* | | *0.46* | | |
| *3* | *Cinnamic acid* | *3.47* | *6.14* | | *0.51* | | | *0.24* | *0.06* | | |
| 4 | Vanillic acid | | | 0.12 | 0.13 | | 2.49 | 0.32 | 0.04 | | |
| 5 | Ellagic acid | | 0.32 | | 0.45 | | 0.22 | | | | |
| 6 | Hydrocoumaric acid | | | | 0.12 | | | | | | |
| 7 | 2-Hydroxy-3-methoxybenzyl alcohol | 0.09 | 0.54 | 0.10 | | | 2.44 | | 0.2 | | |
| 8 | Coniferyl alcohol | 0.50 | | 2.06 | 0.58 | 2.79 | | | 0.15 | | |
| 9 | Coumaric acid | | | | 1.41 | | | | | | |
| 10 | Ferulic acid | | 0.56 | | 0.30 | | | | | | |
| *11* | *Caffeic acid* | *0.13* | *10.16* | *0.96* | *0.33* | *1.58* | | *0.31* | | | |
| *12* | *Eriodictyol* | *1.70* | *2.00* | *0.13* | | *4.70* | | | *0.12* | | |
| 13 | Liquiriteginin | 0.13 | | 0.10 | | 1.96 | | | | | |
| 14 | Myricetin | 2.5 | 34.29 | 0.34 | 0.06 | 5.56 | | 0.18 | 0.24 | | |
| 15 | Luteolin | | 38.74 | 0.67 | 0.96 | 3.66 | | | | 1.58 | 0.43 |
| 16 | Quercetin | 0.28 | | | | 1.36 | 0.07 | 0.73 | 0.15 | | 0.10 |
| 17 | Naringenin | 0.17 | | 0.60 | | *14.5* | | | | | |
| 18 | Pinobankasin | 1.82 | 1.19 | 0.80 | 1.48 | 0.83 | | | | | |
| 19 | Quercetin-3-methylether | 0.16 | 9.35 | 0.15 | 1.25 | 1.33 | | 0.53 | 0.08 | | |
| 20 | Genistein | | | | | 1.88 | | | | | |
| 21 | Hesperetin | 0.22 | 2.78 | | | *3.85* | 0.18 | | | 0.32 | |
| 22 | 8-Methoxykaempferol | | 0.17 | | | 0.75 | 0.23 | | 0.44 | | |
| 23 | Apigenin | 0.14 | 7.50 | 0.44 | 0.37 | 1.02 | 0.47 | 0.48 | 0.05 | | 0.07 |
| 24 | Kaempferol | | | 2.00 | | | 0.86 | | 0.47 | 0.19 | 0.40 |
| 25 | Luteolin-3'-methylether | 0.80 | 12.22 | 0.44 | 2.30 | 5.39 | | 3.37 | 0.13 | 0.79 | 0.38 |
| 26 | Kaempferol-3-methylether | | 5.43 | 0.77 | 12.7 | | | | 1.86 | | |
| 27 | Quercetin-3,3'-dimethylether | 1.57 | 10.31 | 0.73 | 1.00 | *22.8* | 0.03 | 0.44 | 0.42 | | 0.40 |
| *28* | *Formonontin* | *5.45* | | *1.73* | *3.44* | *10.2* | | | | *0.50* | *0.82* |
| 29 | Quercetin-7-methylether | 3.23 | 6.30 | 0.61 | 1.18 | 4.56 | | 3.11 | 0.18 | 0.13 | 0.27 |
| 30 | Dimethylallylcaffeate | 1.52 | 13.04 | 5.07 | 5.11 | 2.42 | 0.09 | 31.1 | 1.43 | | |
| 31 | Pinocembrin | 4.22 | 47.05 | 0.79 | 0.89 | 39.4 | 0.03 | | 0.49 | | |
| 32 | Phenylethylcaffeate | | | | 1.89 | | | | | | |
| 33 | Chrysin | 0.51 | 7.56 | | 1.26 | | | | | | |
| 34 | Pinobankasin-3-acetate | 0.78 | | 1.06 | 2.92 | | | | | | |
| 35 | Prunetin | 0.95 | | | | 2.98 | | | | | |
| 36 | Formononetin | | | | 1.15 | 1.82 | | | | | |
| 37 | Galangin | 0.63 | | | 5.00 | | | | | | |
| *38* | *Acacetin* | | *24.52* | | | *7.00* | | *4.84* | *0.41* | *0.18* | |
| 39 | Quercetin-7,3'- | | | 0.17 | | | | | | | |

| No | Name | F | As | So | D | Sh | Is | El | Is-R | S | M |
|---|---|---|---|---|---|---|---|---|---|---|---|
| | dimethylether | | | | | | | | | | |
| 40 | Biochanin A | 3.18 | 0.64 | 1.19 | 3.15 | 10.2 | 0.07 | | 0.70 | | |
| 41 | Pinostrobin | 0.58 | 0.55 | 0.48 | 2.06 | 1.24 | 1.19 | 2.48 | | | |
| 42 | Galangin-7-methylether | | | | | | 0.12 | 10.7 | | | |

, Fayoum; As, Assiut; So, Souhag; D, Dakahlia; Sh, Sharkia; Is, Ismailia; El, El-Saff and IsR, Ismailia reclaimed ; S, Siwa; M, Matrooh.

### *Matrooh Beach and Siwa Oasis Propolis*

*(S)* Propolis showed the highly significant amount of luteolin. Hesperetin and acacetin were only present in this sample. Quercetin was only present in (M) propolis [21].

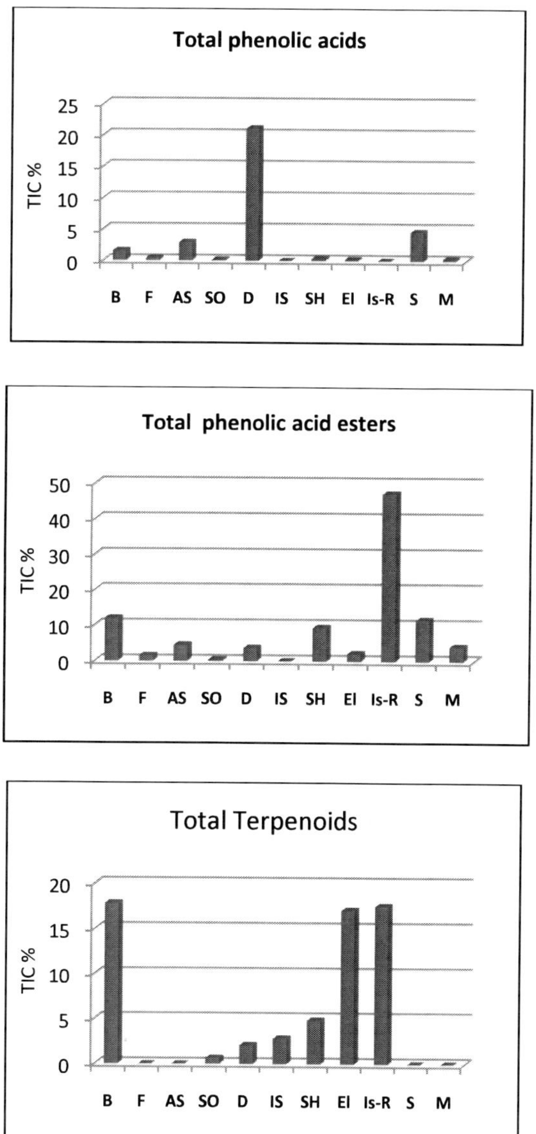


Figure 1. (Continued)

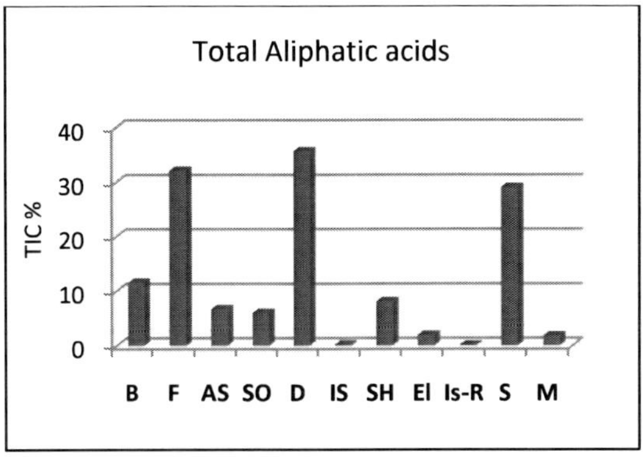
Total Aliphatic acids
TIC %
40
30
20
10
0
B F AS SO D IS SH El Is-R S M

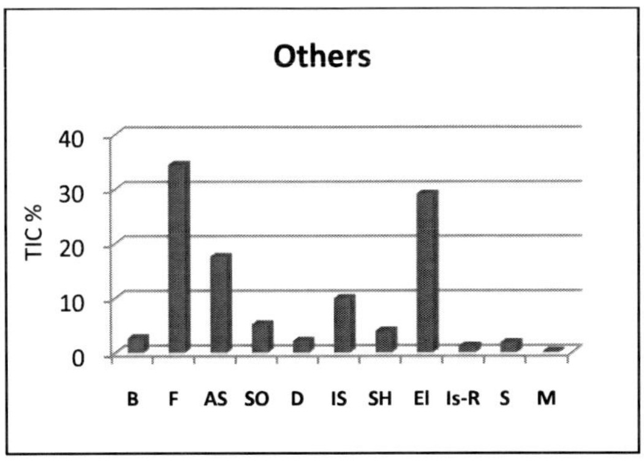
Others
TIC %
40
30
20
10
0
B F AS SO D IS SH El Is-R S M

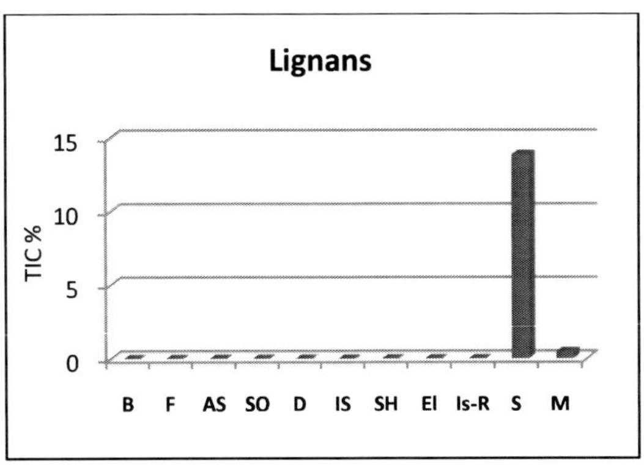
Lignans
TIC %
15
10
5
0
B F AS SO D IS SH El Is-R S M

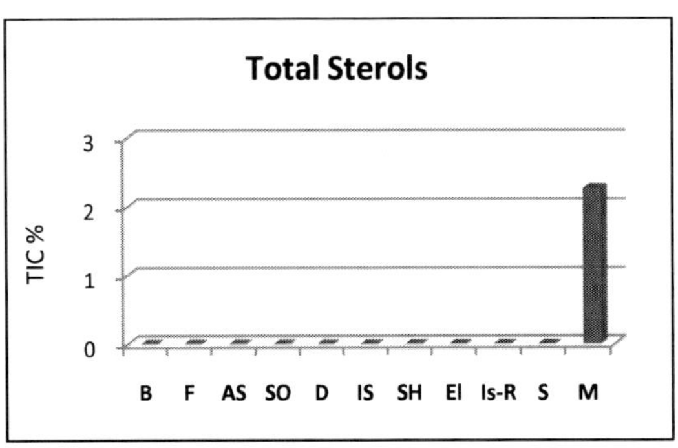
Total Sterols
TIC %
3
2
1
0
B F AS SO D IS SH El Is-R S M

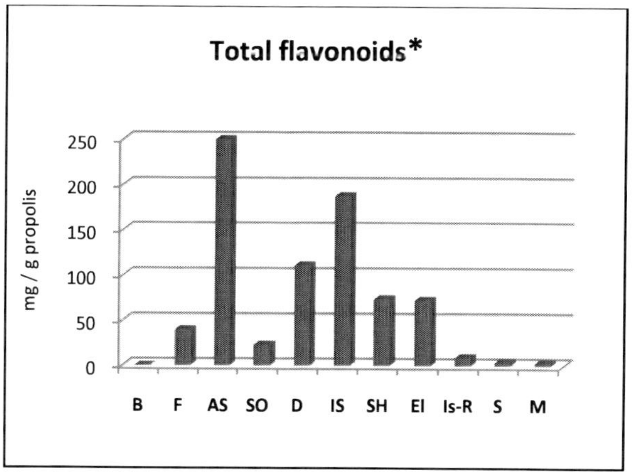


Figure 1. Illustrates the total of each chemical group assessed in propolis samples by GC/MS (TIC% = total ion. current). * Polyphenolic compounds assessed by HPLC of Egyptian propolis (mg/g propolis).

Due to the difference of the Egyptian flora rather than other country's flora from which bees collect propolis, these findings also were observed by Wollenweber and Buchmann who identified in propolis flavonoids typical for leaf exudates of *Ambrosia deltoidea ;* among them 5,7,4'-trihydroxy- 6,8-dimethoxyflavone and sideritiflavone which are also being new for propolis [52].

# 3. Antimicrobial Activity of Egyptian Propolis

## Upper Egypt Propolis

The antimicrobial activity of propolis samples collected from four governorates of Upper Egypt against *Staphylococcus aureus; Escherichia coli,* and *Candida albicans* were recorded in Figure 2.

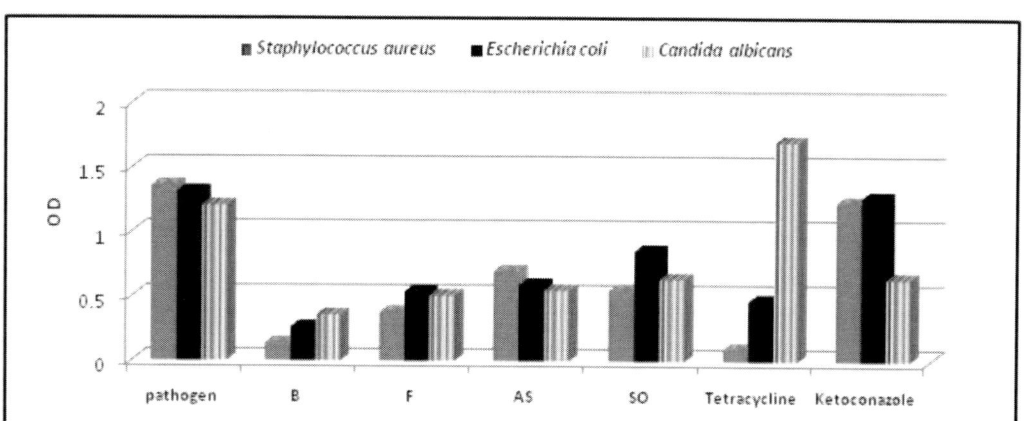


**Figure 2. Antimicrobial activity of Upper Egyptian propolis**

All propolis samples showed inhibition in the growth of all examined bacteria but the inhibition varied according to the propolis origin. It was obvious that propolis collected from Banisweif *(B)* showed the highest antimicrobial activity against *Staphylococcus aureus, Escherichia coli* and *Candida albicans*, while propolis collected from Fayoum province *(F)* had moderate activity against all tested pathogen. Propolis collected from Assiut *(AS)* and Souhag *(SO)* gave lower antimicrobial activity if compared with propolis collected from Banisweif and Fayoum governorates.

The variation in antimicrobial activity seems to be due to the differences in the chemical composition of different propolis samples.

The higher antimicrobial activity of Banisweif propolis probably attributed to the presence of some esters as (isopentenyl caffeate, dimethyl allyl caffeate, benzyl caffeate, dodecyl caffeate, tetradecyl caffeate and tetradecenyl caffeate), triterpenes as (cycloartinol, lanosterol, β-amyrin and triterpene of β-amyrin type) and flavonoids as (pinostrobin, pinocembrin, pinobankasin, pinobankasin-3-acetate, chrysin and galangin) [18].

## Nile Delta Propolis

The antimicrobial activity of propolis collected from three provinces of East Nile Delta, Egypt against *Staphylococcus aureus; Escherichia coli,* and *Candida albicans* (Figure 3). Dakahlia *(D)* propolis had the highest antimicrobial activity against *Escherichia coli* and *Candida albicans*. But Sharkia *(Sh)* propolis had highest antimicrobial activity against *Staphylococcus aureus*. The variation in the antimicrobial activity seems to be due to the variability in the chemical composition of different propolis samples.

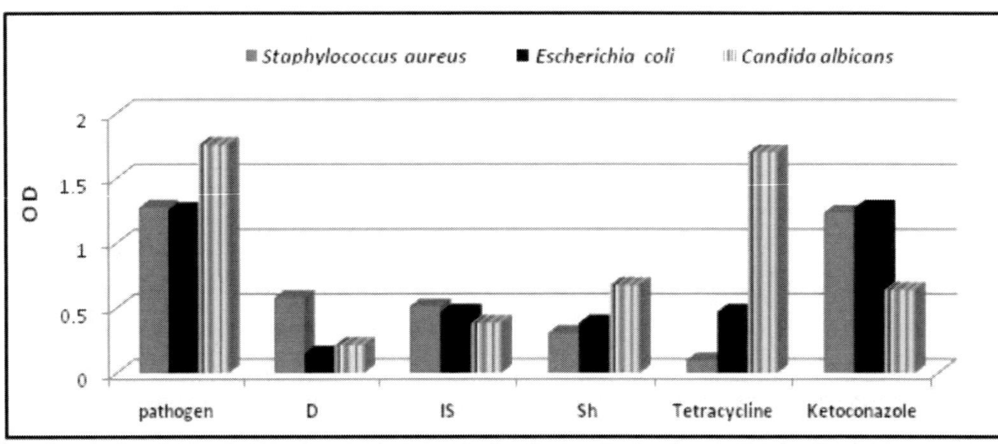


Figure 3. Antimicrobial activity of Nile Delta propolis

The higher antimicrobial activity *(D)* propolis against *Escherichia coli* and *Candida albicans* may be due to the presence of some aliphatic and aromatic acids, eleven caffeate esters, triterpenes as (lupeol, cycloartinol) and flavonoids as (pinostrobin, pinocembrin, pinobankasin, pinobankasin-3-acetate, chrysin, galangin and 5,7- dihydroxy-3-butanoyloxy flavanone). *(Sh)* propolis had the highest antimicrobial activity against *Staphylococcus aureus* probably for the presence of caffeate and di- and triterpenes as (pimaric acid, abietic acid, lanosterol), flavonoids as (pinostrobin chalcone and pinobankasin) and myristicin isomers [19].

## Reclaimed Lands Propolis

The antimicrobial activity of propolis collected from two localities of reclaimed lands, (Egypt) against *Staphylococcus aureus; Escherichia coli,* and *Candida albicans* were recorded in Figure 4. The two propolis samples showed growth inhibition of the examined pathogens but inhibition varied according to the propolis origin. It was clear that propolis collected from *(El)* propolis had the highest antimicrobial activity against *Staph. aureus and Candida albicans*, while *(Is-R)* propolis had the highest antibacterial activity against *Escherichia coli.*

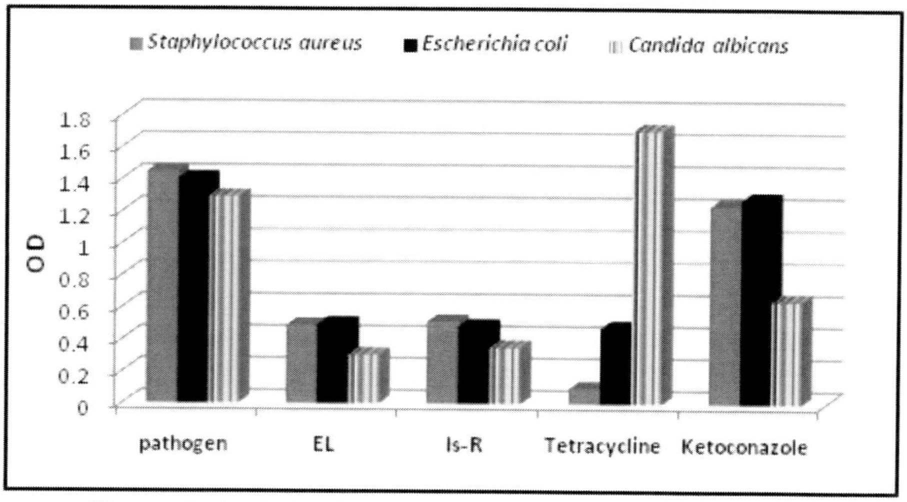


**Figure 4. Antimicrobial activity of Reclaimed lands propolis**

**Table 8. Minimum inhibition concentration (MIC) of different Egyptian propolis samples**

| | *Staphylococcus aureus* | *Escherichia coli* | *Candida albicans* |
|---|---|---|---|
| | MIC (μg/ml) | MIC (μg/ml) | MIC (μg/ml) |
| *Upper Egypt* | | | |
| B | 2600 | 1800 | 1400 |
| F | 3400 | 2300 | 2600 |
| AS | 5400 | 2600 | 2800 |
| SO | 4200 | 3200 | 3200 |
| *Nile delta* | | | |
| D | 3200 | 1200 | 1320 |
| IS | 2800 | 2800 | 1400 |
| Sh | 2400 | 2200 | 3380 |
| *Reclaimed land* | | | |
| EL | 2200 | 1600 | 1420 |
| Is-R | 2600 | 1460 | 1800 |
| Tetracycline (50 μg) | 1000 | 1400 | 4400 |
| Ketoconazole (50 μg) | 5400 | 4600 | 2400 |

The variation in the antimicrobial activity seems to be due to the differences in the chemical composition of different propolis samples. The higher antimicrobial activity of *(El)* propolis to *Staphylococcus aureus and Candida albicans* can probably be attributed to the presence of a very high significant amount of 2,6-bis-(pentanyloxy)- 4-pentanylphenethanol (27 %) and the synergistic effects of the other compounds [20].

The comparison between the activity of different therapeutic agents (against bacteria and fungi) as Tetracycline and Ketoconazole in relation to different propolis samples revealed that the propolis samples were effectively acting to inhibit the pathogens growth. The minimal inhibitory concentration (MIC) of propolis samples was determined by ten-fold dilution in-vitro against *Staphylococcus aureus*, *Escherichia coli* and *Candida albicans,* Table 8 [18-20].

The above mentioned data were in agreement with the findings of *Mohammadzadeh* et al., who found that ethanolic extract of Iranian propolis inhibited the growth of all examined microorganisms including bacteria and fungi with the highest antimicrobial activity against Gram-positive bacteria such as *Staphylococcus aureus* and *Staphylococcus epidermidis* [53]. Popova et al., found that all six Turkish propolis samples investigated were active against the bacterial test strains used; however, samples 1 (Yozgat), 2 (Izmir) and 3 (Kayseri) were more active than samples 4 (Adana), 5 (Erzurum) and 6 (Artvin). All samples were found to contain poplar taxonomic markers but in samples 4 (Adana), 5 (Erzurum) and 6 (Artvin), different substances were observed, which were not present in *P. nigra*L. bud exudates. The results confirm the importance of phenolics for propolis antibacterial activity, and the significance of *P. nigra*L. as a propolis source, which provides the hive with the best defense against microorganisms[54]. Also Kujumgiev et al., (1999) found that all investigated propolis samples were active against the fungal and Gram-positive bacterial strains, and most of them showed antiviral activity. Propolis from the Temperate Zone contains flavonoids and esters of phenolic acids are known to be responsible for antimicrobial activity. Tropical samples did not contain such substances but showed similar activities [55]. The *in vitro* antibacterial activity was verified against several Gram-positive and Gram-negative bacteria and results from synergism between propolis compounds, mainly pinocembrin and galangin flavonoids. Other flavonoids, such as chrysin and kaempferol, have shown antiviral activity with reduction of intracellular proliferation of some viruses, such as herpes simplex [3].

The data included in this chapter confirm the striking variability of the chemical composition of Egyptian propolis and demonstrate the need for further investigation of Egyptian plants possessing resinous exudates as probable source of propolis.

## Matrooh Beach and Siwa Oasis Propolis

The antimicrobial activity of propolis collected from the three localities against *Clostridium oedematiens (Clostridium novyi)* type B were recorded in Figure 5. The three propolis samples showed variable inhibition in the growth of the examined pathogen where it was reduced significantly with *(D)* sample followed by *(S)* and *(M)* propolis samples (0.046, 0.051and 0.060 respectively) if compared with the tested drugs ( 0.730 and 0.095 for Triclabendazole and Tetracycline) respectively. The MIC µg/ml of all different propolis samples was 1000, 2100 and 1600, while it was 2400 and 1100 in Triclabendazole and Tetracycline respectively [21].

It was important to focus on the antimicrobial activity of propolis against *Clostridium oedematiens (Clostridium novyi)* type B, where chronic fascioliasis provided the right environment in the liver for the germination of the spores of the bacterium, *Clostridium novyi* type B, which causes Black disease [56]. It was clear that propolis collected from Dakahlia had the highest antimicrobial activity against *Clostridium oedematiens (Clostridium novyi)* type B. The variation in the antimicrobial activity seemed to be due to the differences in the chemical composition of the different propolis samples. The higher antimicrobial activity of Dakahlia propolis to *Clostridium oedematiens (Clostridium novyi)* type B probably was attributed to the presence of very high significant amount of flavonoids and the synergistic effects of the other compounds. The antimicrobial activity differed according to the differences in the chemical composition [20, 55-58]

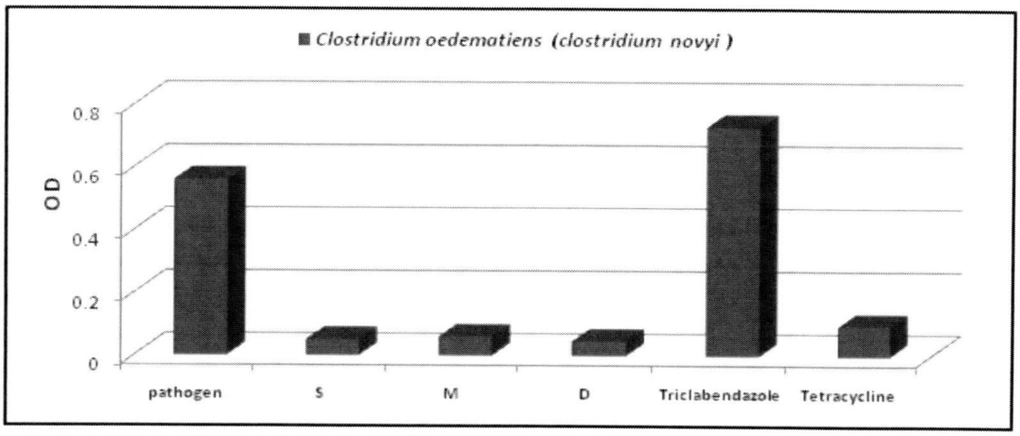


**Figure 5. Antimicrobial activity of Matrooh and Siwa propolis**

# 4. Antiviral Activity of Egyptian Propolis

## The Antiviral Activity against NDV and IBDV Viruses

The antiviral activity of 8 propolis samples was detected by minimum lethal dose on embryonic chicken fibroblasts. The mean tissue culture infective dose fifty ($TCID_{50}$) of Newcastle disease virus *(NDV)* was 3.52X $10^8$/ ml and Infectious Bursal Disease Virus *(IBDV)* was 1.37X $10^9$ (viral particles) / ml (Figures 6 and 7). All propolis samples from different provinces showed reduction in the infectivity mean titers of *NDV* (Figures 6) and *IBDV* (Figures 7). It was obvious that the reduction varied according to propolis origin.

The highest reduction in ($TCID_{50}$) against *NDV* was detected in the case of Dakahlia *(D)* propolis followed by Fayoum *(F),* Assiut *(AS)* and Souhag *(SO)* propolis.

Also the highest reduction was observed in the case of IBDV by Dakahlia propolis followed by El Saff *(EL),* Assiut Souhag and Sharkia *(Sh)* propolis. It was clear that propolis induced variable activities in the inhibitory effect of all viral strains [22].

## The Antiviral Activity against Reo Virus

The minimum lethal dose of the (D), (IS) and (Sh) propolis on embryonated chicken fibroblasts were determined. It is clear that its dilution to 1/100 of the original propolis (100 mg / ml) gave less mortality, no cytopathic effect on chicken embryos fibroblast. The effect of propolis on the infectivity titers as measured by the mean tissue culture infective dose ($TCID_{50}$) of Reo virus is illustrated in (Figures 8). It was clear that the dilution of all propolis samples from different

provinces revealed reduction in the infectivity mean titers of the Reo virus. It was obvious that the reduction varied from propolis sample to another. Ismailia (IS) propolis showed the highest reduction, while (Sh) and (D) propolis showed moderate activity against Reo virus.

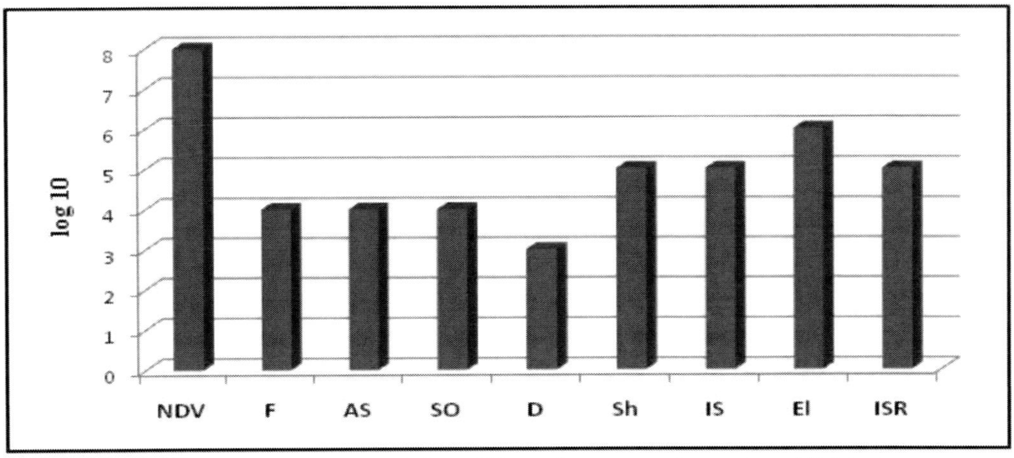


Figure 6. Antiviral activity of Egyptian propolis against NDV virus

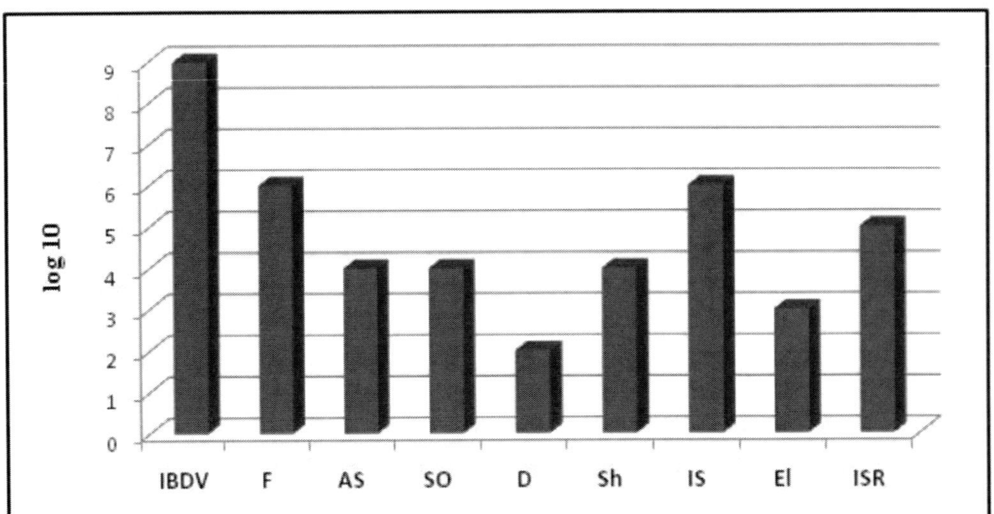


Figure 7. Antiviral activity of Egyptian propolis against IBDV virus

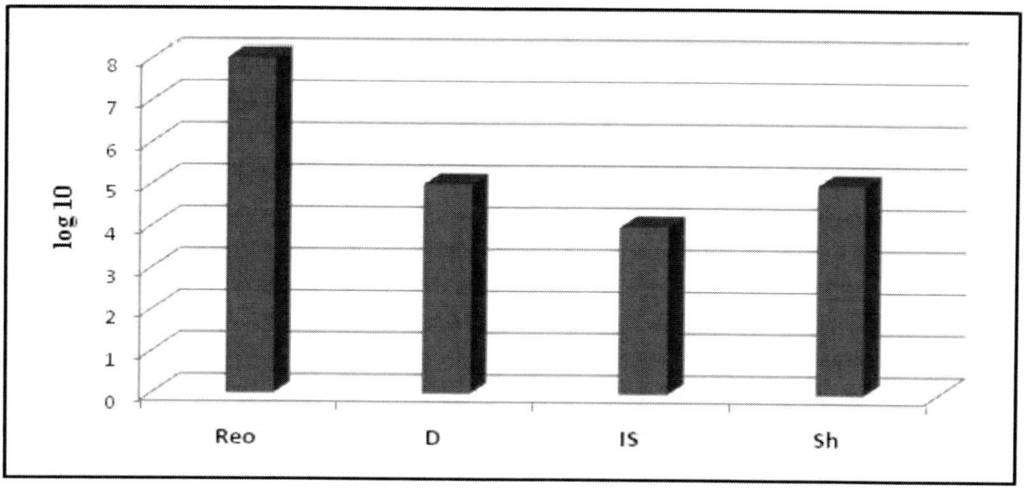


**Figure 8. Antiviral activity of Nile Delta propolis against Reo virus**

Regarding to the inhibitory effect of propolis on replication of NDV, IBVD and Reo viruses, it showed variable inhibitory activity on the mentioned viral strains Similar results were observed previously by Ktivotuchko on small pox vaccine virus [59], Maolova on influenza virus [60], Hegazi on Newcastle disease virus [61],

Amoros on herpes simplex virus [62], Hegazi on rift valley fever virus [63] and Kujumgiev on avian influenza virus [55]. The reduction of the infectivity depends on the chemical composition of different propolis sample collected from the different provinces and confirmed by the chemical analysis (Tables, 1-7).

These findings of the difference in the chemical composition were previously reported as considerable difference in the biological activities [55]. Recently, Schnitzle found that among the compounds they analysed, only galangin and chrysin displayed some antiviral activity. However, the propolis extracts containing many different components exhibited significantly higher antiherpetic effects as well as higher selectivity indices than single isolated constituents. Propolis extracts might be suitable for topical application against herpes infection [64].

## CONCLUSION

Although, the chemical composition is qualitatively and quantitatively variable through the eleven Egyptian propolis samples collected from extremely different areas (Figure 1), most of the Egyptian propolis samples had high antiviral activity against NDV, Reo and IBDV viruses and antimicrobial activity against *Staph. aureus, E. coli. C. albicans* and *Clostridium oedematiens.*

Such comparative studies are extremely valuable with respect to propolis standardization and practical applications in therapy. It is our hope that in the near future their number is going to grow significantly. They will allow scientists to connect a particular chemical propolis type to a specific type of biological activity and formulate recommendations for the practitioners. This could help the general public to make more efficient use of the beneficial properties of propolis with respect to CAM.

## REFERENCES

[1] Abd El Hady FK and Hegazi, AG. Egyptian propolis: 2- Chemical composition, antiviral and antimicrobial activities of East Nile Delta propolis. *Z. Naturforsch,* 2002 57c: 386-394.

[2] Abd El Hady FK, Hegazi, AG and Wollenweber E. Effect of Egyptian propolis on the susceptibility of LDL to oxidative modification and antiviral activity with special emphasis on chemical composition. *Z. Naturforsch,* 2007; 62c: 645-655.

[3] Ackermann T. Fast chromatography study of propolis crudes. *Food Chemistry,* 1991; 42: 135-8.

[4] Aga H, Shibuye T, Sugimoto T, Kurimoto M, Nakagima S. Isolation and identification of antimicrobial compounds Brazilian Propolis. *Biosci. Biotechnol. Biochem.*, 1994; 58: 945-946.

[5] Alcici NMF. Heavy metals in propolis: practical and simple procedures to reduce the lead in the Brazilian propolis. *Chemical Abstracts,* 1996; 127: 236-7.

[6] Almeida EC, Menezes H. Anti-inflammatory activity of propolis extracts: a review. *J. Venom. Anim. Toxins,* 2002; 8: 191-212.

[7] Amoros M, Lurton E, Boustie J, Girre L, Sauvager F and Cormier M. Comparison of anti herpes simplex virus activities of propolis and 3-methyl-but-2-enyl caffeate. *J. Nat. Prod.,* 1994; 57: 644-647.

[8] Bagadi HO and Sewell MM. An epidemiological surveys of infectious necrotic hepatitis (Black disease) of sheep in southern Scotland. *Res. Vet. Sci.,* 1973;15: 49-53.

[9] Bankova V, Christov R, Marcucci C and Popov S. Constituents of Brazilian geopropolis. *Z. Naturforsch,* 1998; 53c: 402-406.

[10] Bankova V, Popov S and Marekov N. Isopentenyl cinnamates From poplar buds and propolis. *Phytochemistry*, 1989; 28: 871-873.

[11] Bankova V. Chemical diversity of propolis and the problem of standardization. *J. Ethnopharmacol*, 2005; 100:114-7.

[12] Bankova VS, Popov SS, Marekov NL. Isopentenyl cinnamates from poplar buds and propolis. *Phytochemistry,* 1989; 28: 871-3.

[13] Banskota AH, Tezuka Y, Midorikawa K, Matsushige K, Kadota S. Two novel cytotoxic benzofuran derivatives from Brazilian Propolis. *J. Nat. Prod.*, 2000; 63: 1277-9.

[14] Banskota AH, Tezuka Y, Prasain J K, Matsushige, K, Saika I, Kadota S H. Chemical constituent of Brazilian propolis and their cytotoxic activities. *J. Nat. Prod.,* 1998; 61: 896-900.

[15] Castaldo S, Capasso F. Propolis, an old remedy used in modern medicine. *Fitoterapia,* 2002, 73, 1-6.

[16] Christov R, Bankova V, Hegazi AG, Abd El-Hady FK and Popov S. Chemical composition of Egyptian propolis. *Z. Naturforsch.,* 1998; 53c: 197-200.

[17] Christov R, Bankova VS, Tsvetkova I, Kujumgiev A, Tejera AD. Antibacterial furofuran lagnans from Canary Islands propolis. *Fitoterapia,* 1999; 70: 89 -92.

[18] Diaz JCQ., Rodrígues OA., Velázquez MD., Miliá NML. Empleo de la tintura de propóleo en la cura de heridas sépticas faciales. *Rev. Cuba Estomatol.*, 1997, 34, 347-51.
[19] Fernandes JA, Sugizaki MF, Fogo ML, Funare SRC, Lopes CAM. *In vitro* activity of propolis against bacterial and yeast pathogens isolated from human infections. *J. Venom. Anim. Toxins,* 1995; 1: 63-9.
[20] Ghisalberti EL. Propolis: a review. *Bee World*, 1979; 60: 59-84.
[21] Greenaway W, English S and Whatley FRS. Phenolic Composition of bud exudates of Populus deltoides. *Z. Naturforsch*, 1990; 45c: 587-593.
[22] Greenaway W, May J and Whatley FRS. Flavonoid aglycone identification by gas chromatography-mass spectrometry in bud exudate of Populus balsamifera. *J. Chromatography.*, 1989; 472:393-400.
[23] Greenaway W, May J, Scaysbrook T and Whatley FRS. Identification by gas chromatography mass spectrometry of 150 compounds in propolis. *Z. Naturforsch.*, 1991; 46c: 111-121.
[24] Greenaway W, Scaysbrook T and Whatley FRS. The analysis of bud exudate of Populus x euramericana, and propolis, by GC/ MS. *Proc. R. Soc. Lond,* 1987; B 232: 249-272.
[25] Greenaway W, Scaysbrook T and Whatley FRS. The composition and plant origin of propolis : A report of work at Oxford. *Bee World.,* 1990; 71: 107-118.
[26] Havsteen BH. The biochemistry and medical significance of the flavonoids. *Pharmacol. Therapeutics*, 2002; 96: 67-202.
[27] Hegazi AG, Abd El Hady FK and Abd Allah FAM. Chemical composition and antimicrobial activity of European propolis. *Z. Naturforsch.,* 2000; 55c: 71-75.
[28] Hegazi AG, Abd El Hady FK and Hatem A. Shalaby. Inhibitory Effect of Egyptian Propolis on Fasciola gigantica Eggs with Reference to its Effect on Clostridium oedematiens and Correlation to Chemical Composition. *Pakistan Journal of Biological Sciences,* 2007; 10: 3295-3305.
[29] Hegazi AG, Awadalla KY and Mansour SM. Influence of honey and propolis on Rift Valley Fever Virus. Proceeding of International Symposium On Apitherapy, Cairo 8-9th, March, 1997; p, 70.
[30] Hegazi AG, El Berdiny F, El Assily S, Khashabah E, Hassan N and Popov S. Studies on some aspects of antiviral activity. 1- Influence of propolis on NDV. *Vet. Med. J. Giza.*, 1993; 41:53-56.
[31] Hegazi, AG and Abd El Hady FK. Egyptian propolis: 1- Antimicrobial activity and chemical composition of Upper Egypt propolis. *Z. Naturforsch,* 2001; 56c: 82-88.
[32] Hegazi, AG and Abd El Hady FK. Egyptian propolis: 3- Antioxidant, antimicrobial activity and chemical composition of propolis from reclaimed land. *Z. Naturforsch,* 2002; 57c: 395-402.
[33] Ktivotuchko VF, Degtyarenko VI, Zaitseva TL and Ganchenko M G. Antiviral effects of propolis. *Vitusy I Virusnye Zabolevaniya*, 1975; 3: 61-64.
[34] Kujumgiev A, Tsvetkova I, Serkedjieva Y, Bankova V, Christov R, Popov S . Antibacterial, antifungal and antiviral activity of propolis of different geographic origin. *J. Ethnopharmacol*, 1999; 64: 235-240.
[35] Kumazawa S, Hamasaka T, Nakayama T. Antioxidant activity of propolis of various geographic origins. *Food Chemistry,* 2004; 84: 329-39.

[36] Maolova NH, Maximova A, Gegova G A, Serlcedjieva Y P, Uzunov ST, Matelcov N Y and Bankova VS. On the antinfluenza action on fractions from propolis. *C. R. Acad. Bulg. Sci.,* 1985; 38: 735-738.

[37] Marcucci M. C., Rodriguez J., Ferreres F., Bankova V., Groto R. and Popov, S. (1998), Chemical composition of Brazilian propolis from Sao Paulo State. *Z. Naturforsch*, 53c, 117-119.

[38] Marcucci MC, Ferreres F, Garca-Viguera C, Bankova V.S, De Castro SL, Dantas A.P, Valente P.H.M, Paulino N. Phenolic compounds from Brazilian Propolis with pharmacological activities. *J. Ethnopharmacology*, 2001; 74: 105-112.

[39] Marcucci MC, Rodriguez J, Ferreres F, Bankova V, Groto R and Popov S. Chemical composition of Brazilian propolis from Sao Paulo state. *Z. Naturforsch.,* 1998; 53c:117-119.

[40] Marcucci MC. Propolis: Chemical composition, biological properties and therapeutic activity. *Apidologie*, 1995; 26: 83-99.

[41] Matsuno T, Jung S.K, Matsumoto Y, Saito M, Morikawa J. Preferential cytotoxicity to tumor cells of 3,5-diprenyl-4-hydroxycinnamic acid (artipillin C). Isolated from propolis. *Anticancer Res.,* 1997; 17: 3565-8.

[42] Menezes H. Própolis: uma revisão dos recentes estudos de suas propriedades farmacológicas. *Arq. Inst. Biol.*, 2005; 72: 405-11.

[43] Mertzner J, Bekemeier H, Paintz M, Schneidewind E. Antimicrobial activity of propolis and its constituents. *Pharmazie*, 1979; 34: 97-102.

[44] Mohammadzadeh S, Shariatpanahi M, Hamedi M, Ahmadkhaniha R, Samadi N, Ostad S N. Chemical composition, oral toxicity and antimicrobial activity of Iranian propolis. *Food Chemistry*, 2007; 103: 1097-1103.

[45] Monti M, Berti E, Carminati G, Cusini M. Occupational and cosmetic dermatitis from propolis. *Contact Dermatitis,* 1983; 9: 163.

[46] Moor WB. Solidified media suitable for the cultivation of clostridium novyi type B. *J. General. Microbiol.,* 1968; 53: 415.

[47] Papay V, Soltesz M, Csizmadia B and Toth L. Chemical and pharmacological study of propolis sample of various locations . *Acta Pharm. Hun.,* 1987; 57: 143-151.

[48] Park YK, Ikegaki M, Abreu JA., Alcici NM. Estudo da preparação dos extratos de própolis e suas aplicações. *Ci. Tecnol. Aliment,* 1998; 18: 313-8.

[49] Park YK, Paredes-Guzman J.F, Aguiar CLSM, Fujiwara FY. Chemical constituents in Baccharis dracunculifolia as the main botanical origin of southeastern Brazilian Propolis. *J. Agric. Food Chem.*, 2004; 52: 1100-3.

[50] Popova M, Silici S, Kaftanoglu O, Bankova V. Antibacterial activity of Turkish propolis and its qualitative and quantitative chemical composition. *Phytomedicine,* 2005; 12: 221-228.

[51] Rubio OC, Cuellar, AC, Rojas N, Castro HV, Rastrelli L, Aquino RA. Polyisoprenylated benzophenones from Cuban propolis. *J. Nat. Prod.*, 1999; 62: 1013-1015.

[52] Salatino A, Teixeira E.W, Negri G, Message D. Origin and chemical variation of Brazilian Propolis. *Evid Based Complement Alternat Med.*, 2005; 2: 33–38.

[53] Schnitzler P, Neuner A, Nolkemper S, Zundel C, Nowack H, Sensch KH, Reichling J. Antiviral activity and mode of action of propolis extracts and selected compounds. *Phytother Res.,* 2010; 1: S20-8.

[54] Sforcin JM, Kaneno R, Funari SRC. Absence of seasonal effect on the immunomodulatory action of Brazilian propolis on natural killer activity. *J. Venom. Anim. Toxins*, 2002; 8: 19-29.

[55] Silici S, Kutluca S. Chemical composition and antibacterial activity of propolis collected by three different races of honeybees in the same region. *J.Ethnopharmacol.*, 2005; 99: 69-73.

[56] Tomas- Barbaran F, Garcia-Viguera C, Vit- Olivier P, Ferreres F, Tomas- Lorente F. Phytochermical evidence for the botanical origin of tropical propolis from Venezuela. *Phytochemistry*, 1993; 34: 191- 196.

[57] Trusheva B, Povova M, Naydenski, H, Tsvetkova I, Rodriguez JG, Bankova V. New polyisoprenylated benzophenones from Venezuela propolis. *Fitoterapia,* 2004; 75: 683-689.

[58] Valcic S, Montenegro G, Timmermann, BN. Lignans from Chilean propolis. *J. Nat. Prod.,* 1998; 61: 771-775.

[59] Valcic, S, Montenegro G, Mujica AM, Avila G, Franzblau S, Singh Maya P, Maiese WM, Timmermann BN. Phytochemical, Morphological and Biological Investigations of propolis from Central Chile. *Z.Naturforsch,* 1999; 54c: 406-416.

[60] Whatley FR, Greenaway W and May J. Populus candicans and the balm of Gilead. *Z. Naturforsch*, 1989; 44c: 353-356.

[61] Wollenweber E and Buchmann S L. Feral honey bees in the Sonoran Desert: propolis soures other than poplars (Populus spp.). *Z. Naturforsch*, 1997; 52c: 530-535.

[62] Wollenweber E, Asakawa Y, Schillo D,Lehmann U and Weigel H. A novel caffeic acid derivative and other constituents of Populus bud excretion and propolis. *Z. Naturforsch,* 1987; 42c: 1030- 1034.

[63] Wollenweber E. Flavonoidmuster als systematisches Merkmal in der Gattung Populus. *Biochem. Syst. Ecol.*, 1975; 3: 35-45.

[64] Youies MG, Amer MS and Sheta AE. Chemical examination of local plants. Part X .VI 9Isolation of α- hydroxyursonic acid from the leaves of Egyptian *Eucalyptus rostrata. Arab Gulf J. Scient. Res.*, 1986; 4: 79-86.

In: Beneficial Effects of Propolis on Human Health ...
Editors: Tahira Farooqui and Akhlaq A. Farooqui
ISBN: 978-1- 62081-440-6


*Chapter 7*

# *MACARANGA TANARIUS*, PLANT ORIGIN OF THE PROPOLIS COLLECTED IN OKINAWA, JAPAN

***Shigenori Kumazawa***
Department of Food and Nutritional Sciences,
University of Shizuoka, Japan

## ABSTRACT

Propolis is a resinous substance collected by honeybees from various plant sources. Poplar and *Baccharis* are well known as the source plants of European and Brazilian propolis, respectively. However, the propolis from Okinawa, Japan, contains some prenylflavonoids not seen in other regions such as Europe and Brazil, suggesting that the plant origin of Okinawan propolis is a particular plant that grows in Okinawa. To identify the plant origin of propolis from Okinawa, Japan, the author observed the behavior of honeybees as they collected material from plants and caulked it inside the hive. Honeybees scraped resinous material from the surface of plant fruits of *Macaranga tanarius* and brought it back to their hive to use it as propolis. The samples of the plant and propolis were collected to compare their constituents by HPLC with a photo-diode array detector (PDA). Their 2,2-diphenyl-1-picryl-hydrazyl (DPPH) radical scavenging activity was also compared. The chemical constituents and radical scavenging activity of the ethanol extracts of the plant did not differ from those of propolis. These results indicate directly that the plant origin of propolis from Okinawa, Japan is *M. tanarius*.

## 1. INTRODUCTION

Propolis, a natural resinous substance collected by honeybees from buds and exudates of plants, is presumably used in the beehive as a protective barrier. Many beneficial biological activities such as antibacterial, antiviral, and anticancer have been reported for propolis [1-3]. For this reason, propolis is extensively used in food and beverages to improve health and to prevent diseases such as inflammation, heart disease, diabetes, and cancer [1-3].

The chemical composition of propolis reportedly depends on the specificity of the local flora at the site of collection [3-5]. Thus, the composition of the plant of origin determines the chemical composition of propolis. Various types of propolis and their plant origins have been studied. It is generally accepted and has been chemically demonstrated that the bud exudates of poplar trees are the main source of propolis in the temperate zone [4]. Thus, European propolis contains the typical 'poplar bud' phenolics such as flavonoid aglycones (flavones and flavanones), phenolic acids and their esters [6]. Poplar trees cannot grow in tropical and subtropical regions. Thus, propolis from these regions has a chemical composition different from that of 'poplar type (poplar bud)' propolis. For example, in the southeast Brazil, there are few poplar trees. In these areas, honeybees have to find other plants as the source of propolis to replace poplar trees [7]. Previously the author reported that the plant origin of Brazilian propolis is *Baccharis dracunculifolia* by the observation of honeybee behavior and phytochemical analysis [8]. Brazilian honeybees collect leaves of this plant and bring it back to their nest to use it as propolis. The main compounds found in the Brazilian propolis were prenylated derivatives of *p*-coumaric acid, acetophenone, diterpenes, lignans and flavonoids. These compounds are different from those in 'poplar type' propolis.

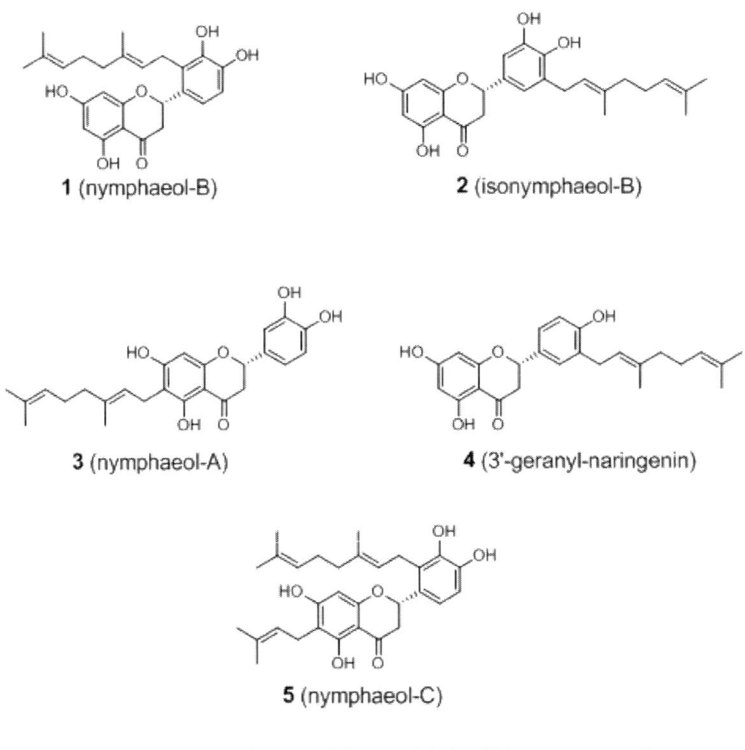


Figure 1. Chemical structures of the main prenylflavonoids in Okinawan propolis.

Our research group has studied the chemistry of not only Brazilian propolis but also the propolis collected in Asian regions such as Japan, Korea, and China [9-11]. Through these studies, we found that the propolis from Okinawa, Japan has constituents not present in propolis from other regions [9]. We isolated and identified several prenylflavonoids with antioxidant activity from this propolis (Figure 1) [12,13]. Okinawa is the southernmost prefecture of Japan and has a subtropical climate. In Okinawa, there are no poplar trees or *Baccharis* plants. Thus, the plant sources of Okinawan propolis are expected to be plants that grow specifically in the region.

The author conducted experiments to identify the plant origin of Okinawan propolis with direct evidence. For this purpose, the behavior of honeybees, *Apis mellifera*, was tracked to determine which plant material they use as the source of propolis. Then the constituents of the plant material and propolis by HPLC with a photo-diode array (PDA) detector were comparatively analyzed. Their 2,2-diphenyl-1-picryl-hydrazyl (DPPH) radical scavenging activity was also compared.

## 2. OBSERVATION OF HONEYBEES

The author used honeybee colonies kept in an apiary in Okinawa, Japan (N26°13′, E127°43′, altitude 76 m), where about 20 hives were located on the rooftop. Various observations were made on 26–29 June 2007.

During research to identify the plant origin of Okinawan propolis, honeybee workers collecting non-food material from the fruits of a certain plant about 500 m east of the apiary were found. Honeybees used their mandibles to scrape the resinous material from the surface of the fruit and made it into a small particle.

They then moved it by their forelegs and pressed it against each of the corbiculae on their hind legs. This series of behaviors on a fruit, from scraping of the surface to packing resinous loads, lasted for several minutes, and bees continued the same behavior on several fruits. This behavior was observed using binoculars and recorded with a digital camera (Figure 2).

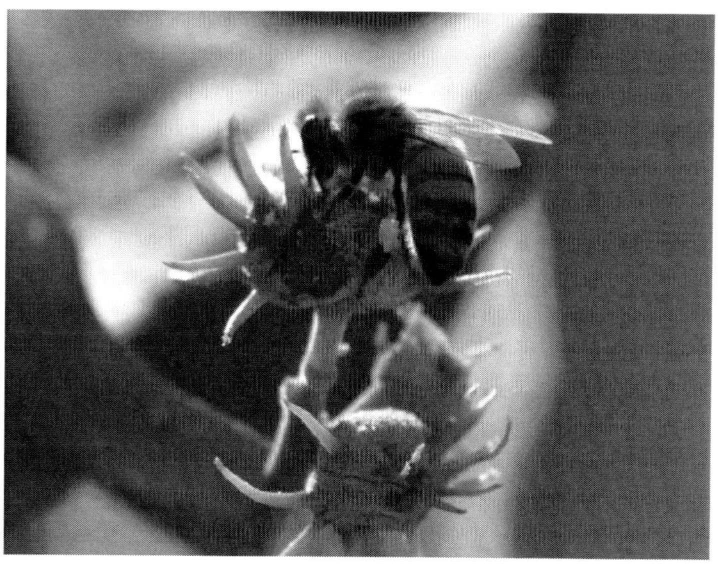

Figure 2. Photograph of a honeybee collecting the surface materials of *M. tanarius* fruit.

The resin collectors inside the hive were also observed. Resin loads brought in were unloaded from the corbiculae by nestmates with mandibles on the comb and frames. Once the worker removed a portion of the resin load, she brought it to the site with cracks requiring caulking, such as cracks in wooden parts and metal meshes covering the ventilation windows of the hive, where similar pieces had already been caulked.

A resin collector with a pollen load sometimes used the resinous material on her mandibles to caulk cracks herself. Honeybee workers collected only resinous material together with the glands on the surface of the fruits and apparently used it as propolis. The plant was sampled after observation. The source plant was identified as *Macaranga tanarius* (L.) Muell. Arg. (Euphorbiaceae).

## 3. HPLC Analysis

The author collected the surface material of *M. tanarius* fruit, which honeybees scraped and packed on their corbiculae (sample **a**), and the propolis from the hive to which a number of resin collectors returned (sample **b**). The samples **a** and **b** were extracted by the following procedure to compare their constituents. One hundred milligrams of the surface material of fruits and propolis were extracted with 5 ml of ethanol at room temperature. After 12 h, extracts were filtered through a 0.45-μm filter prior to injection of 10 μl into an HPLC system with PDA detection. Figures 3**a** and **b** show the HPLC profiles (280 nm) of the extracts. Peaks were assigned by comparing the retention times and UV spectra of authentic compounds isolated previously from Okinawan propolis [13]. The HPLC profiles of samples **a** and **b** showed good correspondence. The existence of five prenylflavonoids, nymphaeol-B (**1**), isonymphaeol-B (**2**), nymphaeol-A (**3**), 3′-geranyl-naringenin (**4**), and nymphaeol-C (**5**) (Figure 1), in both the surface material of *M. tanarius* fruit and propolis, were confirmed.

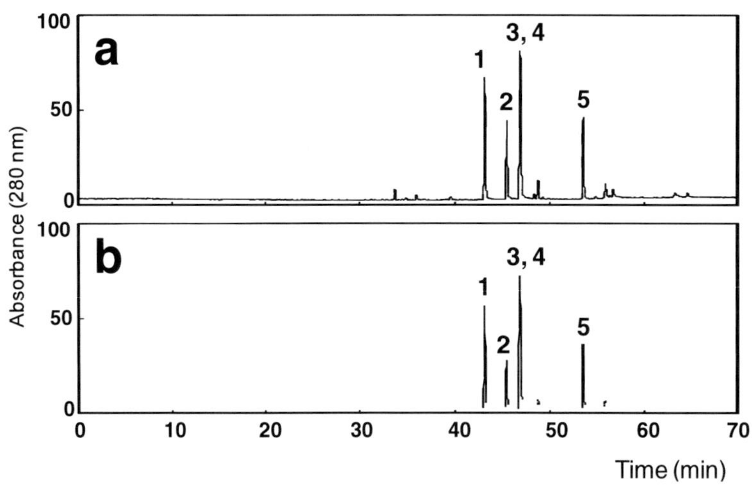


Figure 3. HPLC profiles of the ethanol extracts of the surface materials of *M. tanarius* fruit (a) and propolis (b). Compounds **3** and **4** overlap.

## 4. Radical Scavenging Activity

DPPH radical scavenging activity of the samples **a** and **b** was compared by the following procedure. Reaction mixtures contained 2 ml of ethanol, 125 μM DPPH and a test sample. After 30 min incubation at room temperature, the absorbance was recorded at 517 nm. Control solution contained only ethanol and DPPH. Results were expressed as percentage decrease with respect to control values [14]. The results at 2.0 mg/ml showed that both extracts had potent radical scavenging activity. The activities of the plant and propolis were 91.61 ± 0.28 and 89.80 ± 0.21%, respectively.

## Conclusion and Future Directions

The chemical composition of propolis depends on the specificity at the site of collection and thus on the geographic and climatic characteristics of the site [2]. The author found a new tropical type of propolis from Okinawa, Japan [9,12], and Bankova classified this unique propolis as Pacific propolis [5]. To identify the plant origin of Okinawan propolis, the study of bee behavior in combination with comparative chemical analysis of propolis and plant material was carried out.

Honeybees scraped resinous material from the surface of plant fruits of *Macaranga tanarius* and brought it back to their hive to use it as propolis. The samples of the plant and propolis were collected to compare their constituents and DPPH radical scavenging activity. The chemical constituents and biological activity of the ethanol extracts of the plant did not differ from those of propolis. This indicates directly that the plant origin of propolis from Okinawa, Japan is *M. tanarius*.

There are several reports that the leaves of *M. tanarius* contain prenylflavonoids. Tseng et al. [15,16], Phommart et al. [17], and Guhling et al. [18] isolated the prenylflavonoids nymphaeols-A (**3**), -B (**1**), and -C (**5**) from the leaves of *M. tanarius*. *M. tanarius* is known as a pioneer tree and also as an ant plant. It is defended by ants against herbivores by producing ant-attracting food [19].

This plant can be seen throughout Southeast Asia. In Thailand, a decoction of the root of this plant is drunk as an antipyretic and also as an antitussive [17]. The dried root is used as an emetic agent, whereas the fresh leaves are used to cover wounds as an anti-inflammatory [17]. However, the author first showed that *M. tanarius* is the plant origin of Okinawan propolis.

It is not clear why the honeybees choose this particular plant source. The sticky materials used by honeybees are secreted by plants in order to protect their buds, young leaves and wounded tissues from severe weather conditions and from attack by bacteria, fungi, and viruses. Propolis has similar functions in the hive, and is the main chemical defending the honeybees against infections. The surface material of *M. tanarius* fruit is also thought to be a defensive substance for the plant. In fact, ethanol extracts of the surface material of *M. tanarius* fruit had potent radical scavenging activity similar to propolis, and the prenylflavonoids in the extract had potent antioxidant activity [13], indicating that this surface material is a defensive substance against oxidative stress. It is probable that honeybees, in the course of evolution, found that the particular part of the plant, the surface material of *M. tanarius* fruit, can be used as a source of propolis. The findings that honeybees collected the surface material of plant fruits as the source of propolis are interesting with respect to the ecology of honeybees. Further studies on the biological activities of this interesting plant, *M. tanarius*, are needed.

## ACKNOWLEDGMENTS

The author thanks Mr. Tsutomu Aragaki (Aragaki Beefarm Inc., Okinawa, Japan) for providing his apiary for the research. This work was supported by the Program for Creating Okinawa Innovation of Cabinet Office, Government of Japan and a Grant-in-Aid for Scientific Research of the Japan Society for the Promotion of Science (JSPS).

## REFERENCES

[1] Ahn MR, Kumazawa S, Hamasaka T, Bang KS, Nakayama T. Antioxidant activity and constituents of propolis collected in various areas of Korea. *Journal of Agricultural and Food Chemistry*, 2004; 52: 7286-7292.

[2] Ahn MR, Kumazawa S, Usui Y, Nakamura J, Matsuka M, Zhu F, Nakayama T. Antioxidant activity and constituents of propolis collected in various areas of China. *Food Chemistry*, 2007; 101: 1400-1409.

[3] Bankova V, de Castro SL, Marcucci MC. Propolis: recent advances in chemistry and plant origin. *Apidologie*, 2000; 31: 3-15.

[4] Bankova V, Popova M, Bogdanov S, Sabatini AG. Chemical composition of European propolis: Expected and unexpected results. *Zeitschrift für Naturforschung*, 2002; 57c: 530-533.

[5] Bankova V. Chemical diversity of propolis and the problem of standardization. *Journal of Ethnopharmacology*, 2005; 100: 114-117.

[6] Bankova V. Recent trends and important developments in propolis research. *Evidence-based Complementary and Alternative Medicine*, 2005; 2: 29-32.

[7] Burdock GA. Review of the biological properties and toxicity of bee propolis (propolis). *Food and Chemical Toxicology*, 1998; 36: 347-363.

[8] Guhling O, Kinzler C, Dreyer M, Bringmann G, Jetter R. Surface composition of myrmecophilic plants: Cuticular wax and glandular trichomes on leaves of *Macaranga tanarius*. *Journal of Chemical Ecology*, 2005; 31: 2323-2341.

[9] Hamasaka T, Kumazawa S, Fujimoto T, Nakayama T. Antioxidant activity and constituents of propolis collected in various areas of Japan. *Food Science and Technology Research*, 2004; 10: 86-92.

[10] Heil M, Koch T, Hilpert A, Fiala B, Boland W, Linsenmair K. Extrafloral nectar production of the ant-associated plant, *Macaranga tanarius*, is an induced, indirect, defensive response elicited by jasmonic acid. *Proceedings of the National Academy of Sciences of USA*, 2001; 98: 1083-1088.

[11] Kumazama S, Taniguchi M, Suzuki Y, Shimura M, Kwon M-S, Nakayama T. Antioxidant activity of polyphenols in carob pods. *Journal of Agricultural and Food Chemistry*, 2002; 50: 373-377.

[12] Kumazawa S, Goto H, Hamasaka T, Fukumoto S, Fujimoto T, Nakayama T. A new prenylated flavonoid from propolis collected in Okinawa, Japan. *Bioscience, Biotechnology, and Biochemistry*, 2004; 68: 260-262.

[13] Kumazawa S, Ueda R, Hamasaka T, Fukumoto S, Fujimoto T, Nakayama T. Antioxidant prenylated flavonoids from propolis collected in Okinawa, Japan. *Journal of Agricultural and Food Chemistry*, 2007; 55: 7722-7725.

[14] Kumazawa S, Yoneda M, Shibata I, Kanaeda J, Hamasaka T, Nakayama T. Direct evidence for the plant origin of Brazilian propolis by the observation of honeybee behavior and phytochemical analysis. *Chemical and Pharmaceutical Bulletin*, 2003; 51: 740-742.

[15] Marcucci MC, Bankova V. Chemical composition, plant origin and biological activity of Brazilian propolis. *Current Topics in Phytochemistry*, 1999; 2: 115-123.

[16] Phommart S, Sutthivaiyakit P, Chimnoi N, Ruchirawat S, Sutthivaiyakit S. Constituents of the leaves of *Macaranga tanarius*. *Journal of Natural Products*, 2005; 68: 927-930.

[17] Salatino A, Fernandes-Silva CC, Righi AA, Salatino MLF. Propolis research and the chemistry of plant products. *Natural Product Reports*, 2011; 28: 925-936.

[18] Tseng MH, Chou CH, Chen YM, Kuo YH. Allelopathic prenylflavanones from the fallen leaves of *Macaranga tanarius*. *Journal of Natural Products*, 2001; 64: 827-828.

[19] Tseng MH, Kuo YH, Chen YM, Chou CH. Allelopathic potential of *Macaranga tanarius* (L.) Muell.-Arg. *Journal of Chemical Ecology*, 2003; 29: 1269-1285.

In: Beneficial Effects of Propolis on Human Health ... ISBN: 978-1- 62081-440-6
Editors: Tahira Farooqui and Akhlaq A. Farooqui 

*Chapter 8*

# ARGENTINE PROPOLIS: FLAVONOID AND CHALCONE CONTENT AND ITS RELATION WITH THE FUNCTIONAL PROPERTIES

***María Inés Isla, María Inés Nieva Moreno, Iris Catiana Zampini, Eliana Solórzano, Fatima Carolina Danert, Ana Salas, Nancy Vera, Jorge Sayago, Enrique Bedascarrabure, Luis Maldonado and Roxana Mabel Ordoñez***

Instituto de Química del Noroeste Argentino (INQUINOA), CONICET-UNT; INTA Famailla, Argentina

## ABSTRACT

In recent years, there has been a renewed interest in Argentina about the chemical composition and biological properties of Argentinean propolis, a resinous material collected by the honey bee that can be regarded as a potential natural source of bioactivity in folk medicine and in the food industry. Argentina has a diverse climate that is evidenced in multiple phytogeographical regions. Hence, propolis from the Northwest, West, Center and South of Argentina would have different chemical compositions and consequently, different biological properties. Furthermore, propolis quality is intimately related to harvesting time and methods, and storage tasks performed by the beekeper.

Various studies have shown that the propolis from Argentina contains a high level of polyphenolic compounds, principally, flavonoids and its derivates, phenolic acid and lignans. Antibacterial, antifungal, antioxidant, free radical scavenging and antimutagenic activities were demonstrated in propolis from different Argentinean regions (provinces of Catamarca, Chaco, Entre Rios, Jujuy, Mendoza, Misiones, Rio Negro, Salta, San Juan, Santiago del Estero and Tucumán). It has recently been reported that the chemical components responsible for some of the functional properties of Argentinean Northwest propolis are flavonoids, principally chalcones and flavones, with different degrees of hydroxylation and methoxylation while the principal bioactive components in the propolis from the province of San Juan are lignans and flavonoids.

The findings on the bioactivity and chemical composition of Argentinean propolis support its potential use in functional food and complementary medicine.

## INTRODUCTION

Propolis (bee glue) is a natural product bees make by collecting resin and other substances from some plants and trees. Much of the current literature concerning propolis has focused on its chemical constituents, biological activity and botanical origin (Banskota et al., 2001; Bankova et al., 2008). Preparations containing propolis have been used to treat human diseases for centuries. It has been proven to possess a wide range of biological activities such as an antimicrobial (antibacterial, antifungal and antiviral), anti-inflammatory, anti-tumor and antioxidant substances due to different propolis constituents (Banskota et al., 2001; Isla et al., 2001; 2005; 2009). The chemical composition of propolis is highly variable and depends mainly on botanical origin (Bankova et al., 2000). For this reason, numerous studies led to differentiation of two propolis groups with a completely different chemistry: propolis from temperate regions and propolis from tropical regions. As the bee glue from different tropical regions is chemically diverse, different phenolics, prenylated p-coumaric acid, flavonoids and benzophenones, and terpenes have been found (Kumazawa et al., 2008; Bankova et al., 2008). In tropical climates, honey bees collect resins from *Clusia minor* and *Clusia rosea* flowers (Tomás Barberán et al., 1993; Cuesta-Rubio et al., 1999) and from *Baccharis dracuncufolia* (alecrim plants) (Kumazawa et al., 2004). Recently, a leguminous species (*Dalbergia* sp.) has also been identified as a common source in tropical regions (Silva et al., 2008). Propolis samples originating from temperate zones are characterized by a similar composition, being the main constituents biologically active phenolic compounds like flavonoids, aromatic acids and their esters (Bankova et al., 2008), and the plant sources are *Populus* sp., mainly *Populus nigra* and their hybrids (Bankova et al., 2000; 2006; Markham et al., 1996; Salatino et al., 2005). However, it is clear that other trees, like pine, birch, elm, alder, beech and horse-chestnut species, are adequate resin sources, particularly when poplar species are unavailable (Crane, 1990). Additionally, honey bees in Uganda appear to forage for resins selectively on *Alnus* sp. and can actually defoliate these trees; whether there are other possible sources in the region remains unclear (Nyeko et al., 2002).

Honeybees will forage for resins from droplets appearing on the bark of the trunks or limbs of trees, from the surfaces of some fruits (i.e. *Macaranga tanarius*; Kumazawa et al., 2008), or more typically on the vegetative apices (buds, leaf primordia and young leaves).

Thus, characterization of propolis from different areas is necessary to assess its pharmacological properties as well as the natural compounds involved in such disease-preventing activity.

## PROPOLIS IN ARGENTINA

A cluster of public institutions (Ministerio de Ciencia, Tecnología e Innovación Productiva, Universidad Nacional de Tucumán, Universidad Nacional de Jujuy, INTA-Famaillá), beekeepers and government, have been working together in the characterization of Argentinean hive products to obtain differentiated products. Since propolis chemical composition depends on the phytogeographic characteristics of the site of collection and Argentina has a wide biodiversity, propolis obtained in different regions (Northwest, Northeast, Cuyo, Center and Patagonia) at different times of the year were characterized from the physicochemical point of view (Maldonado, 2000). The analytical methodology was developed and the production methods were evaluated (Bedascarrasbure et al., 2000a, 2000b, 2004, 2006). With this information, IRAM-INTA15935-1 and -2 regulations applicable to raw propolis and extracts were developed and propolis has been incorporated since May 2008 into the Argentine Food Code as a dietary supplement by decission of the Secretaría de Agricultura, Ganadería, Pesca y Alimentos and the Ministerio de Salud.

Different techniques were used to determine the chemical profile of bioactive compounds in Argentine propolis: HPLC-DAD, HPLC-MS, RMN and GC–MS. Quantifications of total phenolics, total flavons/ flavonols and total flavanones/dihydroflavonols were used as a measure for the active principles (Isla et al., 2005; Vera et al., 2011). Because of the chemical variability of propolis, our study was not limited to a single specimen in each area. In addition, the studies on biological activities were realized using different experimental models.

## Propolis from Northwestern Argentina

### *Chemical Composition*

Isla and co-workers (2005) reported the chemical composition of northern argentine propolis (Tucumán, Santiago del Estero, Salta, Chaco and Catamarca). The samples analyzed showed a phenolic content ranging from 35 to 358 mg GAE/g of propolis (Table 1). The phenolic constituents were identified in ethanolic extract by HPLC with a photodiode array (PDA) detector and coumaric acid, ferulic acid, cinnamic acid, pinobanksin, quercetin, kaempferol, apigenin, pinocembrin, 1,1, dimethylalylcaffeic acid, chrysin, galangin, kaempferide and tectochrysin (Isla et al., 2005; Chaillou and Nazareno, 2009) were identified. The presence of coumaric acid, ferulic acid and apigenin (Isla et al., 2005) was demonstrated in Chaco propolis. In the same year, Nieva Moreno and co-workers isolated and identified 2'4' dihydroxychalcone (13 mg/g of propolis) in propolis from an arid region of Tucuman (Amaicha del Valle). The compound showed antibacterial activity against methicillin-resistant *Staphylococcus aureus* (MRSA). It also proved to be cytotoxic ($LC_{50}$ values of 0.5 μg/mL), but it was not genotoxic or mutagenic. Furthermore, this compound was able to inhibit IQ mutagenicity ($ID_{50}$ values of 1 μg/plate) but was unable to inhibit NPD mutagenicity (Nieva Moreno et al., 2005). Agüero and co-workers, confirmed the presence of 2', 4'-dihydroxychalcone and isolated 2',4'-dihydroxy-3'-methoxychalcone in Tucumán propolis (Amaicha del Valle) later. The authors demonstrated that both compounds displayed strong activity against clinical isolates of *Trichophyton rubrum* and *T. mentagrophytes* (MICs and MFCs between 1.9 and 2.9 μg/ml) (Aguero et al., 2010). It has recently been demonstrated that the main bioactive compounds of Catamarca propolis (Monte phytogeographic region), are 2',4'-dihydroxy-3-methoxychalcone, 2', 4'-dihydroxychalcone, 2',4',4-trihydroxy-6'-methoxychalcone, 5 hydroxy- 4',7 dimethoxy flavone, *4',5-dihydroxy-3,7,8-trimethoxyflavone and* **7-** hidroxy- 5, 8- dimethoxyflavone (Figure 1), (Vera et al., 2011).

**Table 1. Collection sites, total polyphenol and flavonoid content of propolis ethanolic extracts**

| | Collection site | Total polyphenol (mg GAE.$g^{-1}$ of propolis) | Flavonoid (mg QE. $g^{-1}$ of propolis) |
|---|---|---|---|
| Cuyo | Mendoza | 181-348<br>Kumazawa et al., 2010<br>Lozina et al., 2010 | 106-255<br>Kumazawa et al., 2010 |
| | San Juan | 227-363<br>Isla et al., 2009 | 116-238<br>Isla et al., 2009 |
| | Rio Negro | 244.5-290<br>Kumazawa et al., 2010 | 93.7-290<br>Kumazawa et al., 2010 |
| Center-South | La Pampa | 14.3-215.2<br>Kumazawa et al., 2010 | 0-65<br>Kumazawa et al., 2010 |
| | Entre Rios | 72.4-171.1<br>Kumazawa et al., 2010 | 29-100<br>Kumazawa et al., 2010 |
| North | Tucumán | 32-358<br>Isla et al., 2005<br>Nieva Moreno et al., 2000<br>Isla et al., 2001 | 120-200<br>Isla et al., 2005<br>Nieva Moreno et al., 2000<br>Isla et al., 2001 |
| | Catamarca | 200-330<br>Isla et al., 2005<br>Vera et al., 2011 | 212<br>Isla et al., 2005<br>Vera et al., 2011 |
| | Santiago del Estero | 42-288<br>Isla et al., 2005<br>Chaillou and Nazareno, 2009<br>Lozina et al., 2010 | 0.48-30<br>Chaillou and Nazareno, 2009<br>Lozina et al., 2010 |
| | Salta | 101-210<br>Isla et al., 2005 | Not reported |
| | Chaco | 10.9-145<br>Lozina et al., 2010<br>Isla et al., 2005 | 0.12-3.87<br>Lozina et al., 2010 |
| | Corrientes | 1.43-103<br>Lozina et al., 2010 | 0.79-1.51<br>Lozina et al., 2010 |

All of these compounds displayed activity against clinical isolates of MRSA ($MIC_{50}$ 10 μg/ml) and antioxidant activity on $ABTS^{\bullet +}$ ($SC_{50}$ values of 20 μg/ml). According to our results, a new biologically active natural compound was detected in propolis from Northern Argentina, principally in some regions of Tucumán and Catamarca.

Recently, 2',4',4-trihydroxy-chalcone (isoliquiritigenin) was identified in Brazilian red propolis and it was active against *Staphylococcus aureus*, *Streptococcus mutans*, and *Actinomyces naeslundii* with MIC values from 15.6 to 62.5 μg/ml (Oldoni et al., 2011).

Up to now, no chalcones have been reported in propolis from other Argentinean regions.

## Biological Activities

Propolis samples from Salta (600 meters above sea level, masl), Tucumán (600 to 1700 masl), Santiago del Estero (100 masl) and Catamarca (1300 masl) have been characterized, in previous works for their biological properties. All of the Argentinean regions mentioned above are phytogeographically and altitudinally different.

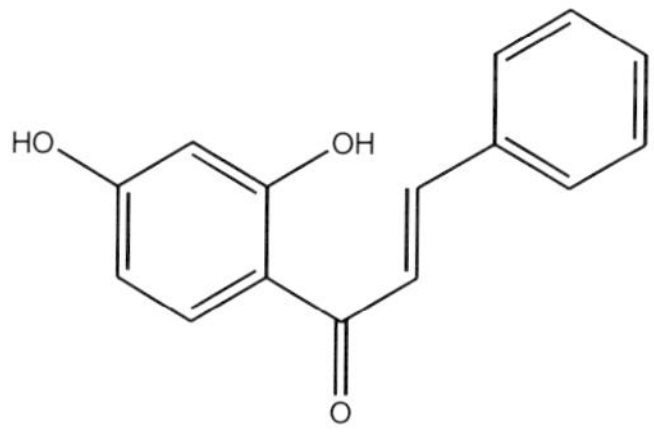


2’, 4’-dihydroxychalcone

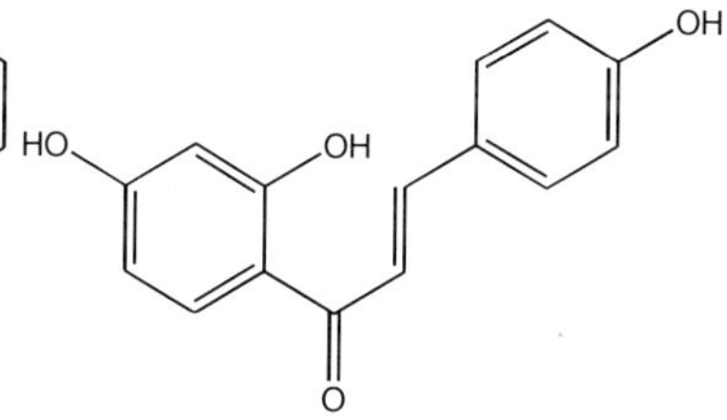


2’,4’,4-trihydroxychalcone

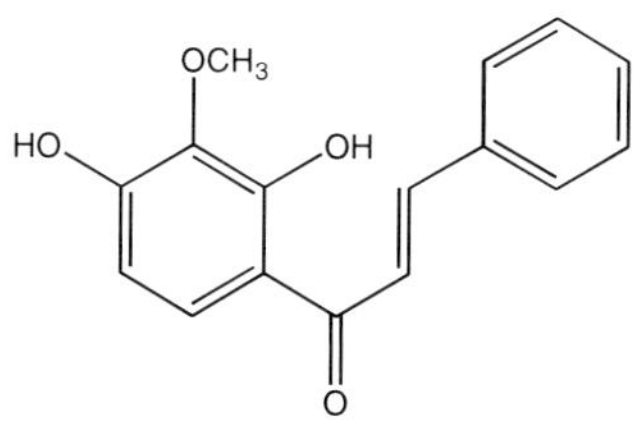


2’,4’-dihydroxy-3-methoxychalcone

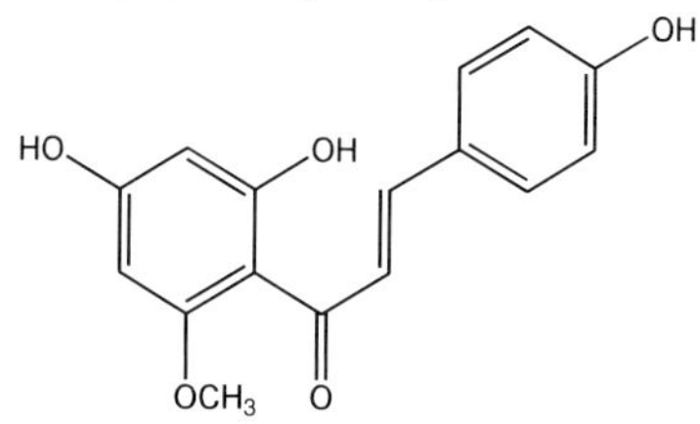


2’,4’,4-trihydroxy-6’- methoxychalcone.

Figure 1. Chalcones isolated from propolis of Northern Argentine.

All Tucumán propolis samples showed antibacterial activity against MRSA (Nieva Moreno et al., 1999) and phytopathogenic bacteria (Ordoñez et al., 2011). They also proved to have free radical-scavenging (Nieva Moreno et al., 2000; Isla et al., 2005), antioxidants (using the assay of the oxidation of lipid in unfractionated serum), antimutagenicity (Isla et al., 2001, Nieva Moreno et al., 2005) and antifungal activities (Quiroga et al., 2006; Agüero et al., 2010).

Vera et al., 2011 have demonstrated antibacterial and antioxidant activities for propolis collected from *Rincón,* in the beekeeping production area of the province of Catamarca (Monte phytogeographical region, Prepuna), at high altitude (1300 masl) and arid and dry climatic conditions.

Antibacterial and antioxidant activities were also demonstrated in the ethanolic extracts from Santiago del Estero (samples collected in seven places from the center of Santiago del Estero province) (Isla et al., 2005). These results were confirmed by Chaillou and Nazareno, 2009.

## Botanical Origin

*Zuccagnia punctata* Cav. has been assigned as the botanical origin of propolis from Amaicha del Valle, Tucumán (Gurini et al., 2004; Zampini et al., 2004; Agüero et al., 2010).

## Propolis from Cuyo Region

### *Chemical Composition*

The chemical characterization, as well as the assessment of the geographical origin of propolis from different districts of the San Juan province, was reported (Lima et al., 2009).

Six main flavonoids were isolated, identified and quantified from the propolis samples: the flavanones 7-hydroxy- 8-methoxyflavanone, pinocembrin, and pinobanksin, the flavones chrysin and tectochrysin, and the flavonol galangin (Lima et al., 2009; Isla et al., 2009). Other authors identified lignans (3´-methyl-nordihydroguaiaretic acid and nordihydroguaiaretic acid) in samples from the mountain valleys of Iglesia and Calingasta (province of San Juan) (Agüero et al., 2011).

Caffeic acid, ferulic acid and caffeic acid phenethyl ester as well as the flavonoids pinocembrin, chrysin, galangin and tectochrysin (Kumazawa et al., 2010) were detected in ethanolic extracts of propolis from Mendoza and Rio Negro. These components are similar to those identified by Isla et al. in propolis from northwestern Argentina in 2005.

### *Biological Activities*

The effect of seasonal variations and harvesting form on the chemical parameters and antioxidant capacity of propolis samples of hives from Calingasta (San Juan) was determined (Isla et al., 2009). Those obtained from October to December showed the highest antioxidant activity. Flavones and flavonol content of each analyzed extract showed a positive correlation with antioxidant activity. Galangin, a major flavonol in propolis samples, protected against linoleic acid peroxidation suggesting that galangin can play a role in the antioxidant activity of propolis extracts from San Juan in a synergistic effect with other compounds (Isla et al., 2009). Also, propolis from San Juan was active against different fungi (Agüero et al., 2011).

The propolis from Mendoza and Rio Negro also showed antioxidant activity (Kumazawa et al., 2010).

## Botanical Origin

Two plant species (*Baccharis* sp, and *Larrea nitida*) have been assigned as the botanical origin of San Juan propolis (Isla et al., 2009; Agüero et al., 2011).

## Propolis from Entre Rios and La Pampa (Center-South of Argentina)

### *Chemical Composition and Biological Activity*

Caffeic acid, ferulic acid and caffeic acid phenethyl ester as well as the flavonoids, pinocembrin, chrysin, galangin and tectochrysin were detected in the ethanolic extract of propolis from Entre Rios (Kumazawa et al., 2010). These components are similar to those identified by Isla et al. in propolis from northwestern Argentina in 2005.

Free radical scavenging activity was demonstrated in all samples of Entre Rios propolis. No flavonoids were detected in samples from La Pampa propolis and antioxidant activity was not confirmed (Kumazawa et al., 2010).

## References

Agüero, M.B., González, M., Lima, B., Svetaz, L., Sanchez, M., Zacchino, S., Feresin, G., Schmeda-Hirschmann, G., Palermo, J., Wunderlin, D., Tapia, A. (2010) Argentinean propolis from *Zuccagnia punctata* Cav. (Caesalpinieae) exudates: Phytochemical characterization and antifungal activity. *Journal of Agriculture and Food Chemistry*, 58, 194–201.

Agüero, M.B., Svetaz, L., Sánchez, M., Luna, M., Lima, B., López, M., Zacchino, S., Palermo, J., Wunderlin, D., Feresin, G., Tapia, A. (2011) Argentinean Andean propolis associated with the medicinal plant *Larrea nitida* Cav. (Zygophyllaceae). HPLC–MS and GC–MS characterization and antifungal activity. *Food and Chemical Toxicology*, 49, 1970-1978.

Bankova, V., Marcucci, M. (2000). Standardization of propolis. Present status and perspectives. *Bee World*, 81, 182-183.

Bankova, V., Popova, M., Trusheva, B. (2006) Plant sources of propolis: an update from a chemist's point of view. *Natural Product Communications*, 1, 1023-1028.

Bankova, V., Trusheva, B., Popova, M. (2008). New developments in propolis chemical diversity studies (since 2000). In Ethnomedicine 1–13, Orsolich N, Basic I. (Eds). Transworld Research Network, Trivandrum.

Banskota, A.H., Tezuka, Y., Kadota, S. (2001) Recent progress in pharmacological research of propolis. *Phytoteraphy Research* 15, 561-571.

Bedascarrasbure, E., Maldonado, L., Gurini, L., Álvarez, A., Van Der Horst, A., Tabera, A. (2000a) Caracterización de propóleos Argentinos. I- Delta del Río Paraná. Congreso Internacional de propóleos. Argentina.

Bedascarrasbure, E., Maldonado, L., Álvarez, A., Van der Horst, A., Tabera, A. (2000b) Caracterización de propóleos Argentinos. III- Mendoza. Congreso Internacional de propóleos. Argentina.

Bedascarrasbure, E., Maldonado, L., Álvarez, A., Rodríguez, E. (2004) Contenido de fenoles y flavonoides de propóleos argentinos. *Acta Farmacéutica Bonaerense*, 23 (3) 369-372.

Bedascarrasbure, E., Maldonado, L., Fierro Morales, W., Álvarez, A. (2006) Propóleos. Caracterización y normalización de propóleos argentinos. Revisión y actualización de composición y propiedades. Ediciones Magna. Argentina. 1-213.

Boletín Oficial de la República Argentina Nº 29.162 (1999) Disponible en ANMAT. http://www.anmat.gov.ar/principal.html.

Chaillou, L., Nazareno, M. (2009) Bioactivity of propolis from Santiago del Estero, Argentina, related to their chemical composition LWT. *Food Science and Technology*, 42, 1422–1427.

Crane, E. (1990) Bees and beekeeping, Cornell Univ. Press, Ithaca, N.Y.

Cuesta Rubio, O., Cuellar, A., Rojas, N., Castro, H.V., Rastrelli, L., Aquino, R. (1999) A polyisoprenylated benzophenone from Cuban propolis. *Journal of Natural Product* 62, 1013-1015.

Gurini, L., Segura, C., Maldonado, L., Alvarez, A., Torné, C., Rodríguez, D., Bedascarrasbure, E. (2004) Origen botánico de propóleos obtenidos en dos zonas de la República Argentina. 1º Encuentro Latinoamericano de apicultores y 1º Congreso Cubano de Apicultura. La Habana. Cuba.

Isla, M.I., Nieva Moreno, M.I., Vattuone, M.A., Sampietro, A.R. (2001) Antioxidant activity of argentine propolis extracts. *Journal of Etnopharmacology*, 76, 165-170.

Isla, M.I., Paredes Guzman, J.F., Nieva Moreno, M.I., Koo, H., Park, Y.K. (2005) Some chemical composition and biological activity of Northern Argentine. Propolis. *Journal of Agricultural and Food Chemistry*, 53, 1166-1172.

Isla, M.I., Carrasco Juárez, B., Nieva Moreno, M.I., Zampini, I., Ordóñez, R., Sayago, J., Cuello, S., Alberto, M.R., Bedascarrabure, E., Alvarez, A., Cioccini, F., Maldonado, L.M. (2009) Effect of seasonal variations and collection form on antioxidant activity of propolis from San Juan, Argentina. *Journal of Medicinal Food*, 12(6), 1334-1342.

Kumazawa, S., Yoneda, M., Nakayama, T. (2004) Constituents in Brazilian Propolis and its Plant Origin. *Foods Food Ingredients J. Jpn.*, 209 (2).

Kumazawa, S., Nakamura, J., Murase, M., Miyadawa, M., Ahn, M.R., Fukumoto, S. (2008) Plant origin of Okinawan propolis: honeybee behavior observation and phytochemical analysis. *Naturwissenschaften*, 95, 781–786.

Kumazawa, S., Ahna, M., Fujimoto, T., Kato, M. (2010) Radical-scavenging activity and phenolic constituents of propolis from different regions of Argentina. *Natural Product Research*, 24, 804–812.

Lima, B., Tapia, A., Luna, L., Fabani, M.P., Schmeda-Hirschmann, G., Podio, N.S., Wunderlin, D.A., Feresin Main, G.E. (2009) Flavonoids, DPPH activity, and metal content allow determination of the geographical origin of propolis from the Province of San Juan (Argentina). *Journal Agriculture and Food Chemistry*, 57, 2691-2698.

Lozina, L., Peichoto, M., Acosta, O., Granero, G. (2010) Standarization and organoleptic and physicochemical characterization of 15 Argentinean Propolis. *Latin American Journal of Pharmacy*, 29 (1),102-110.

Maldonado, L. (2000) Perfil de los propóleos argentinos. Congreso Internacional de propóleos. Argentina.

Markham, K.R., Mitchell, K.A., Wilkins, A.L., Daldy, J.A., Lu, Y. (1996) HPLC and GC-MS identification of the major organic constituents in New Zealand propolis, *Phytochemistry*, 42, 205–211.

Nieva Moreno, M.I., Isla, M.I., Cudmani, N.G., Vattuone, M.A., Sampietro, A.R. (1999) Screening of antibacterial activity of Amaicha del Valle (Tucumán, Argentina). Propolis. *Journal of Ethnopharmacology*, 68, 97-102.

Nieva Moreno, M.I., Isla, M.I., Vattuone, M.A., Sampietro, A.R. (2000). Comparison of the free radical-scavenging activity of propolis from several regions. *Journal of Ethnopharmacology*, 71, 109-114.

Nieva Moreno, M.I., Zampini, I.C., Ordoñez, R.M., Vattuone, M.A., Isla, M.I. (2005) Evaluation of the cytotoxicity, mutagenicity and antimutagenicity of propolis from Amaicha del Valle, Tucumán, Argentina. *Journal of Agricultural and Food Chemistry*, 53, 8957-8962.

Norma IRAM-INTA 15935-2. (2008) Extractos de Propóleos. Instituto Argentino de Normalización -Buenos Aires, Argentina.

Nyeko, P., Edwards-Jones, G., Day, R.K. (2002) Honeybee, *Apis mellifera* (Hymenoptera: Apidae), leaf damage on *Alnus* species in Uganda: a blessing or curse in agroforestry? *Bulletin of Entomology Research*, 92, 405–412..

Oldoni, T., Cabral, I., Regitano d'Arce, M., Rosalen, P., Ikegaki, M., Nascimento, A., Alencar, S. (2011) Isolation and analysis of bioactive isoflavonoids and chalcone from a new type of Brazilian propolis. Separation and Purification Technology, 77, 208-213.

Ordoñez, R., Zampini, I.C., Nieva Moreno, M.I., Isla, M.I. (2011) Potential application of Argentine propolis to control some phytopathogenic bacteria. *Microbiological Research*, 166, 578-584.

Quiroga, E.N., Sampietro, D.A., Soberón, J.R., Sgariglia, M.A., Vattuone, M.A.(2006) Propolis from the northwest of Argentina as a source of antifungal principles. Journal of Applied Microbiology, 101,103-110.

Salatino, A., Teixeira, E.W., Negri, G., Message, D. (2005) Origin and chemical variation of Brazilian propolis, *eCAM* 2, 33–38.

Silva, B.B., Rosalen, P.L., Cury, J.A., Ikegaki, M., Souza, V.C., Esteves, A., Alencar, S.M. (2008) Chemical composition and botanical origin of red propolis a new type of Brazilian propolis, eCAM 5, 313–316.

Tomás-Barberán, F.A., García-Viguera, C., Vit-Oliver, P., Ferreres, F., Tomás-Lorente, F. (1993) Phytochemical evidence for the botanical origin of tropical propolis from Venezuela. *Phytochemistry*, 34, 191-196.

Vera, N., Solorzano, E., Ordoñez, R., Maldonado, L., Bedascarrasbure, E., Isla, M.I. (2011) Chemical composition of Argentinean propolis collected in extreme regions and its relation with antimicrobial and antioxidant activities. *Natural Product Communications*, (6) 823-827.

Zampini, I.C., Nieva Moreno, M.I., Vattuone, M., Isla, M.I. (2004) Botanical origin of propolis from Amaicha del Valle Tucuman, Argentina. *Bio Cell*, 28(1) 1.

In: Beneficial Effects of Propolis on Human Health ... ISBN: 978-1- 62081-440-6
Editors: Tahira Farooqui and Akhlaq A. Farooqui 

*Chapter 9*

# STRUCTURAL BASIS OF ANTIMICROBIAL ACTIVITY OF MEDITERRANEAN PROPOLIS

***Milena P. Popova****
Institute of Organic Chemistry with Centre of Phytochemistry,
Bulgarian Academy of Sciences, Bulgaria

## ABSTRACT

Propolis, or bee glue, is a resinous material collected by honeybees from buds and leaves of certain plant species. The bees use propolis as a protective agent; they cover the internal walls of the hives and thus increase their mechanical stability and stability against pathogenic microorganisms. Propolis possesses a broad spectrum of biological activity which is the reason for its use by man since ancient times. Nowadays, it is still a popular remedy and exceptional suitable constituent in different pharmaceutical preparations, mainly due to its antimicrobial properties. The action against bacteria, fungi and viruses is the main characteristic of propolis but its active principles are different for propolis samples originating from different geographic and climatic regions. The reason is that propolis chemical composition depends strongly on the specific local flora at the site of collection and bees' preference to certain plant exudates. Till now, several types of propolis are formulated on the basis of its plant and/or geographic origin, among them is the Mediterranean propolis. Samples from the subtropical areas, like Southern Greece, Greek islands (Andros, Skopelos, Tinos, Crete), Malta, Southern Italy (Sicily), Turkish Anatolia and Algeria, display specific chemical profile, rich in diterpene compounds.

Here, the current data are summarized about the structural basis of antimicrobial activity of that new propolis type. Its plant origin is also discussed.

**Keywords:** Mediterranean propolis, diterpenes, plant origin, antimicrobial activity

* Correspondence concerning this chapter should be addressed to: Milena P. Popova, Dr. Institute of Organic Chemistry with Centre of Phytochemistry, Bulgarian Academy of Sciences, Acad. G. Boncev str., bl. 9, 1113 Sofia. Email: popova@orgchm.bas.bg.

# Introduction

Propolis (bee glue) is one of the most valuable and enigmatic bee products with healing properties. It is a plant-derived mixture of plant exudates and beeswax. The bees (*Apis mellifera*) collect resinous material from leaf buds, young leaves and bark, which protect the plants from bacteria, viruses and damages [1]. These substances, actively secreted by plants, are the source of propolis biological activity [1,2]. The term "propolis" is connected with the role of propolis in the hive, translated from Greek it means defence of the city or the hive [1].

Being the most important barrier of bees against pathogenic microorganisms, propolis has been used as a remedy by man since ancient times [2]. Nowadays, there is a substantional evidence indicating that propolis possesses antimicrobial, anti-inflammatory, antioxidant, antiviral, antitumor activities, etc. [reviewed by 3-9]. Due to its healing properties propolis is still a popular product, used in many preparations in medicine, cosmetics and food industry, to promote health and prevent diseases [3,4,7,10-12].

Along with the healing properties, the scientists' interest is focused on revealing of the structural basis of its biological activity. Currently, it is well known that propolis is a bioactive complex of many structurally different constituents [13-15] and more than several hundred natural compounds have been identified in propolis from different locations [16,17]. The reason for the propolis chemical diversity is that, as a plant derived product, its chemical composition depends on the local flora and thus on the climatic characteristic at the site in which it is collected [3]. Thanks to the bees' preference to certain plant species in different geographic regions it became possible "local" propolis types to be formulated on the basis of its plant and/or geographic origin. The knowledge of the propolis type allows defining the type of the main active propolis constituents, which is of great importance to their quantification in respect to propolis standardization and quality control [18]. Till now, several propolis types are formulated as all they are characterized by distinct chemical profile [reviewed by 15,18]. For example, flavonoids and esters of aromatic acids are the main bioactive constituents in poplar type propolis [16,19], prenylated *p*-coumaric acids and diterpenic acids in Brazilian green (6,20-23), isoflavonoids, lignans, polyisoprenylated benzophenones, pterocarpans in red propolis from Brazil [24-26], Cuba [27,28], Venezuela [29-31] and Mexico [32], C-prenylflavanones in "Pacific" type (33-37), furofuran lignans in "Canarian" type [38]. Antibacterial activity has been shown for all of these propolis types and some isolated constituents.

Undoubtedly, the poplar propolis is one of the most studied and the most widespread propolis type. The reason is that in temperate zone the bees visit *Populus* spp. for collecting resin and as a result samples from temperate regions of Europe, North and South America, Asia and even New Zealand have similar qualitative chemical composition. Flavonoids, aromatic acids and their esters such as pinocembrin, chrysin, pinobanksin 3-*O*-acetate, caffeic and *p*-coumaric acids, phenethyl and prenyl caffeates are among the active principles, especially against bacteria and fungi [3,13,15,16,18,39-41]. In Europe bees have preference to *Populus* spp. (mainly *Populus nigra*), but in border areas where poplars are rarely distributed they visit other alternative plants to collect resin [18]. During the last decade chemical investigations of propolis from different Mediterranean regions led to revealing of a new specific chemical profile, different from the typical poplar type. The land borders nearby the region of Mediterranean Sea is characterized by subtropical climate and its high degree of floral biodiversity results in distinct propolis chemistry and thus in isolation of new natural compounds with valuable activity. In this chapter, the current data about the structural basis of antimicrobial activity of that new propolis type are reviewed.

## Mediterranean Type Propolis and Area of Its Distribution

As mentioned above, the European propolis is the most studied one. The intensive investigations of its chemistry, dating back to 1980, show that the bioactive compounds are "poplar" phenols (flavonoids, aromatic acids and their esters). The first data about unusual chemical profile of European propolis appeared in 2002, when Bankova et al. [41] reported very low phenolic content and diterpenic acids as main constituents for Mediterranean propolis from South Italy (Sicily). At that time, diterpenic acids were characteristic for tropical propolis from South Brazil [20,21]. In 2004 diterpenes have also been found in propolis from West Greece [42]. Some years later two research groups detected diterpenes in a number of samples from different regions of Greece and Greek islands [43-45].

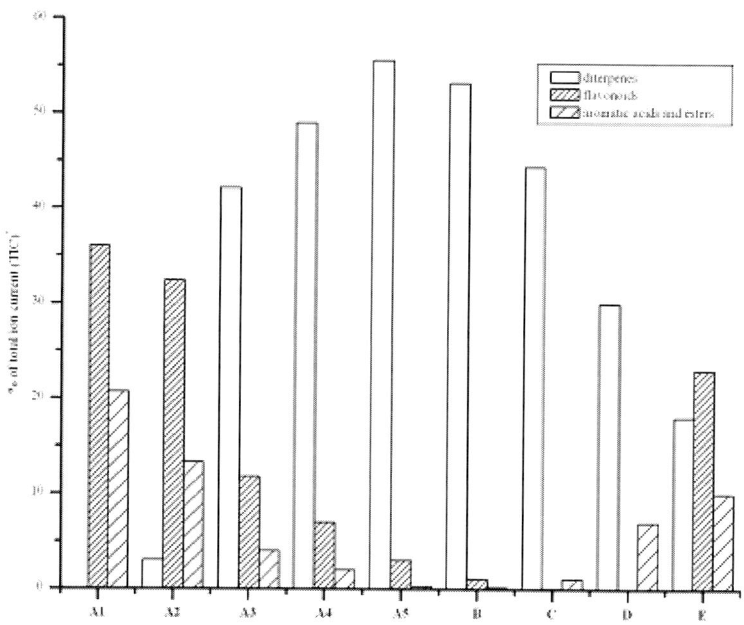


Figure 1. Chemical profile of Mediterranean propolis: *A1* North Greece (Nigrita) [48]. *A2* Central Greece (2 samples of Thessaly) and Central Peloponnesus (Arcadia) [43]; *A3* Peloponnese: East Peloponnese (Epidavros, Argolida) [45], North Peloponnese (Kalavryta, Achaia) and Southern Peloponnese (Messinia) [43] and (Laconia, Mani) [45]; *A4* Greek Aegean islands – Skopelos (NW Aegean Sea) [43], Andros [45] and Tinos (Central Aegean sea) [43]; *A5* Greek island of Crete: Aloides [43], Sfakia, Chania and Zaros [45]; *B* Italy (Sicily) [41]; *C* island of Malta (17 samples from different localities incl. 3 samples of island of Gozo) [46]; *D* Turkey (2 samples from Central and South-western Anatolia)) [47]; *E* Algeria (2 samples from North-Central Algeria) [48]. *The ion current generated depends on the characteristics of the compounds concerned and it is not a true quantification. Nevertheless, it is useful for comparing of the qualitative composition of similar models like propolis samples.

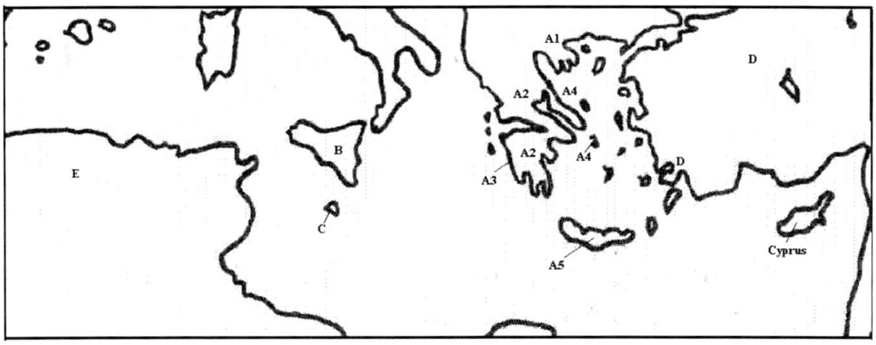


Figure 2. Map of Mediterranean countries.

Recently, the same specific chemical profile was established for propolis from Malta [46]. Diterpenes are the characteristic compounds also for propolis from Western Asian and North African Mediterranean regions as Turkish Anatolia [47] and Algeria [48]. The chemical profile of propolis from different Mediterranean localities, presented by diterpenes, as characteristic for Mediterranean propolis constituents, and "poplar" phenolics, is shown on Figure 1.

The chemical composition of a typical poplar type propolis (presented by a sample from North Greece) is also included. The data are based on the percentage of total ion current (TIC), obtained by gas chromatography-mass spectrometry (GC-MS) analysis of 70% ethanolic propolis extracts, studied by several groups [41,43,45-48].

As it is obvious, diterpenes have been found in propolis from different regions in the Central and East Mediterranean area. Moreover, typical Mediterranean propolis type, with diterpenes as major group of compounds, display samples originating from the islands and coastal regions within the Mediterranean climate area (Figure 2).

It is interesting to note that in the case of Greek propolis, its chemical composition changes from "poplar" from North Greece to typical Mediterranean type in South Greece. This is an example of the phytogeographic and climatic influence on the propolis chemical composition. The area around Mediterranean basin is characterized by subtropical climate, where the characteristic for temperate zone *Populus* spp. are rarely distributed.

## Chemical Composition of Mediterranean Type Propolis

### Diterpenes

Diterpenes are the characteristic class of Mediterranean type propolis constituents. The diterpenes identified are summarized in Table 1 and structures of selected compounds are shown on Figure 3. Compounds with valuable antimicrobial activity have been isolated. Among the diterpenes detected, two main groups may be distinguished: bicyclic diterpenes of labdane type and tricyclic diterpenes of abietane and pimarane type.

**Table 1. Diterpenes found in Mediterranean type propolis**

| | Diterpenes | Geographic origin | References |
|---|---|---|---|
| | Isolated diterpenes | | |
| | *Bicyclic diterpenes (labdane type)* | | |
| **1**[b] | Communic acid | Italy (Sicily)<br>Greece | [49]<br>[44] |
| **2**[b] | Isocupressic acid | Italy (Sicily)<br>Greece | [49]<br>[42,44] |
| **3**[b] | Acetylisocupressic acid | Italy (Sicily)<br>Greece | [49]<br>[44] |
| **4**[b] | 13-*epi*-Cupressic acid | Greece | [42,44] |
| **5**[c] | Junicedric acid | Greece | [44] |
| **6**[c] | Mixture of 15-oxolabda-8(17),13*E*-dien-19-oic acid and 15-oxolabda-8(17),13*Z*-dien-19-oic acid | Greece | [44] |
| **7**[a] | 14,15-Dinor-13-oxo-8(17)-labden-19-oic acid | Greece | [44] |
| **8**[a] | Mixture of labda-8(17),13*E*-dien-19-carboxy-15-yl oleate and palmitate. | Greece | [44] |
| **9**[a] | Copalol (labd-8(17),13*E*-diene-15-ol) | Italy (Sicily)<br>Greece | [49]<br>[42,44] |
| **10**[c] | 13-*epi*-Manool | Greece | [44,50] |
| **11**[c] | 13-*epi*-Torulosol | Greece | [42,44] |
| **12**[c] | Agathadiol | Greece | [42,44] |
| **13**[c] | 13-*epi*-Torulosal | Greece | [42,44] |
| **14**[c] | Isoagatholal | Greece | [42,44] |
| **15**[c] | *trans*-Communal | Greece | [44] |
| | *Tricyclic diterpenes* | | |
| **16** | Totarol | Greece | [42,44] |
| **17**[c] | Totarolone (3-oxototarol) | Greece | [44] |
| **18**[c] | Pimaric acid | Greece | [44] |
| **19**[c] | 18-Succinyloxyabieta-8,11,13-triene | Greece | [45] |
| | Diterpenes identified by GC/MS | | |
| | *Bicyclic diterpenes (labdane type)* | | |
| | **1-5**, **7**, **9-15** | Greece<br>Malta | [45]<br>[46] |
| **20** | Manoyl oxide | Greece<br>Malta | [45]<br>[46] |
| **21** | Labda-8(17),12,13-triene | Greece<br>Malta | [45]<br>[46] |
| **22**[b] | 13(14)-Dehydrojunicedric acid (agathic acid) | Greece<br>Malta | [45]<br>[46] |
| **23** | Imbricataloic acid | Greece<br>Malta | [45]<br>[46] |
| **24**[b] | Imbricatoloic acid | Greece<br>Malta | [45]<br>[46] |
| | *Tricyclic diterpenes* | | |
| | **16** | Greece<br>Malta<br>Cyprus | [43,45]<br>[46]<br>[43] |

**Table 1. (Continued)**

| | Diterpenes | Geographic origin | References |
|---|---|---|---|
| | **17** | Greece<br>Malta | [45]<br>[46] |
| | **18** | Greece<br>Malta<br>Cyprus | [43,45]<br>[46]<br>[43] |
| | **19** | Greece | [45] |
| **25**[c] | Sempervirol | Greece<br>Malta | [45]<br>[46] |
| **26**[c] | Ferruginol | Greece<br>Malta | [42,45]<br>[46] |
| **27**[c] | Ferruginolon | Greece<br>Malta | [45]<br>[46] |
| **28**[c] | 2-Hydroxyferruginol | Greece<br>Malta | [45]<br>[46] |
| **29**[c] | 6/7-Hydroxyferruginol | Greece<br>Malta | [45]<br>[46] |
| **30** | Abietic acid | Greece<br>Malta<br>Cyprus<br>Turkey<br>Algeria | [43,45]<br>[46]<br>[43]<br>[47]<br>[48] |
| **31** | Neoabietic acid | Greece<br>Malta | [45]<br>[46] |
| **32** | Dehydroabietic acid | Greece<br>Malta<br>Cyprus<br>Turkey<br>Algeria | [43,45]<br>[46]<br>[43]<br>[47]<br>[48] |
| **33**[c] | 18-Hydroxyabieta-8,11,13-triene | Greece | [45] |
| **34** | Isopimaric acid | Greece, Cyprus<br>Turkey<br>Algeria | [43]<br>[47]<br>[48] |
| | *Tentative structures* | | |
| **35**[c] | Dihydroxyabieta-8,11,13-triene | Greece | [45] |
| **36**[c] | Hydroxydehydroabietic acid | Greece<br>Malta | [45]<br>[46] |
| **37**[c] | 18-Succinyloxyabietadiene | Greece | [45] |
| **38**[c] | 18-Succinyloxyabietadiene (isomer) | Greece | [45] |
| **39**[c] | 18-Succinyloxyhydroxyabietatriene | Greece | [45] |
| **40** | Diterpenic acid M=302 | Greece | [45] |
| **41** | Diterpenic hydroxyacid M=322 | Algeria | [48] |
| | *Others* | | |
| **42** | Phytol | Greece, Cyprus | [43] |

[a] New natural compounds [44,49].

[b] Isolated also from Brazilian propolis [20,21].

[c] Identified for the first time in propolis [42,44].

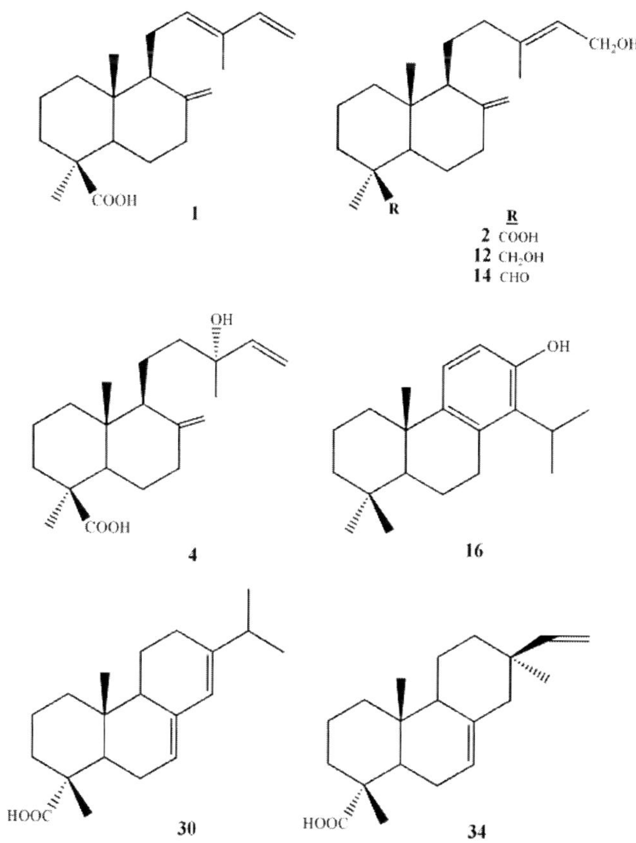


Figure 3. Structures of selected compounds found in Mediterranean propolis.

Specific chemical profile of European propolis, rich in diterpenes, has been described for sample from Sicily (South Italy) [41]. Its main constituents further have been isolated and identified by Trusheva et al. [49], as labdane derivatives: E/Z communic acid **1**, isocupressic acid **2**, acetylisocupressic acid **3** and new diterpene alcohol labd-8(17),13*E*-diene-15-ol (copalol) **9**. Later, from a Greek propolis sample (Northwest Greece, Preveza region), Melliou et al. [42] characterized eight diterpenic acids and alcohols: isocupressic acid **2**, 13-*epi*-cupressic acid **4**, copalol **9**, totarol **16**, and new for propolis 13-*epi*-torulosol **11**, agathadiol **12**, 13-*epi*-torulosal **13** and isoagatholal **14**. All mentioned acids have previously been isolated from tropical propolis from Brazil [20,21] (Table 1).

Compounds from the same class were reported for other 6 propolis samples from different regions of Greece (East and South Peloponnesus) and the Greek islands Andros and Crete (Sfakia, Chania and Zaros) [45]. Firstly, from one of the Cretan propolis samples (Chania), Popova et al. [44] isolated a total of 19 diterpenes, 10 of them (**1-4**, **9**, **11-14**, **16**) found also in Sicilian and Western Greek propolis. Among the rest, 14,15-dinor-13-oxo-8(17)-labden-19-oic acid **7** and a mixture of labda-8(17),13*E*-dien-19-carboxy-15-yl oleate and palmitate **8** were new natural compounds and seven were isolated for the first time from propolis: junicedric acid **5**, mixture of 15-oxolabda-8(17),13*E*-dien-19-oic acid and 15-oxolabda-8(17),13*Z* dien-19-oic acid **6**, 13-*epi*-manool **10**, *trans*-communal **15**, totarolone (3-oxototarol) **17** and pimaric acid **18**. A new propolis constituent, 18-succinyloxyabieta-8,11,13-triene **19** from a sample from East Peloponnesus (Epidavros), has also been characterized [45]. Using the isolated compounds as authentic standards as well as literature reference spectra, Popova et al. [45] recognized a total of 37 diterpenes (presented 46 – 86% of TIC) by GC-MS in the sixth Greek propolis samples (Table 1; Figure 1 and 2) [45]. Among the diterpenes identified, 21 were presented in all samples analysed and 20 were new propolis constituents (sempervirol and abietane derivatives). Substantial amounts of the labdane diterpenes **1**, **2**, **4**, **12** and **14** have been detected in all samples, as the isocupressic acid **2** is presented in the highest amounts (16 - 29% of TIC) (except of a samples from East Peloponnese, Epidavros). Tricyclic diterpene alcohol, totarol **16**, is also pointed out as a characteristic constituent in the samples. Recently, similar chemical profile has been established for propolis from Malta [46]. A total of 32 diterpenes have been detected by GC-MS in 17 propolis samples from different locations in Malta (incl. island of Gozo) as all of them have been found in the Greek propolis. Analogically, diterpenic acids such as isocupressic **2**, communic **1** and imbricatoloic **24** acids were shown among the most abundant constituents. It is interesting to note that the Greek samples (from South Peloponnesus and Greek islands) and Malta are characterized by similar diterpenic composition, rich in labdane type diterpenes. Tricyclic diterpenes (abietane derivatives) in low amounts (<5% of TIC) have been found, which are the main fraction (>29% of TIC) in the distinct Greek propolis sample, gathered from the hives situated in Epidavros, East Peloponnesus. In this sample, abietic **30** and dehydroabietic acids **32** and their derivatives (mainly succinyl esters) in high amounts have been found [45].

Tricyclic diterpenes of abietane and pimarane type are characteristic constituents for the Greek propolis samples, analysed by Kalogeropoulos et al. [43]. Using GC-MS, the authors identified abietic **30**, dehydroabietic **32**, pimaric **18** and isopimaric acids **34** and totarol **16**, and no labdanes, in a total of 12 samples from mainland Greece, Creek islands and Cyprus. The diterpenes are the main constituent (20 - 40% of TIC) in six samples displaying a pattern of a Mediterranean type propolis (Figure 1). In addition, the resin acids **30**, **32** and **34** have been quantified by GC-MS using abietic acid as a standard. The authors estimated higher values of the resin acids for North Peloponnesus propolis (374 mg/g dry ethanolic extract), mainly due to the presence of abietic acid **30** (345 mg/g), followed by the rest 5 samples from Southern Peloponnesus and Creek islands (Crete, Tinos, Skopelos), in which isopimaric acid **34** is the major constituent (62 - 260 mg/g). Although, no labdanes have been detected in North Peloponnesus propolis sample, its chemical composition is somewhat similar to those of propolis from east part of the peninsula, Epidavros, studied by Popova et al. [45].

It should be notice that in the case of Greek propolis both scientific groups [43,45] analysed samples originating from different localities but in close geographic area. The chemical composition of 70% ethanol extracts after derivatization have been analysed by both groups using HP5-MS capillary column at the same chromatographic conditions. Similar chemical composition, but different diterpenic profile is found for the samples from Southern Peloponnesus and Crete as well as from two Central Aegean islands Andros [45] and Tinos [43]. Kalogeropoulos et al. [43] identified diterpenic acids (except of abietic acid) by means of Wiley 275 mass spectra library and isopimaric acid **34** as a major constituent (15 - 29% of TIC) and no labdane derivatives were detected. In contrast, in samples analysed by Popova et al. [45] isocupressic acid **2** was the most abundant diterpene (16 - 29% of TIC), identified by GC/MS with authentic sample. The differences could be explained by incorrectly identification of isopimaric acid **34**, taking into account the same relative retention time of the major diterpenes toward totarol **16**, detected by both groups. On the other hand, the mass spectral fragmentation pattern of the labdane derivatives, in particular of **2**, is very similar to those of tricyclic acids like **18** and **34** [45,51]. The isocupressic acid **2** is characterized by very low intensive $[M-15]^+$ ion and characteristic peak at m/z 374, due to $[M-90(HOSi(CH_3)_3]^+$ ion, which corresponds to the molecular ion $M^{+\cdot}$ (at m/z 374) at diterpene acid **34**. That is why it is difficult to recognize the labdane acids without authentic spectra.

Specific chemical profile, rich in terpenes, has also been established for propolis from Cyprus [43]. Diterpenes **16**, **18**, **30**, **32** and **34** were recognized by GC/MS, but the main fraction (>24% of TIC) was due to co-eluted terpenes (one shown as caryophyllene based diterpene). This fraction has not been observed in the second Cypriot sample, collected from the same place, a year later.

Tricyclic resin acids (abietic acid **30**, dehydroabietic acid **32** and isopimaric acid **34**), as predominant group of constituents, have been detected in propolis from Turkish Anatolia Mugla-Marmaris (Southwestern Anatolia) and Ankara-Kazan (Central Anatolia) [47]. The same acids as well as high amounts of unidentified hydroxyditerpenic acid were the main constituents in Algerian propolis samples [48]. These samples are shown as a "mixed" type, in respect to the presence of relatively high amounts of diterpenes and "poplar" markers (Figure 1).

## Phenolic Compounds

As it is presented on Figure 1 "poplar" phenolic compounds (flavonoids, phenolic acids and their esters) are minor group of compounds, identified in the Mediterranean propolis samples.

Among the detected phenolics are pinocembrin, pinobanksin-3-*O*-acetate, caffeic acid, phenetyl and penthenyl caffeates, which are typical bioactive constituent for *Populus* spp. [16,40]. They are more abundant in propolis from Algeria (the samples with "mixed origin"), followed by those from Peloponnesus (Greece) and Greek islands (Skopelos and Tinos). In propolis from Sicily, Crete, Malta and Turkey traces or no "poplar" phenolics have been found. Among the Greek propolis samples, lower amounts of phenolics have been detected in Cretan propolis by both scientific groups [43,45].

For some Mediterranean propolis samples other phenolics that may be regarded as "specific" constituents have been reported, due to ability of a "specific" plant source at the side of propolis collection. For example, new prenylated flavonoid 7-prenylstrobopinin together with the new propolis constituent 7-prenylpinocembrin have been isolated from a Greek propolis sample [42].

Mono- and sesquiterpenyl esters of substituted benzoic acids have been detected in almost all Maltese samples: ferutinin (ferutinol *p*-hydroxybenzoate), teferine (ferutinol vanillate) and the new for propolis 2-acetoxy-6-*p*-methoxybenzoyl jaeschkeanadiol and 2-acetoxy-6-*p*-hydroxybenzoyl jaeschkeanadiol [46]. The first two esters have previously been isolated from Iranian propolis [52].

In propolis samples from Greece and Cyprus anthraquinones, mainly chrysophanol and emodin have been detected [43]. Chrysophanol has also been found in propolis from Egypt [53] and Turkey [54] as in all cases anthraquinones were detected only by GC/MS.

### Other Constituents

Other groups of constituents of all Mediterranean samples are aliphatic hydroxyacids, fatty acids and esters, sugars and sugar derivatives. Triterpenes (mainly amyrine and its alcohols) have also been found [43,45-48]. Moreover, two new cycloartane triterpenes 3,4-seco-cycloart-12-hydroxy-4(28),24-dien-3-oic acid and cycloart-3,7-dixydroxy-24-en-28-oic acid have been isolated from Cretan propolis [44]. Triterpenes have also been isolated for tropical propolis [55-57].

## Plant Sources

The botanical origin of the Mediterranean propolis is yet unidentified as there are no data about directly comparison between propolis and plant resin extracts. Despite of this, based on the terpenic profile different scientific groups proposed one suggestion that the plant source should be some conifer plant [42-44,47,49].

It is noteworthy, that the diterpenes detected are typical oleoresin constituents of different Conifer (mainly Pinaceae and Cupressaceae) species, which are widespread in the Mediterranean region [45,49]. Similarities in the chemical profile of propolis from Sicily, Southern Greece, Crete and Malta, in which the labdane type of diterpenes are predominant compounds, show the presence of the same propolis plant source, different from that of samples rich in tricyclic resin acids. Representatives of Cupressaceae family, Cupressus sempervirens (Italian cypress) or/and Juniperus phoeniciana (Phoenician juniper), were shown as possible plant sources for Sicilian propolis [49], while Pinus spp. for the Greek one [42]. Pinus spp. are also proposed as a source of the Cypriot [43] and Turkish propolis [47] because of the richness in resin acids such as abietic **30**, dehydroabietic **32** and isopimaric **34** acids. However, according to Popova et al. [45,46], for propolis samples from Greece and Malta it is seems more likely that the plant source belongs to the Cupressaceae family (e.g. Cupressus sempervirens), based on the fact that the propolis samples contain totarol **16**, ferruginol **26** and their derivatives, which are characteristic for Cupressaceae, but not for the Pinaceae. From the other side, participation of two plant sources of Pinaceae and Cupressaceae was proposed for propolis from East Peloponnesus (Epidavros), in which succinyl esters of abietic acids, found in representatives of Pinaceae, have also been detected [45]. The same could be valid for samples, analysed by Kalogeropoulos et al. [43], since tricyclic acids and totarol **16** were found.

Representatives of the genus *Ferula* are shown as a secondary plant source of propolis from Malta, although not the basic one [46]. The conclusion is based on the fact that sesquiterpene esters of benzoic acids are characteristic secondary metabolites of the genus *Ferula*, in particular of *Ferula communis*, which is typical of the island's flora. Moreover, it is interesting that *Ferula* was chosen by bees as a secondary propolis source in two different phytogeographic regions: Iran and Malta [46]. Analogically, the bees' preference to *Populus* spp. is obvious from the detected "poplar" markers, even in traces, in almost all Mediterranean samples. *Platanus acerifolia* could be the source of the prenylated flavonoids in the Greek propolis [42], and nothing was suggested for the plant source of antraquinones.

## ANTIMICROBIAL ACTIVITY

Antimicrobial activity is the main and essential characteristic of propolis which is associated with its role in the bee hive [3]. That is why many articles discussed the chemical composition and the corresponding plant sources along with its action against bacteria and fungi [58]. Although, the antimicrobial properties of Mediterranean propolis have been studied (Table 2), it is difficult to compare the results, due to different methods used for the evaluation of its antimicrobial activity.

**Table 2. Antimicrobial activity of Mediterranean propolis**

| Propolis – Geographic origin | Tested extracts and compounds | Method | Tested microorganism | References |
|---|---|---|---|---|
| Italy (Sicily) | Ethanol, 70% diterpenes | Agar cup | *S. aureus* | [49] |
| Malta | Ethanol, 70% | Agar cup | *S. aureus, E. coli, C. albicans* | [46] |
| Greece | | | | |
| Preveza region (West Greece)<br><br>Chania (Crete) | n-Butanol Diterpenes, flavonoids, aromatic acid<br>Ethanol, 70% Diterpenes, triterpenes | Disc diffusion and dilution | *S. aureus* (ATCC 25923), *S. epidermidis* (ATCC 12228), *E. coli* (ATCC 25922), *Enterobacter cloacae* (ATCC 13047), *Klebsiella pneumoniae* (ATCC 13883), *Pseudomonas aeruginosa*, *Streptococcus mutans*, *S. viridans*, *Candida albicans* (ATCC 10231), *C. tropocalis* (ATCC 13801), *C. glabrata* (ATCC 28838) | [42]<br><br>[44] |
| Central Greece, Greek islands and Cyprus | Ethanol, 70% | Agar diffusion | *S. aureus* (NCTC 6571), *S. aureus* (ATCC 25923), *S. epidermidis* (NCTC 11047), *Bacillus cereus* (NCTC 7464), *B. cereus* (ATCC 9139), *Listeria monocytogenes* (NCTC 10357), *L. monocytogenes* (ATCC 7644), *Lactobacillus bulgaricus* (ACA-DC 101), *L. fermentum* F 12, *L. casei* LC 14, *L. delbrueckii* sup. *delbrueckii* LDD-C1, *L. plantarum* LP 101, *L. helveticus* LH 09, *Shigella dysenteriae* (NCTC 2966), *Salmonella typhimurium* (NCTC 12023), *E.coli* (NCTC 09001), *Yersinia enterocolitica* (NCTC 10460), *Enterobacter aerogenes* (NCTC 10006), *Candida albicans* (ATCC 10231), *C. tropocalis* (ATCC 13801) | [43] |
| Algeria (M'Sila) | Ethanol, 70% | Agar cup | *S. aureus, E. coli, C. albicans* | [48] |

### Antibacterial Activity

The *in vitro* inhibitory activity of propolis ethanolic extracts from West Greece and Crete as well as of isolated compounds has been evaluated by Melliou et al. [42] and Popova et al. [44]. The sensitivity of eight bacteria, two Gram-positive and four Gram-negative, and two oral pathogenic Gram-positive bacteria (*Streptococcus mutans* and *Streptococcus viridans*) were assayed using both disc diffusion and dilution methods. The extracts and almost all individual constituents showed activity against all strain tested. High inhibition against the Gram-positive bacteria was noticed for both samples (MIC values 0.05 - 0.80 mg/ml). For Cretan propolis (Chania) lowest concentration (0.05 mg/ml) was found using *S. epidermis* strains and the Creek sample inhibited at lower concentrations the oral pathogenic bacteria *S. mutans* (MIC 0.50 mg/ml). Both samples displayed activity against the Gram-negative bacteria *P. aeruginosa*, *E. cloacae*, *E. coli* and *K. pneumoniae* as for the diterpene-rich Cretan propolis highest zone of inhibition and lowest MIC were observed against *P. aeruginosa* (22 mm, MIC 0.24 mg/ml). The total propolis extract possessed higher activity than the isolated constituents. Among the tested individual diterpenes, totarane (**16** and **17**) and labdane (**5-7** and **10**) derivatives, were pointed out as the most active constituents against all tested strains [44]. Lower concentrations of all diterpenes were needed to inhibit *S. aureus* and *S. epidermis* strains (0.07-0.75 mg/ml). *S. aureus* were also susceptible to Sicilian propolis, in which the main constituents like isocupressic and acetylisocupressic acids (**2** and **3**) displayed higher activity than copalol **9** and communic acid **1** [49]. Diterpenic acids of labdane type were found to contribute also to the antibacterial activity of Brazilian propolis [20]. Using the agar cup method, the antibacterial activity against *S. aureus* and *E. coli* of Maltese propolis has been assessed [46]. All samples were inactive against Gram-negative bacteria, whereas their activity against Gram-positive was significant and somewhat higher than that of a typical poplar propolis sample (Bulgarian sample). Inhibition of *S. aureus* and no activity against *E. coli* were recorded for Algerian propolis by agar cup method [48].

Similar approach to investigation of chemical composition and antibacterial activity of Greek and Cypriot propolis samples describes Kalogeropoulos et al. [43]. A large panel of pathogenic and non-pathogenic bacteria (thirteen Gram positive and five Gram negative bacteria) was tested using the agar diffusion assay. The authors noticed that almost all samples (except of two from North Peloponnesus and Cyprus, which inhibited most of the strain used at lower concentrations) were characterized by similar antibacterial activity. All extracts inhibited the growth of Gram-positive bacteria used (except of four *Lactobacillus* strains). The authors detected the lowest MIC (0.04 – 0.15 mg/ml) against *L. monocytogenes* and both *B. cereus* strains, followed by *S. aureus* strains (0.15 – 0.60 mg/ml), while the highest concentrations were needed to be inhibited the non-pathogenic *S. epidermis*. The Gram-negative pathogenic bacteria *S. dysenteriae, S. typhimurium, E. coli* and *E. aerogenes* are sensitive only to the ethanolic extracts of the samples from East Cyprus and the sample with the highest amounts of diterpenes (mainly abietic acid), from North Peloponnese, at the same concentration (MIC 2.50 – 5.00 mg/ml). Interestingly, the authors [43] assayed also the inhibitory activity of the samples against six strains of lactic acid bacteria. All extracts inhibited *L. fermentum* and *L. helveticus*, while *L. bulgaris* and *L. casei* were susceptible only to both most active samples.

The biological activity of the diterpene-rich propolis from Turkish Anatolia has not been studied. However, a year later, the same group Kartal et al. [59] evaluated the antimicrobial properties of two samples, collected from the same localities (Marmaris and Kazan). Using agar cup method, 11 bacteria have been tested and activity against *S. aureus*, *S. epidermis* and *B. subtilis* was detected for both samples. The authors mentioned higher activity for the sample from Central Anatolia (Kazan) contributed mainly to isolated mixture of caffeic acid esters (poplar markers). No other chemical data are given or referred, but based on their previous results [47] the inhibition could be also due to the presence of diterpene constituents.

Despite the differences in the diterpene composition, all Mediterranean samples possess high antibacterial activity, mainly against Gram-positive bacterial test strains. Their action against Gram-negative was lower or no activity was detected. The same results have been shown for poplar type European propolis [60,61], Brazilian propolis [62] and other samples from different geographical and climatic zones [63]. The propolis extracts displayed high activity due to the action of many individual compounds.

## Antifungal Activity

Along with antibacterial activity, the action against fungi has also been studied (Table 2). The same methods (mentioned above) have been used to evaluate the antifungal activity of the Mediterranean propolis against several clinically important yeasts belonging to *Candida* genera. Similar and moderate activity against pathogenic fungi *C. albicans*, *C. tropicalis* and *C. glabrata* displayed propolis extracts from West Greece and Crete, as both samples inhibited *C. glabrata* at lower concentrations [42,44]. Concerning the individual constituents, diterpenic alcohols **10**, **16** and **17** as well as triterpenic acid 3,4-seco-cycloart-12-hydroxy-4(28),24-dien-3-oic acid showed strongest activity, especially against *C. tropicalis* and *C. glabrata* [44].

Sensitivity of *C. albicans* only to 6 of a total 17 Maltese samples have been observed by agar cup method, as all of the active samples were characterized by high present of terpenyl esters of hydroxybenzoic acids [46]. The pathogenic fungi *C. albicans* and *C. tropicalis* were susceptible to the ethanolic propolis extracts of Greek and Cypriot origin, even at low concentrations (MIC 0.02 mg/ml) [43]. Antifungal activity against *C. albicans* has also been detected for propolis from Turkey (Kazan sample) [58] and Algeria [48].

The presence of significant amounts of terpenoids seemed to enhance the antimicrobial activity of propolis from Greece and Cyprus [43]. Abietane and pimarane type resin acids are known to possess antimicrobial properties [64]. Synergistic effect between terpenes and aromatic compounds (flavonoids and acids) has also been proposed for selective and strong antimicrobial activity [42,43], especially for the antifungal activity. The most active samples inhibited the *Candida* strains and *B. cereus* bacteria at the same concentration; whereas all the rest of the samples displayed stronger antifungal than antibacterial activity. For the sample, in which phenolic compounds were presented only in traces (Chania, Crete) lower antifungal activity was evaluated. All diterpenes isolated are more active against bacteria (especially against *S. aureus* and *S. epidermis*) than assayed fungi [44].

For the Maltese samples the antifungal activity was attributed mainly to terpenyl esters of hydroxybenzoic acids [46]. It was shown also by statistically significant Pearson's correlation between the amounts of the esters and the antifungal activity. On the basis of these data the authors [46] suggested that the terpenyl hydroxybenzoates play an important role in the antifungal properties of Maltese propolis, while the diterpene constituents are of grater significance for the antibacterial properties.

## OTHER BIOLOGICAL ACTIVITIES

Antiproliferate activity of Greek propolis (a sample from North Greece, Preveza region) has been evaluated [63]. The authors tested butanolic extract and nine isolated compounds (diterpenes **2**, **4**, **10**, **12-14,** and flavonoids pinostrobin, 7-prenylpinocembrin and 7-prenylstrobopinin) for their cytotoxic activities against human malignant and normal cell strains. As a result, the extract and the diterpenes, especially 13-*epi*-manool **10**, were found as the most active against HT-29 human colon adenocarcinoma cells.

Antioxidant activity of Greek and Cypriot propolis extracts has been evaluated by their radical scavenging activity (DPPH assay) and ferric reducing/antioxidant potential (FRAP) assay [43]. The authors found very good correlation ($p<0.01$) between DPPH˙assayed values and total polyphenols (quantified by GC/MS) as well as with reducing power values ($p<0.01$, $R=0.838$). As a propolis characterized by diterpenes as major constituents and low amounts of phenols, the samples displaying typical Mediterranean type propolis showed lower antioxidant activity among the all samples tested.

## CONCLUSION

The Mediterranean propolis is a specific propolis type in which diterpenic alcohols, aldehydes and acids are the main group of compounds. They are also the structural basis of its antimicrobial activity which makes this type different from most of the other propolis types, where the action is associated mainly with polyphenolic fraction. For Mediterranean type, high activity against different bacteria and fungi has been proved and new natural and propolis constituents have been characterized. Revealing of a new propolis type is an example for the increasing interest on this valuable natural product which is also result of its medical application due to its beneficial effects on human health.

## REFERENCES

[1] Crane E. *Beekeeping: Science, Practice and World Recourses.* Heinemmann, London 1988.

[2] Ghisalberti EL. Propolis: a review. *Bee World*, 1979;60:59-84.

[3] Marcicci MC. Propolis: chemical composition, biological properties and therapeutical activity. *Apidologie*, 1995;26:83-99.

[4] Burdock GA. Review of the biological properties and toxicity of bee propolis (propolis). *Food Chemistry and Toxicol*ogy, 1998;36:347-363.

[5] Hegazi AG. Propolis: An Overview, Part II. *Journal of Bee Informed*, 1998;6:723-728.

[6] Marcucci MC, Bankova VS. Chemical composition, plant origin and biological activity of Brazilian propolis. *Current topics in Phytochemistr,*. 1999;2:115-123.

[7] Banskota AH, Tezuka Y, Kadota Sh. Resent Progress in Pharmacological Research of Propolis. *Phytotherapy Research,* 2001;15:561-571.

[8] Farré R, Frasquet I, Sánchez A. Propolis and human health. *Ars Pharmaceutica,* 2004;45(1):21-43.

[9] Lofty M. Biological activity of Bee Propolis in Health and Disease. *Asian Pasific Journal of Cancer Prevention*, 2006;7:22-31.
[10] Matsuda Sh. Propolis-health care food. *Foods and Food Ingredients Journal of Japan*, 1994;160:64-73.
[11] Suarez D, Zayas D, Guisado F. Propolis: Patents and technology trends for health applications. *Journal of Business Chemistry,* 2005;2(3):119-125.
[12] Viuda-Martos M, Ruiz-Navajas Y, Fernandes-Lopez J, Perez-Alvarez JA. Functional properties of Honey, Propolis, and royal jelly. J*ournal of Food Science,* 2008;73(9):R117-R124.
[13] Farooqui T, Farooqui AA. Molecular Mechanism Underlying the Therapeutic Activities of Propolis: A Critical Review. *Current Nutrition and Food Science,* 2010;6:186-199.
[14] Oršolić N. A review of propolis antitumour action *in vivo* and *in vitro*. *Journal of ApiProduct and ApiMedical Science*, 2010;2(1):1-20.
[15] Salatino A, Fernandes-Silva CC, Righi AA, Salatino MLS. Propolis research and the chemistry of plant products. *Natural Product Reports*, 2011;28:925-936.
[16] Bankova V, de Castro SL, Marcucci MC. Propolis and recent advances in chemistry and plant origin. *Apidologie*, 2000;31:3-15.
[17] Bankova V, Trusheva B, Popova M. New developments in propolis chemical diversity studies (since 2000). In Oršolić N, Bašić I, eds. *Scientific Evidence of the Use of Propolis in Ethnomedicine,* Kerala: Transworld Research Network. 2008;1-13.
[18] Bankova V. Chemical diversity of propolis and the problem of standardization. *Journal of Ethnopharmacology*, 2005;100:114-117.
[19] Popova MP, Bankova VS, Bogdanov S, Tsvetkova I, Naydenski C, Marcazzan GL, Sabatini A-G. Chemical characteristics of poplar type propolis from different geographic origin. *Apidologie*, 2007;38:306-311.
[20] Bankova V, Marcucci MC, Simova S, Nikolova N, Kujumgiev A, Popov S. Antibacterial diterpenic acids from Brazilian propolis. *Zeitschrift fuer Naturforschung*, 1996;51c:277-280.
[21] Banskota AH, Tezuka Y, Prasian JK, Matsushige K, Saiki I, Kadota Sh. Chemical constituents of Brazilian propolis and their cytotoxic activities. *Journal of Natural Products*, 1998;61:896-900.
[22] Kumazawa Sh, Yoneda M, Shibata I, Kanaeda J, Hamasaka T, Nakayama T. Direct Evidence for the Plant Origin of Brazilian Propolis by the Observation of Honeybee Behavior and Phytochemical Analysis. *Chemical and Pharmaceutical Bulletin*, 2003;51:740-742.
[23] Salatino A, Teixeira EW, Negri G, Message D. Origin and chemical variation of Brazilian propolis. *Evidence Based Complementary and Alternative Medicine*, 2005;**2:**33–38.
[24] Trusheva B, Popova M, Bankova V, Simova S, Marcucci MC, Miorin PL, da Rocha Pasin F, Tsvetkova I. Bioactive Constituents of Brazilian Red Propolis. *Evidence Based Complementary and Alternative medicine (eCAM)*, 2006;3(2);249–254.
[25] Daugsch A, Moraes CS, Fort P, Park YK. Brazilian Red Propolis-Chemical Composition and Botanical origin. *Evidence Based Complementary and Alternative medicine (eCAM)*, 2007;5:434-441.
[26] Awale A, Li F, Onozuka H, Esumi H, Tezuka Y, Kadota S. Constituents of Brazilian red propolis and their preferential cytotoxic activity against human pancreatic PANC-1

cancer cell line in nutrient-deprived condition. *Bioorganic and Medicinal Chemistry*, 2008;16:181-189.

[27] Cuesta-Rubio O, Frontana-Uriba BA, Ramirez-Apan T, Cardenas J. Polyisoprenylated benzophenones in Cuban propolis; biological activity of nemorosone. *Zeitschrift fuer Naturforschung*, 2002;57c:372-378.

[28] Piccinelli AL, Fenandez MC, Cuesta-Rubio O, Harández IM, De Simone F, Rastrelli L. Isoflavonoids isolated from Cuban propolis. *Journal of Agricultural and Food Chemistr,*. 2005;53:9010-9016.

[29] Tomás-Barberán FA, García-Viguera C, Vit-Olivier P, Ferreres F, Tomás-Lorente F. Phytochemical evidence for the botanical origin of tropical propolis from Venezuela. *Phytochemistry*, 1993;34:191-196.

[30] Trusheva B, Popova M, Naydensky C, Tsvetkova I, Rodriguez JG, Bankova V. New polyisoprenylated benzophenones from Venezuelan propolis. *Fitoterapia,* 2004;75:683-689.

[31] Hernández M, Fernandez MC, Cuesta-Rubio O, Piccinelli AL, Rastrelli L. Polyprenylated benzophenone derivatives from Cuban propolis. *Journal of Natural Products*, 2005;68:931–934.

[32] Lotti C, Fernandez MC, Piccinelli AL, Cuesta-Rubio O, Hernández IM, Rastrelli L. Chemical constituents of Red Mexican propolis. *Journal of Agricultural and Food Chemistry*, 2010;58:2209-2213.

[33] Chen Ch, Wu Chi, Shy H, Lin J. Cytotoxic prenylflavones from Taiwanese propoli. *Journal of Natural Products,* 2003;66:503-506.

[34] Yang H-Y, Ho W-L, Chang C-M, Chou C-C. Antibacterial activity of Propolis Ethanol Extract against *Streptococcus mutans* as Influenced by Concentration, Temperature, pH and Cell Age. *Journal of Food and Drug Analysis,* 2007;15(1):75-81.

[35] Kumazawa Sh, Ueda R, Hamasaka T, Fukumoto S, Fujimoto T, Nakayama T. Antioxidant Prenylated Flavonoids from Propolis Collected in Okinawa, Japan. *Journal of Agricultural and Food Chemistry*, 2007;55(19):7722-7725.

[36] Huang W-J, Huang C-H, Wu C-L, Lin J-K, Chen Y-W, Lin C-L, Chuang S-E, Huang C-Y, Chen C-N. Propolis G, a Prenylflavanones, Isolated from Taiwanese Propolis, Induces Caspase-Dependent Apoptosis in Brain Cancer Cells. *Journal of Agricultural and Food Chemistr,*. 2007;55:7366-7376.

[37] Raghukumar R, Vali L, Watson D, Fearnley J, Seidel V. Antimethicillin-resistant Staphylococcus aureus (MRSA) activity of "pacific propolis" and isolated prenylflavones. *Phytotherapy Research,* 2010;24(8):1181-1187.

[38] Christov R, Bankova V, Tsvetkova I, Kujumgiev A, Delago Tejera A. Antibacterial furofuran lignans from Canary Islands propolis. *Fitoterapia*, 1999;70:89-92.

[39] Greenaway W, Scaysbrook T, Whatley ER. The composition and plant origins of propolis: a report of work at Oxford. *Bee World*, 1990;71:107-118.

[40] Kujumgiev A, Bankova V, Ignatova A, Popov S. Antibacterial activity of propolis, some of its components and their analogs. *Pharmazie,* 1993;48(10):785-786.

[41] Bankova V, Popova M, Bogdanov S, Sabatini AG. Chemical composition of European Propolis: Expected and Unexpected Results. *Zeitschrift fuer Naturforschung*, 2002;57c:530-533.

[42] Melliou E, Chinou I. Chemical analysis and antimicrobial activity of Greek propolis. *Planta Medica*, 2004;70:1-5.

[43] Kalogeropoulos N, Konteles SJ, Troullidou E, Mourtzinos I, Karathanos VT. Chemical composition, antioxidant activity and antimicrobial properties of propolis extracts from Greece and Cyprus. *Food Chemistry*, 2009;116:452-461.

[44] Popova M, Chinou I, Marekov I, Bankova V. Terpenes with antimicrobial activity from Cretan propolis. *Phytochemistry*, 2009;70:1262-1271.

[45] Popova M, Graikou K, Chinou I, Bankova V. GC-MS Profiling of diterpene compounds in Mediterranean propolis from Greece. *Journal of Agricultural and Food Chemistry*, 2010;58:3167-3176.

[46] Popova M, Trusheva B, Antonova D, Cutajar S, Mifsud D, Farrugia C, Tsvetkova I, Najdenski H, Bankova V. The specific chemical profile of Mediterranean propolis from Malta. *Food Chemistry*, 2011;126:1431-1435.

[47] Kartal M, Kaya S, Kurucu S. GC-MS Analysis of propolis samples from two different regions of Turkey. *Zeitschrift fuer Naturforschung*, 2002;57c:950-909.

[48] Velikova M, Bankova V, Sorkun K, Houcine S, Tsvetkova I, Kujumgiev A. Propolis from the Mediterranean Region: Chemical Composition and Antimicrobial Activity. *Zeitschrift fuer Naturforschung*, 2000;55c:790-793.

[49] Trusheva B, Popova M, Bankova V, Tsvetkova I, Najdenski C, Sabatini AG. A new type of European propolis, containing bioactive labdanes. *Rivista Italiana EPPOS*, 2003;3-7.

[50] Pratsinis H, Kletsas D, Melliou E, Chinou I. Antiproliferative activity of Greek propolis. *Journal of Medicinal Food*, 2010;13(2):286-190.

[51] Cox RE, Yamamoto S, Otto A, Simoneit BRT. Oxygenated di- and tricyclic diterpenoids of southern hemisphere conifers. *Biochemical systematics and ecology*, 2007;35:342-362.

[52] Trusheva B, Todorov I, Ninova M, Najdenski H, Daneshmand A, Bankova V. Antibacterial mono- and sesquiterpene esters of benzoic acids from Iranian propolis. *Chemistry Central Journal*, 2010;4:8.

[53] Abd Ei-Hady FK, Hegazi AG. Egyptian propolis: 2. Chemical Composition, Antiviral and Antimicrobial Activities of East Nile Delta Propolis. *Zeitschrift fuer Naturforschung*, 2002;57c:386-394.

[54] Silici S, Ünlü M, Vardar-Ünlü G. Antibacterial activity and phytochemical evidence for the plant origin of Turkish propolis from different regions. *World Journal of Microbiology and Biotechnology*, 2007;23:1797-1803.

[55] Da Silva MSS, Citó AMGL, Chaves MH, Dantas JA. Cycloarthane triterpenoids of propolis from Teresina. Pl. *Química Nova*, 2005;28:801-804.

[56] Li F, Awale S, Zhang H, Tezuka Y, Esumi H, Kadota Sh. Chemical consituents of propolis from Myanmar and their preferential cytotoxicity against a human pancreatic cancer cell line. *Journal of Natural Products*, 2009;72:1283-1287.

[57] Hernandez IM, Cuesta-Rubio O, Fernandez MC, Pérez AR, de Oca Porto RM, Piccinelli AL, Rastrelli L. Studies on the Constituents of Yellow Cuban propolis: GC/MS Determination of Triterpenoids and Flavonoids. *Journal of Agricultural and Food Chemistry*, 2010;58:4725-4730.

[58] Kosalec I, Pepeljnjak S. Antimicrobial activity of propolis: A review. In Oršolić N, Bašić I, eds. *Scientific Evidence of the Use of Propolis in Ethnomedicine*, Kerala: Transworld Research Network. 2008;149-173.

[59] Kartal M, Yildiz S, Kaya S, Kurucu S, Topçu. Antimicrobial activity of propolis samples from two different regions of Anatolia. *Journal of Ethnopharmacology*, 2003;86(1):69-73.

[60] Grange JM, Davey RW. Antibacterial properties of propolis (bee glue). *Journal of the Royal Society of Medicine,* 1990;83:159-160.

[61] Drago L, Mombelli B, De Vecchi E, Fasina MC, Tocalli L, Gismondo MR. In vitro antimicrobial activity of propolis dry extract. *Journal of Chemotherapy,* 2000;12:390-395.

[62] Sforcin JM, Fernandes JA, Lopes CAM, Bankova V, Funari SRC. Seasonal effect on Brazilian propolis antibacterial activity. *Journal of Ethnopharmacology*, 2000;73:243-249.

[63] Seidel V, Peyfoon E, Watson DG, Fearnley J. Comparative study of the antibacterial activity of propolis from different geographical and climatic zones. *Phytotherapy research,* 2008;22:1256-1263.

[64] Savluchinske-Feio S, Marcelo Curto MJ, Gigante B, Carlos Roseiro J. Antimicrobial activity of resin acid derivatives. *Applied Microbiology and Biotechnology*, 2006;72:430-436.

In: Beneficial Effects of Propolis on Human Health ... ISBN: 978-1- 62081-440-6
Editors: Tahira Farooqui and Akhlaq A. Farooqui 

*Chapter 10*

# THE ANTIMICROBIAL PROPERTIES OF PROPOLIS

***Yuva Bellik[1] and Laïd Boukraâ[2,*]***
[1]Faculty of Life and Nature Sciences, University A. Mira, Bejaia, Algeria
[2]Veterinary Institute, Ibn-Khaldun University of Tiaret, Tiaret, Algeria

## ABSTRACT

The action against microorganisms is an essential characteristic of propolis and that's why it has been applied as a remedy by men since ancient times. Bees collect resins from numerous different plant species, thus the chemical composition of propolis varies greatly and depends directly on the local flora and phenology of the host plants and indirectly on the locality and time of collection.

It is believed that part of the substances collected undergoes chemical alteration by bee enzymes prior to incorporation in propolis, making propolis a substance considered to be of both plant and animal origin. While chemical composition varies, propolis is generally composed of about 45% resin, 35% wax and 20% inert material. More specifically, propolis constituents include about 10% essential oils, 5% pollen, and 15% various organic polyphenolic compounds including, flavonoids and phenolic acids. A multi-step extraction with ethanol can result in dewaxed propolis extracts rich in polyphenolic components.

There is substantial evidence that propolis has antiseptic, antifungal, antibacterial, antiviral, anti-inflammatory and antioxidant properties. The polyphenolic content of propolis is considered to contribute more to the observed healing effects than other propolis constituents. Its antimicrobial property has been widely investigated, and several authors have demonstrated its antibacterial action. Propolis also shows antiviral, antifungal and antiparasite activities. Many therapeutic and cosmetic formulations containing Propolis have been described.

**Keywords:** Propolis, chemical composition, antibacterial, antifungal, antiviral, formulations

* Corresponding author, Dr Laïd Boukraâ, Institute of Veterinary Sciences, Ibn-Khaldoun University of Tiaret, 14000, Tiaret, Algeria, Tel: +213 7 95 306930, Email: laid_bouk@hotmail.com.

# INRODUCTION

The term propolis was used by authors in Ancient Greece: *pro* (for, in front of, e.g., at the entrance to) and *polis* (city or community); a substance that is for or in defense of the city or hive [1]. Bees apply propolis in a thin layer on the internal walls of their hive or other cavity they inhabit. It is used to block holes and cracks, to repair combs, to strengthen the thin borders of the comb, and for making the entrance of the hive weathertight or easier to defend [2]. Propolis also is used as an "embalming" substance to cover hive invaders which bees have killed but cannot transport out of the hive [1]. Bees use the mechanical properties of propolis and of its biological action; bee glue contains the putrefaction of the embalm intruders which is responsible for the lower incidence of bacteria and molds within the hive [1]. The action against micro-organisms is an essential characteristic of propolis and it has been used by human beings since ancient times for its pharmaceutical properties [2]. Propolis possesses antibacterial, antifungal and antiviral properties [3,4] and many other beneficial biological activities [5,6].

Undoubtedly, propolis is in no way a new discovery since its use goes back to ancient times, at least to 300 BC, and it has been used as an ethno-medicine in many parts of the world, both internally and externally [7]. Nevertheless, its use continues today in remedies and personal products, and the list of preparations and uses is endless. It is still one of the most frequently used remedies in the Balkan States [8], and, only, during the last decades, scientists have investigated its constituents and biological properties [7]. The present chapter will focus on the description of antibacterial, antifungal and antiviral properties of propolis, and he main involved chemical constituents as well as to discuss some mechanisms of action of this bee product. Finally, initiatives regarding many formulations including propolis that is increasingly requested to meet a very specific need will be developed.

# PROPOLIS CHARACTERISTICS AND CHEMICAL COMPOSITION

Propolis (bee glue) is a natural resinous substance collected by bees from parts of plants, buds and exudates [1]. This resin is masticated, added of the 13-glicosidase enzyme of their saliva, causing the hydrolysis of the glucosyl flavonoids, originating flavonoids aglycones [9], and then it is mixed with beeswax and probably with other compounds of bee metabolism [6].

Bees use it as a sealer for their hives [10] and, more importantly, to prevent the decomposition of creatures which have been killed by bees after an invasion of the hive [11].

The first scientific work on propolis, reporting its chemical properties and composition, was published in 1908 [12]. Later, in 1968, the first patent [13] was obtained to produce bath lotions in Romania. The following years have shown an increase in international patents, predominantly from the former USSR and satellite countries during the 1980s. From 2000 about half of the commercial licenses were Japanese [9], but in the last decades there were patents registered worldwide [14].

Characteristically, propolis is a lipophilic material, hard and brittle when cold but soft, pliable, and very sticky when warm, hence the name bee glue [15]. It possesses a pleasant aromatic smell, and varies in color, depending on its source and age [16].

Propolis shows a complex chemical composition. More than 300 components have already been identified in different samples [17], and new ones are still being recognized during chemical characterization of new types of propolis [2,18,19].

Among the types of chemical substances found in propolis are 50% resins, 30% waxes, 10% essential oils, 5% pollen and 5% of various organic compounds [6,20]. The proportion of these types of substances varies and depends on the season and local flora at the site of collection as well as on the type of bees foraging [5,21, 22].

Vast array of analytical techniques have been used for separation and identification of propolis components and the substances identified belong to the following groups of chemically similar compounds: flavonoids; benzoic acids and derivatives; benzaldehyde derivatives; cinnamyl alcohol, and cinnamic acid and its derivatives; other acids and respective derivatives; alcohols, ketones, phenols and heteroaromatic compounds; terpene and sesquiterpene alcohols and their derivatives; sesquiterpene and triterpene hydrocarbons; aliphatic hydrocarbons; sterols and steroid hydrocarbons; sugars and amino acids [23]. Volatile compounds mainly sesquiterpenoids are present in low concentrations [17]. Sugars are thought to be introduced accidentally during the elaboration of propolis and/or passage of bees over the resin [14].

Propolis contains some minerals such as Mg, Ca, I, K, Na, Cu, Zn, Mn and Fe as well as some vitamins like B1, B2, B6, C and E, and a number of fatty acids.

In addition, it contains some enzymes as succinic dehydrogenase, glucose- 6-phosphatase, adenosine triphosphatase and acid phosphatase [24]. Propolis contains copper (26.5 mg/kg), manganese (40 mg/kg) and the ash residue contains iron, calcium, aluminum, vanadium, strontium, manganese and silicon [25]. Some compounds are probably present in all propolis samples and contribute to its characteristic properties. Others are represented in many samples of different origins, but a few others only occur in propolis from particular plant species [1].

## BIOLOGICAL PROPERTIES OF PROPOLIS

Among the several bee products, propolis has been highlighted due to its chemical composition, several therapeutic and biological properties, mentioned in numerous scientific works, all over the world, particularly the antimicrobial activity.

This is probably the reason why bee glue plays such an important role in the hive: it is a "chemical weapon" against pathogenic microorganisms, a constant threat to the vital sanitary status of this crowded and busy "city", vulnerable to the invasion of an array of enemies and to the proliferation of diseases [14]. In spite of this universal function and due to plant diversity, there are different propolis types, which contain numerous chemical constituents (Figure 1) responsible not only for the antimicrobial property but also for other valuable bioactivities [26]. These biological activities include: antibacterial [3,4,20,27], antifungal [4, 48], antiviral [29, 30], antiprotozoan [31-32], antitumour [33, 34], anti-inflammatory [35-36], local-anesthetic [37], antioxidant [38-39], immunostimulating [40-41], and hepatoprotective [42, 43].

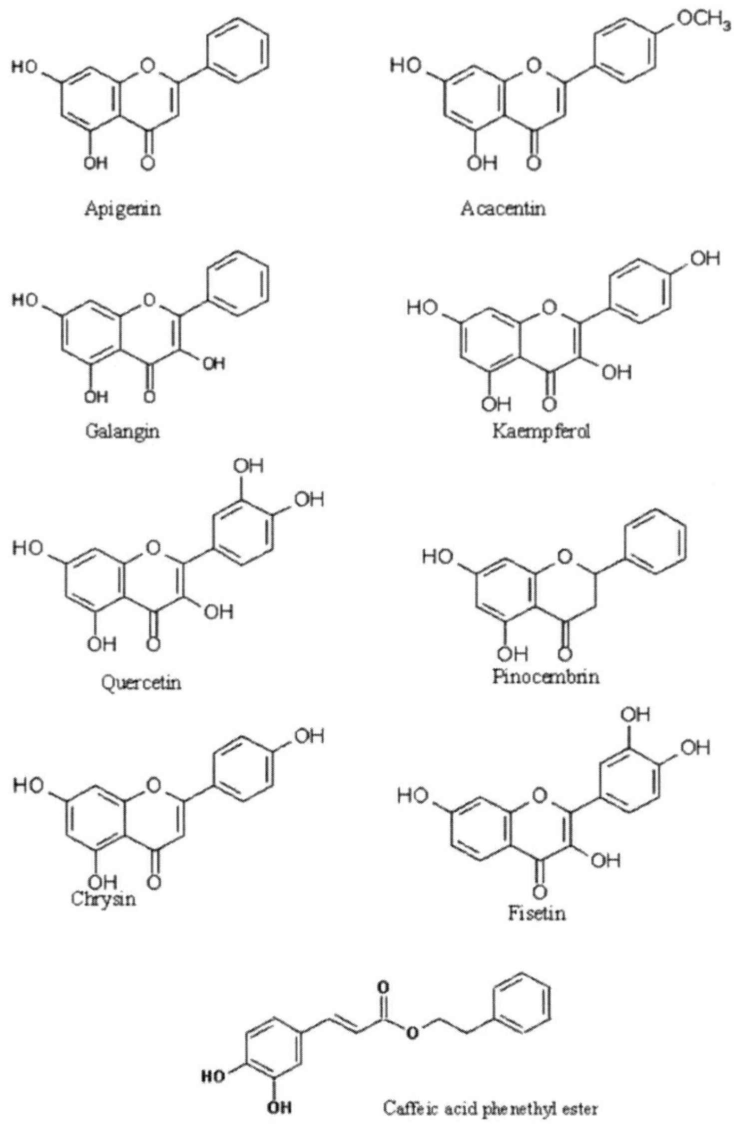


Figure 1. Chemical structures of the most important flavonoids found in propolis [44].

## Antibacterial Activity

Propolis antimicrobial activity is one of the most extensively investigated biological actions [3,4,20,45,46]. Certainly, one of the first biological activities to be recognized and probably one of the most important properties of propolis is the antimicrobial activity. Many researchers had investigated the antibacterial activity of propolis and its extracts against Gram-positive and Gram-negative strains (Table 1), either aerobic or anaerobic from laboratory collections or isolated from clinical samples, and found that propolis had antibacterial activity against a wide range of Gram-positive rods but had a limited activity against Gram-negative bacilli [20,47, 48,49].

**Table 1. Bacteria screened for sensitivity to propolis in antimicrobial tests**

| Gram Positive | References | Gram Negative | References |
|---|---|---|---|
| *Staphylococcus* spp (*S. auricularis, S. capitis, S.epidermidis, S. haemolyticus, S. hominis, S. mutans, S. pneumoniae, S. warnerii*) | [46,48,49,51,52,53,54,55,56,57,58,59,60,61] | *Escherichia coli*<br>*Pseudomonas aeruginosa* | [4,20,48,51,54,57,58,60,61,63,66,67,84,]<br>[3,20,54,57,58,60,63,68,77,78,85] |
| *Staphylococcus aureus* | [4,20,46,54,57,58,59,60,61,62,63,64,65,66,67,68,69,70] | *Salmonella sp* (*S. enteritidis, S. typhi, S. typhimurium*) | [20,48,57,66,67,77,78,79,85] |
| *Streptococcus* spp (*S. cricetus, S. faecalis, S. pneumioniae S. pyogenes, S.* β-*haemolyticus, S. mutans, S. sobrinus, S. viridians*) | [19,60,46,51,56,57,66,71,72,73,74,] | *Helicobacter pylori*<br>*Klebsiella pneumoniae* | [86,87]<br>[3,57,58] |
| *Enterococcus* spp (*Enterococcus faecalis*) | [3,60,68,79] | *Proteus vulgaris*<br>*Proteus mirabilis* | [57,58,77] |
| *Bacillus cereus*<br>*Bacillus subtilis* | [3,54,57,60,63,80,81]<br>[57,60,82,83] | *Brucella abortus*<br>*Shigella spp* (*S. dysenteriae, S. sonnei*) | [67,78] |
| *Micrococcus luteus* | [61] | Bacillus larvae | [1,88] |
| *Nocardia asteroids* | [77] | | |
| *Rhodococcus equi* | [77] | *Mycobacterium sp* (*M. tuberculosis*) | [3,89,90] |
| | | *Corynebacterium sp.* (*C. pseudotuberculosis*) | [66] |
| | | *Aeromonas hydrophila* | |
| | | *Enterobacter aerogenous* | [81] |
| *Actinomyces naeslundii*<br>*Lactobacillus acidophilus*<br>*Peptostreptococcus micros* | [89] | *Shiga Bacillus*<br>*Pyocanic Bacillus*<br>*Sonne Bacillus* | [48] |
| | | *Enterobacter cloacae*<br>*Serratia marcescens*<br>*Serratia sp* | [57] |
| | | *Fusobacterium nucleatum*<br>*Porphyromonas gingivalis*<br>*Prevotella melaninogenica* | [91,92] |
| | | *Actinobacillus actinomycetemcomitans*<br>*Capnocytophaga gingivalis*<br>*Porphyromonas anaerobius*<br>*Prevotella intermedia* | [92] |
| | | *Prevotella oralis*<br>*Veillonella parvula* | [89] |
| | | *Brucella melitensis* | [78] |

Propolis is known as Nature's Antibiotic, capable of fighting bacteria, as opposed to conventional antibiotics which destroy all the body's natural flora. In addition, bacteria do not become resistant because many natural factors (the sap source, climate and geographical region) all indiscernibly yet significantly continually alter the natural composition [50]. The mechanism of antibacterial action of propolis has been the subject of only a few publications. It was evidenced that the mechanism of action of propolis on bacterial cell is complex and a simple analogy cannot be made to the mode of action of any classic antibiotics. Valdez Gonzales et al. [71] stated that several UV-absorbing substances inhibiting the DNA-dependent RNA polymerases of *Escherichia coli* and *Streptomyces aureofaciens*, as well as the restriction endonucleases Eco RI have been isolated from the water-soluble extract of propolis by two dimensional paper chromatography. The inhibition of bacterial RNA-polymerase by the components of propolis was probably due to the loss of their ability to bind to DNA [93]. Takaisi-Kikuni and Schilcher [73] showed through electron microscopy and micro-calorimetric assays that ethanolic extract of propolis (EEP) interferes with the division of *Streptococcus agalactie* through the formation of pseudo-multicellular forms, cytoplasm disorganization, inhibition of protein synthesis, leading to lysis of bacteria.Takaisi and Schilcher [73] attributes this capacity to the presence of aromatic acids and esters, while Burdock [6] suggest that it is due to the action of the flavonone pinocembrin and the flavonol galangin, and caffeic acid phenethyl ester, whose action mechanism is based on the inhibition of bacterial RNA polymerase. In addition, the bactericidal effect of flavonoids may be originated from a metabolic perturbation in ion channels as a result of impairment in phosphorylation/dephosphorylation reactions [61, 94]. Caffeic acid, benzoic acid, and cinnamic acid probably act on the microbial membrane or cell wall sites as well, causing functional and structural damages [83,94]. Mirzoeva et al. [94] found that EEP and some phenolics components affect the bioenergetical status of the membrane by inhibition of the membrane potential leading to increased permeability of the membrane to ions and to immobility of *Bacillus subtilis.*

Among the most potent microbicidal compounds in propolis are flavanone pinocembrin (5,7-dihydroxyflavanone) [95] and its 3-OH analogue flavonol galangin (3,5,7-trihydroxyflavon) [83,96]. Caffeic acid (3,4-dihydroxycinnamic acid) and its esters, volatile fractions with phenols and/or terpenoids [97] and chrysin (5,7-dihydroxyflavone) possess notable antimicrobial activities as well [6].

The action mechanism involves degrading the cytoplasmmembrane of the bacteria, which leads to a loss of potassium ions and the damage caused provoking cell autolysis [44].

## ANTIFUNGAL ACTIVITY

In recent years, there has been an increasing search for new antifungal agents, since many of the available antifungal drugs have undesirable side effects or are very toxic (amphotericin B), produce recurrence, show drug-drug interactions (azoles) or lead to the development of resistance (fluconazole, 5-flucytosine), some shows ineffectiveness [98] and have become therefore less successful in therapeutic strategies.

Therefore it is necessary to search for more effective and less toxic novel antifungal agents that would overcome these disadvantages. Interestingly, propolis is widely employed in folk medicine, mainly in communities with inadequate conditions of public health and sanitation [99].

Although antibacterial activity is more relevant than the antifungal properties of propolis, many studies have reported the susceptibility of clinically important yeasts belonging to *Candida* genera [4,79,100] such as *Candida albicans* [66, 84], as well as the sensitivity of some filamentous fungi, mainly dermatophites.

Propolis samples have a fungicidal effect against *Candida, Microsporum, Trichophyton, Fusarium* and other dermatophytes [17] (Table 2). An antifungal activity of propolis was also observed in some plant fungi *in vitro*. The fungicidal effect was associated with the presence of flavonoids and other phenolic components [101,102] such as for antibacteria properties. Differences in antifungal activity of propolis extracts can again be attributed to the differences in chemical composition and concentration of propolis compounds [27, 103].

As for antibiotics, a synergistic effect with conventional antimycotic drugs was observed [79,104].

**Table 2. Fungi screened for sensitivity to propolis in antifungal tests**

| Fungi | References |
|---|---|
| *Candida*<br>*(C. albicans, C. glabrata, C. tropicali, C. krusei, C. guilliermondii, C. parapsilosis)* | [27,28,54,56,66,82,102,105,106,107,108,109,110,111,112,113,114] |
| *Trichophyton sp*<br>*(T. verrucosum, T. mentagrophytes, T. rubrum)* | [81,106,115,116,117] |
| *Aspergillus spp*<br>*(A. flavus, A. ochraceus, A. sulphureus, A. fusariumA. tamarii, A. versicolor, parasiticus)* | [82,94,108,118,119] |
| *Penicilium sp*<br>*(P. viridicatum, P. notatum, P. digitatum, P. italicum)* | [82,96,108] |
| *Cryptococcus neoformans* | [111,120] |
| *Trichosporon spp.* | [27,113] |
| *Scopulariopsis brevicaulis* | [108] |
| *Cladosporium sphaerospermum* | [96] |
| *Rhodotorula sp.* | [27] |
| *Epidermophyton floccosum* | [116] |
| *Microsporum* | [106] |

## Antiviral Activity

Propolis and its derivates have the capacity to inhibit virus propagation. Several *in vitro* studies have shown that propolis interferes with the reproduction of different virus such as those causing influenza and hepatitis B and also against Herpes simplex type 1, Herpes simplex type 2, vesicular stomatitis virus, adenovirus type 2, poliovirus type 2, avian and herpes zoster viruses (Table 3), reviewed in Amoros et al. [29]. It has also been claimed that various propolis fractions affect the replication of viruses such as vaccine virus and the virus responsible for Newcastle disease [121]. Substances isolated from propolis have also been seen to have antiviral activity. For example, isopentyl ferulate inhibits the infectious activity of Hong Kong virus A [122]. Compounds with the molecular moiety of ceffeic acid were considered as new family of natural antiviral compounds [122]. Two of the flavonoids present in propolis (chrysin and campherol) have also been studied and were seen to be very active in the inhibition of replications of several herpes viruses, adenovirus, and rotavirus [123], while other flavonoids, which are responsible for antioxidant activity (galangin and acacentin) had no effect on these viruses [30,124]. However, other studies have pointed to the antiviral effect of galangin on herpes simplex virus (HSV) and Coxsackie b virus [125]. Flavonoids such as quercetin and rutin show antiviral activity against HSV, syncytial virus, poliovirus, and Sindbis virus. The action mechanisms proposed for these compounds are related with the inhibition of viral polymerase and the binding of viral nucleic acid or viral capsid proteins [44].Further studies showed that propolis, flavonoids (quercetin and kaempferol) and the caffeolics (CAPE and isoprenyl caffeate) interfere with the replication of human immunodeficiency virus (HIV-1), inhibiting the enzyme HIV-1 integrase [126,127].

**Table 3. Viruses screened for sensitivity to propolis in antiviral tests**

| Viruses | References |
|---|---|
| RNA viruses<br>*(Poliovirus type 1, Poliovirus type 2, vesicular stomatitis virus (VSV), newcastle disease virus (NDV)* | [29,121,128,129] |
| DNA viruses<br>*(Adenovirus type 2)* | [29] |
| HIV-1 | [127,138] |
| Herpes simplex virus<br>*(HSV-1, HSV1-R, HSV-2)* | [29,125,130,131,132] |
| Influenza virus (A and B) | [4,122,135,136,137] |
| Avian herpes | [132,133,134] |
| vaccine virus | [121] |
| Coxsackie B virus type 1 (Cox B1) | [125] |

# Formulations Including Propolis

In recent years the focus on propolis led to the development of formulations that have improved some features of the product. Nowadays, there are many products that contain propolis on the market, and these include ethanolic extracts (with or without other plant extracts, vitamins, honey, *etc.*), syrups, sprays, tablets and capsules [139]. Propolis mixed with other bee products is usually found in retail markets – honey with propolis being the most common. Due to the acidic taste of propolis, it is usually mixed with honey to increase consumer acceptance. Worldwide, the propolis is used broadly in the formulation of several drugs, supplements or food additives, to improve the health, treatment of minor ulcers in the mouth, angina, thrush or skin infections [139], and to prevent some inflammatory diseases, cardiovascular and liver diseases, diabetes and even some cancers. Of course, different combinations of substances are essential for the biological activity of propolis. It 'felt therefore that the pharmacological properties of propolis are due to the synergy among all its known and unknown compounds, as naturally balanced and not for the isolated component.

Propolis preparations have also seen rapid development, from propolis liquid and ointment in the 1980s, to propolis spray and capsules in the 1990s. After the year 2000, there has been development of propolis soft capsule products, and cosmetic products have seen dramatic growth. Currently, a wide variety of propolis products can be found in supermarkets, shopping malls, specialty shops including propolis tincture, propolis dental liquid, propolis tablets, propolis capsule, propolis liquid, propolis oral membrane, propolis honey, propolis spray and ointment, etc.

## APPLICATION FORMS

### Tinctures

Due to its rich biological properties, propolis tinctures and extracts have become more and more used in the industry, founding utility in a wide range of nutritional, pharmaceutical and cosmetic applications [140,141,142]. The most widely used form as 10 or 20 % tinctures in 70 to 100 % ethanol. The percentage of the propolis tinctures is calculated according to the amount of propolis used. However the actual concentration of the propolis components is only half of that as the alcohol soluble resin is about 50 % of the total propolis.

An intake of 3 times 20 drops of 20 % tincture a day corresponds to about 1 g tincture (from a standard 30 ml eye drop bottle) or about 200 mg of propolis per day [143]. Propolis is well known for its anti-styptic, anaesthetic and astringent qualities – providing quick wound healing properties and suitable for use in the treatment of ulcers; in particular, *helicobacter pylori* and germs, which cause stomach upsets and discomfort. It is also well known for its immunogenic properties; it stimulates the body to manufacture immune T-cells, which protects the body against viral and bacterial attack. By taking propolis regularly, one is able to protect oneself against these viruses and germs and the ravages of winter 'flu and ills.

### Toothpaste

Propolis toothpaste with a pleasant tasting is a mouth deodorizer, eliminates bad breath and halitosis. Propolis kills bacteria which resides in the oral cavity that feeds on food particles and residue. Propolis inhibits the activity of several streptococcal bacteria species that cause dental caries [146,147]. It prevents and stops bleeding gums which are usually due to food particles which normal brushing cannot remove. The food particles decay causing irritation to the gums, resulting in bleeding. Propolis toothpaste protects teeth from decay and also has a strong anti-inflammatory effect which quickly heals the irritated gums and stops further bleeding [148]. It prevents and heals cold sores and mouth ulcerations and sores caused by bacteria or accidental scuffing. The benefit is especially enhanced in older people whose teeth usually shrink away from the gums due to ageing and usually suffer more from bleeding gums than usual.*Soap*

Propolis soap contains an adequate level of propolis which prevent and assists in mild vaginal infections from fungal and bacterial pathogens [149]. It is a well-known fact that the skin often suffers from small cuts and nicks from daily exposure to the environment which allows germs and bacteria to enter into the skin which may lead to serious infections.

By using propolis soap regularly this risk is reduced, as it has a strong natural antibacterial effect [4,144]. Blemishes can sometimes be caused by a cold sore virus, herpes simplex, which causes cold sores on the face which are often difficult to heal. Propolis is known to be effective against this virus [150]. The use of propolis soap can also assist in the treatment of acne vulgaris which is basically caused by bacterial action on excessive oily skin. The mildness of the soap, combined with the antibacterial effect and stimulation of the growth of skin cells assists in the elimination of acne.

### Cream

Its powerful antibacterial and antifungal properties protects the skin from germs and pathogens which are present in the atmosphere. Infections are less likely and if infections occur it prevents the skin from being broken and causing scarring and blemishes [144,145].

### Tablets

Propolis extract paste can easily be included in tablets or sweets. Tablet contains generally about 50 mg of propolis, 3 to 6 pills per day are recommended, in total 300 mg of propolis [143]. According to US Patent several recipes of propolis tablet forms were described [151,152].

## Conclusion

The current prevalence of emerging and remerging diseases resisting to conventional treatment has led to a re-evaluation of the therapeutic use of ancient remedies, including propolis. It is a natural product which has no adverse effect on tissues, so it can safely be used on wounds and inserted into cavities, including sinuses, to clear infection.

The use of propolis for the 1972-2000 period has been dedicated to the development of new products, especially in those products related to their medicinal and nutraceutical properties and with dermatological applications [153]. The growing number of filings for the 1995-2000 period shows that propolis is a natural product of interest for the scientific and technological world at the present time, since the innovation capability shows an ascending trend in the fields (drugs, cosmetics or nutritional supplements).

Around the world, Japan and the United States appear in the first and second place as source and destination country, so both countries are innovators and tributary of the inventions. Japan appears as the country with the most innovative strength in the field of propolis [153].

Official records on current world propolis production are not available, although it was estimated that in 1984 approximately 200 tonnes was traded on the world market [154] (Crane, 1990.) Major producers include China, Brazil, USA, Australia and Uruguay. In fact, Brazil is the more important supplier of propolis on the world market [9]. Importers and processing companies in Japan report that Brazil is the largest exporter of propolis to Japan, accounting in volume for 80% of its total imports, followed by China with around 10%. It is believed that the propolis coming from Brazil, where the natural environment is harsh, has the largest content of beneficial ingredients, resulting in increased imports to Japan.

## REFERENCES

[1] Ghisalberti EL. Propolis: a review. *Bee World* 1979;60:59-84.

[2] Garcia-Viguera C, Greenaway W, Whatley FR. Composition of propolis from two different Spanish regions. *Zeitschrift für Naturforschung,* 1992;47C:634-637.

[3] Karptal M, Yildiz S, Kaya S, Kurucu S, Topcu G. Antimicrobial activity of propolis samples from two different regions of Anatolia. *Journal of Ethnopharmacology*, 2003;86:69-73.

[4] Metzner J, Schneidewind EM, Friedrich E. Effect of propolis and pinocembrin on fungi.*Pharmazie*,1977;32:730.

[5] Ravn H, Andray C, Kovacs G, Moelgaard P. Caffeic acid esters as in vitro inhibitors of plant pathogenic bacteria and fungi. *Biochemical Systematics and Ecology,* 1989;17:175-184.

[6] Fernandes JA, Sugizaki MF, Fogo ML, Funari SRC, Lopes CAM. *In vitro* activity of propolis against bacteria and yeast pathogens isolated from human infections. *Journal of Venomous Animals and Toxins,* 1995;1:63-69.

[7] Holderna E, Kedzia B. Investigations upon the combined action of propolis and antimycotic drugs on Candida albicans. *Herba Polonica*, 1987;33:145-151.

[8] Kovalik, PV. Use of propolis for treatment of chronic sinusitis of fungal etiology. *Vestnik otorinolaringologii,* 1979;6:60-62.

[9] Millet-Clerc J, Michel D, Simeray J, Chaumont JP. Étude préliminaire des propriétés fongistatiques de la propolis comparées à celles de quelques produits commerciaux. *Plantes Médiciales et Phytothérapie*, 1987;21:3-7.

[10] Valdés G, Rojas NM, Morales C. Ensayo preliminar de la acción antifúngica de extractos de propóleo sobre Candida albicans. *Ciencia y Técnica en la Agricultura. Apicultura*, 1987;3:41-49.

[11] Milena L, Leifertova I, Boloun I. Fungistatic effect of propolis. *Folia Pharmaceutica Universitatis Carolinae*, 1989;13:29-44.

[12] Cafarchia C, De Laurentis N, Milillo MA, Losacco V, Puccini V. Antifungal activity of Apulia region propolis. *Parassitologia*, 1999;41:587-590.

[13] Brumfitt W, Hamilton-Miller JTM, Franklin I. Antibiotic activity of natural products: 1. Propolis. *Microbios*, 1990; 62:19-22.

[14] Santos VR, Pimenta FJGS, Aguiar MCF, do Carmo MAV, Naves MD, Mesquita RA. Oral candidiasis treatment with Brazilian ehtanol propolis extract *Phytotherapy Research,* 2005;19:652-654.

[15] Chee HY. *In vitro* evaluation of the antifungal activity of propolis extract on *Cryptococcus neoformans* and *Candida albicans. Mycobiology,* 2002;30:93-95.

[16] Sawaya AC, Palma AM, Caetano FM, Marcucci MC, da Silva Cunha IB, Araujo CE, Shimizu MT. Comparative study of in vitro methods used to analyse the activity of propolis extracts with different compositions against species of Candida. Letters in *Applied Microbiology,* 2002;35:203-207.[113].

[17] Oliveira ACP, Shinobu CS, Longhini R, Franco SL, Svidzinzki TIE. Antifungal activity of propolis extract against yeasts isolated from onychomycosis lesions. *Memórias do Instituto Oswaldo Cruz,* 2006;101:493-497.

[18] Dota KFD, Consolaro MEL, Svidzinski TIE, Bruschi ML. Antifungal activity of Brazilian propolis microparticles against yeasts isolated from vulvovaginal candidiasis. *Evidence-Based Complementary and Alternative Medicine,* 2011:1-8.

[19] Lori GA. Fungicidal effect of propolis in bovine dermatomycosis. *Industria Apícola,* 1990;1:38-43.

[20] Soares MMSR, Cury AE. *In vitro* activity of antifungal and antiseptic agents against dermatophyte isolates from patients with tinea pedis. *Brazilian Journal of Microbiology,* 2001;32:130-134.

[21] Koc AN, Silici S, Ayangil D, Ferahbaş A, Cankaya S. Comparison of in vitro activities of antifungal drugs and ethanolic extract of propolis against Trichophyton rubrum and T. mentagrophytes by using a microdilution assay. *Mycoses,* 2005;48:205-210.

[22] Ozcan M. Inhibition of Aspergillus parasiticus NRRL 2999 by pollen and propolis extracts. *Journal of Medicinal Food,* 2004;7:114-116.

[23] Aly SA, Elewa NA. The effect of Egyptian honeybee propolis on the growth of Aspergillus versicolor and sterigmatocystin biosynthesis in Ras cheese. *Journal of Dairy Research,* 2007;74:74-78.

[24] Helfenberg KD. *Chemiker Zeitung,* 1908;31:987.

[25] [120 AM, Franco MC. The "in vitro" antifungal activity evaluation of propolis G12 ethanol extract on Cryptococcus neoformans. *Revista do Instituto de Medicina Tropical de São Paulo,* 2007;49:93-95.

[26] Maksimova-Todorova V, Manolova N, Gegova G, Serkedzhieva Iu, Uzunov S. Antiviral action of fractions isolated from propolis. *Acta Microbiologica Bulgarica,* 1985;17:79-85.

[27] Serkedjieva J, Manolova N, Bankova V. Antiinfluenza virus effect of some propolis constituents and their analogues (esters of substituted cinnamic acids). *Journal of Natural Product,* 1992;55:294-297.

[28] Cheng PC, Wong G. *Honey bee propolis: prospects in medicine. Bee World,* 1996;77:8-15.

[29] Debiaggi M, Tateo F, Pagani L, Luini M, Romero E. Effects of propolis flavonoids on virus infectivity and replication. *Microbiologica,* 1990;13:207-213.

[30] Meyer JJ, Afolayan AJ, Taylor MB, Erasmus D. Antiviral activity of galangin isolated from the aerial parts of Helichrysum aureonitens. *Journal of Ethnopharmacology,* 1997;56:165-169.

[31] Fesen MR, Kohn KW, Leteurtre F, Pommier Y. *Inhibitors of human immunodeficiency virus integrase. Proceedings of the National Academy of Science (USA), 1993*;90:2399-2403.

[32] Harish Z, Rubinstein A, Golodner M, Elmaliah M, Mizrachi Y. Suppression of HIV-1 replication by propolis and its immunoregulatory effect. *Drugs under Experimental and Clinical Res*earch, 1997;23:89-96.

[33] Hegazi AG, El Berdiny F, El Assily S, Khashabah E, Hassan N, Popov S. Studies on some aspects of antiviral activity. 1- Influence of propolis on Newcastle Disease Virus. *Veterinary* Medical *Journal Giza,* 1993;41:53-56.

[34] Búfalo MC, Figueiredo AS, de Sousa JP, Candeias JM, Bastos JK, Sforcin JM. Anti-poliovirus activity of Baccharis dracunculifolia and propolis by cell viability determination and real-time PCR. *Journal of Applied Microbiology*, 2009;107:1669-1680.

[35] Iuliu P. *Patente No. RO, 4810.* 1965.

[36] Amoros M, Lurton E, Boustie J, Girre L, Sauvager F, Cormier M. Comparison of the anti-herpes simplex virus activities of propolis and 3-methyl-but-2-enyl caffeate. *Journal of Natural Product*, 1994;57:644-647.

[37] Vynograd N, Vynograd I, Sosnowski Z. A comparative multi-centre study of the efficacy of propolis, acyclovir and placebo in the treatment of genital herpes (HSV). *Phytomedicine*, 2000;7:1-6.

[38] Shimizu T, Takeshita Y, Takamori Y, Kai H, Sawamura R, Yoshida H, Watanabe W, Tsutsumi A, Park YK, Yasukawa K, Matsuno K, Shiraki K, Kurokawa M. Efficacy of Brazilian propolis against herpes simplex virus type 1 infection in mice and their modes of antiherpetic efficacies. *Evidence-Based Complementary and Alternative Medicine*, 2011:1-9.

[39] König B, Dustmann JH. The caffeoylics as a new family of natural antiviral compounds. *Naturwissenschaften*, 1985;72:659-661.

[40] Vilelal CO, Fischer G, Castro CC, Nunes CF, Hübner SO, Raffi MB, Salles SE, Anciuti MA, Vargas GD. Virucidal activity of green propolis against *avipoxvirus* in chorioallantoic membrane of embryonated chicken eggs. *African Journal of Microbiology Research,*2011;5:1075-1082.

[41] Eşanu V, Prahoveanu E, Crişan I, Cioca A. The effect of an aqueous propolis extract, of rutin and of a rutin-quercetin mixture on experimental influenza virus infection in mice. *Virologie*, 1981;32:213-215.

[42] Shimizu T, Hino A, Tsutsumi A, Park YK, Watanabe W, Kurokawa M. Anti-influenza virus activity of propolis in vitro and its efficacy against influenza infection in mice. Antiviral Chemistry and *Chemotherapy*, 2008;19:7-13.

[43] Urushisaki T, Takemura T, Tazawa S, Fukuoka M, Hosokawa-Muto J, Araki Y, Kuwata K. Caffeoylquinic acids aremajor constituents with potent anti-influenza effects in Brazilian green propoliswater. *Evidence-Based Complementary and Alternative Medicine*, 2011:1-7.

[44] Gekker G, Hu S, Spivak M, Lokensgard JR, Peterson PK. Anti-HIV-1 activity of propolis in CD4+ lymphocyte and microglial cell cultures. *Journal of Ethnopharmacology*, 2005;102:158 163.

[45] Kosalec I, Pepeljnjak S, Bakmaz M, Vladimir-Knezević S. Flavonoid analysis and antimicrobial activity of commercially available propolis products. *Acta Pharmaceutica*, 2005;55:423-30.

[46] Fokt H, Pereira A, Ferreira AM, Cunha A, Aguiar C. How do bees prevent hive infections? The antimicrobial properties of propolis. *Current Research, Technology and Education Topics in Applied Microbiology and Microbial Biotechnology,* 2010:481-493.

[47] Krell R. 1996. Value-added products from beekeeping. FAO agricultural services bulletin No. 124, Food and Agriculture Organization of the United Nations, Rome, Italy, ISBN: 92-5-103819-8.

[48] Catchpole OJ, Grey JB, Mitchell KA, Lan JS. Supercritical antisolvent fractionation of propolis tincture. *The Journal of Supercritical Fluids*, 2004;29:97-106.

[49] Dantas TNC, Silva HSRC, NetoAAD, Marcucci MC, Maciel MAM. Development of a new propolis microemulsion system for topical applications. *Brazilian Journal of Pharmacognosy*, 2010;20:368-375.

[50] Shakespeare HK. Propolis: composition, health, medicine: a review. *Bee Product Science*, 2011:1-29.

[51] Vennat B, Arvouet-Grand A, Pourrat A. Skin healing preparations: compared in vitro diffusion of the active ingredients. *Drug Development and Industrial Pharmacy,* 1998;24:253-260.

[52] Gregory SR, Piccolo N, Piccolo MT, Piccolo MS, Heggers JP. Comparison of propolis skin cream to silver sulfadiazine: a naturopathic alternative to antibiotics in treatment of minor burns. *Journal of Alternative and Complementary Medicine*, 2002;8:77-83.

[53] Erde GB. Inhibitory effect of bursa propolis on dental caries formation in rats inoculated with streptococcus sobrinus. *Turkish Journal of Zoology,* 2004;28:29-36.

[54] Duarte S, Rosalen PL, Hayacibara MF, Cury JA, Bowen WH, Marquis RE, Rehder VL, Sartoratto A, Ikegaki M, Koo H. The influence of a novel propolis on mutans streptococci biofilms and caries development in rats. *Archives of Oral Biology,* 2006;51:15-22.

[55] Botushanov PI, Grigorov GI, Aleksandrov GA. A clinical study of a silicate toothpaste with extract from propolis. *Folia Medica (Plovdiv)*, 2001;43:28-30.

[56] Santana Pérez E, Lugones Botell M, Pérez Stuart O, Castillo Brito B. Vaginal parasites and acute cervicitis: local treatment with propolis. Preliminary report Revista *cubana* de enfermería. 1995;11:51-56.[150] Giurcăneanu F, Crişan I, Eşanu V, Cioca V, Cajal N. Treatment of cutaneous herpes and herpes zoster with Nivcrisol-D. *Virologie*, 1988;39:21-24.

[57] Hausen BM, Wollenweber E, Senff H, Post B. Propolis allergy. I. Origin, properties, usage and literature review. *Contact Dermatitis,* 1987;17:163-170.

[58] Busciglio JA. Topical composition. US patent No. 4748022. 1988

[59] Corvi Mora P. Quaternary compounds comprising propolis as the active substance. US patent No. 7763282B2. 2010.

[60] Suárez D, Zayas D, Guisado F. Propolis: Patents and technology trends for health applications. *Journal of Business Chemistry*, 2005;2:P119-125.

[61] Crane E. Bees and beekeeping: Science, Practice and World Resources. Cornstock Publ., Ithaca, NY., USA. 1990:593 pp.

[62] Brown R. Hive products: pollen, propolis and royal jelly. *Bee World,* 1989;70:109-117.

[63] de Castro SL. Propolis: biological and pharmacological activities. Therapeutic uses of this bee-product. *Annual Review Biomedical Sciences,* 2001;3:49-83.

[64] Banskota AH, Tezuka Y, Prasain JK, Matsushige K, Saiki I, Kadota S. Chemical constituents of Brazilian propolis and their cytotoxic activities. *Journal of Natural Products*, 1998;61:896-900.

[65] Alencar SM, Oldoni TLC, Castro ML, Cabral ISR, Costa-Neto CM, Cury JA, Rosalen PL, Ikegakid M. Chemical composition and biological activity of a new type of Brazilian propolis: Red propolis. *Journal of Ethnopharmacology,* 2007;113:278–283.

[66] Bankova VS, Castro DSL, Marcucci MC. Propolis: recent advances in chemistry and plant origin. *Apidologie*, 2000;31:3-15.

[67] Sforcin JM, Fernandes Jr A, Lopes CAM, Bankova V, Funari SRC. Seasonal effect on Brazilian propolis antibacterial activity. *Journal of Ethnopharmacology,* 2000;73:243-249.

[68] Ghisalberti EL, Jefferies PR, Lanteri R, Matisons J. Constituents of propolis. *Experientia,* 1978;34:157-158.

[69] Bankova V, Dyulgerov A, Popov S, Evstatieva L, Kuleva L, Pureb O, Zamjansan Z. Propolis produced in Bulgaria and Mongolia: phenolic composition and plant origin, *Apidologie*, 1992;23:79-85.

[70] Walker P, Crane E. Constituents of propolis. *Apidologie,* 1987;18:327-334.

[71] Tikhonov AI, Mamontova INS. Production and study of a lyophilized phenolic polysaccharide preparation from propolis. *Farmatsevtichnii Zhurnal*, 1987;3:67-68.

[72] Moreira TF. Chemical composition of propolis: Vitamins and amino acids. *Revista Brasileira de Farmacognosia,* 1986;1:12-19.

[73] Bankova V. Chemical diversity of propolis and problem of standardization. *Journal of Ethnopharmacology,* 2005;100:114-117.

[74] Silici S, Kutluca S. Chemical composition and antibacterial activity of propolis collected by three different races of honeybees in the same region. *Journal of Ethnopharmacology,* 2005;99:69-73.

[75] Ota C, Unterkircher C, Fantinato V, Shimizu MT. Antifungal activity of propolis on different species of *Candida*. *Mycoses,* 2001;44:375-378.

[76] Amoros M, Sauvager F, Girre L, Cormier M. *In vitro* antiviral activity of propolis. *Apidologie*, 1992;23:231-240.

[77] Grange JM, Davey RW. Antibacterial properties of propolis (bee glue). *Journal of the Royal Society of Medicine*, 1990;83:159-160.

[78] Amoros M, Simoes CMO, Girre L. Synergistic effect of flavones and flavonols against *Herpes simplex* virus type I in cell culture. Comparison with the antiviral activity of propolis. *Journal of Natural Products,* 1992;55:1732-1740.

[79] Freitas SF, Shinohara L, Sforcin JM, Guimaraes S. *In vitro* effects of propolis on *Giardia duodenalis* trophozoites. *Phytomedicine*, 2006;13:170-175.

[80] Dantas AP, Salomao K, Barbosa HS, de Castro SL. The effect of Bulgarian propolis against Trypanosoma cruzi and during its interaction with host cells. *Memórias do Instituto Oswaldo Cruz*, 2006;101:207-11.

[81] Banskota AH, Tezuka Y, Adnyana IK, Midorikawa K, Matsushige K, Message D, Huertas AAG, Kadota S. Cytotoxic, hepatoprotective and free radical scavenging effects of propolis from Brazil, Peru, the Netherlands and China. *Journal of Ethnopharmacology*, 2000;72:239-246.

[82] Su ZZ, Lin J, Prewett M, Goldstein NI, Fisher PB. Apoptosis mediates the selective toxicity of caffeic acid phenethyl ester (CAPE) toward oncogene-transformed rat embryo fibroblast cells. *Anticancer Research,* 1995;15:1841-1848.

[83] Khayyal MT, El-Ghazaly MA, El-Khatib AS. Mechanisms involved in the antiinflammatory effect of propolis extract. *Drugs under Experimental and Clinical Research*, 1993;19:197-203.

[84] Park E-K, Kim S-H, Park S-S. Anti-inflammatory activity of propolis. *Archives of Pharmacal Research*, 1996; 19:337-341.

[85] Paintz M, Metzner J. Zur lokalanasthetischen Wirkung von Propolis und einigen Inhaltsstoffen. *Pharmazie*, 1979;34:839-841.

[86] Russo A, Longo R, Vanella A. Antioxidant activity of propolis: role of caffeic acid phenethyl ester and galangin. *Fitoterapia,* 2002;73:S21-S29.

[87] Ahn M, Kumazawa S, Hamasaka T, Bang K, Nakayama T. Antioxidant activity and constituents of propolis collected in various areas of Korea. *Journal of Agricultural and Food Chemistry*, 2004;52:7286-7292.

[88] Kujumgiev A, Tsvetkova I, Serkedjieva Y, Bankova V, Christov R, Popov S. Antibacterial, antifungal and antiviral activity of propolis from different geographic origins. *Journal of Ethnopharmacology,* 1999; 64:235-40.

[89] Dimov V, Ivanovska N, Bankova V, Popov S. Immunomodulatory action of propolis: IV. Prophylactic activity against Gram negative infections and adjuvant effect of the water soluble derivative. *Vaccine*, 1992;10:817-823.

[90] Orsolic N, Knezevic AH, Sver L, Terzic S, Basic I. Immunomodulatory and antimetastatic action of Propolis and related polyphenolic compounds. *Journal of Ethnopharmacology*, 2004;94:307-315.

[91] Banskota AH, Tezuka Y, Adnyana IK, Ishii E, Midorikawa K, Matsushige K, Kadota S. Hepatoprotective and anti- Helicobacter pylori activities of constituents from Brazilian propolis. *Phytomedicine*, 2001;8:16-23.

[92] Seo KW, Park M, Song Y.J, Kim S, Yoon KR. The protective effects of propolis on hepatic injury and its mechanism. *Phytotherapy Research*, 2003;17:250-253.

[93] Viuda-Martos M, Ruiz-Navajas Y, Fernandez-Lopez J, Perez-Alvarez JA. Functional properties of honey, propolis, and royal jelly. *Journal of Food Science*, 2008;73: R117-R124.

[94] Orsi RO, Sforcin JM, Funari SRC, Junior AF, Bankova V; Synergistic effect of propolis and antibiotics on the *Salmonella typhi. Brazilian Journal of Microbiology,* 2006;37:108-112.

[95] Scazzocchio F, D'Auria, FD, Alessandrini D, Pantanella F. Multifactorial aspects of antimicrobial activity of propolis. *Microbiolgy Research,* 2006;161:327-333.

[96] Scheller S, Rogala D, Stasiak E, Zurek H. Antibacterial properties of propolis. *Polskie Archwm Wet*, 1968;11:391-398.

[97] Akopyan ZM, Shakaryan GA, Danielyan SG. Sensitivity of microorganism to propolis in some districts of the Armenian S.S.R. *Biol Zh Armeniya*, 1970;23:70-4.

[98] Spataru C, Frasinel N; Actinunesbactericida a peopolisului asupra citerva bacteril patogene pentru om si animal. *Lucrari Scientifice. Ins. Agronomie Timisoara*, 1963.

[99] Drago L, De Vecchi E, Nicola L, Gismondo MR. *In vitro* antimicrobial activity of a novel propolis formulation (actichelated propolis). *Journal of Applied Microbiology,* 2007;103:1914-1921.

[100] Marcucci MC. Propolis: Chemical composition, biological properties and therapeutic activity. *Apidologie,* 1995;26:83-99.
[101] Suárez D, Zayas D, Guisado F. Propolis: Patents and technology trends for health applications. *Journal of Business Chemistry,* 2005;2:119-125.
[102] Chernyak, NF. On synergistic effect of propolis and some anti-bacterial drugs. *Antibiotiki*, 1973;18:259-261.
[103] Scheller S, Szaflaraki J, Tuanowski J, Nolewajka E, Stojko A. Biological properties and clinical application of propolis. I. Some physical properties of propolis. *Arznein Forsch,* 1977;27:889.
[104] Scheller S, Tustanowski J. Kurylo B, Paradowski Z, Obuszko Z. Biological proparties and clinical application of propolis. Investigation of sensitivity of staphylococci isolated from pathological cases to ethanolic extract of propolis. Attempts on inducing resistance in laboratory staphyllococci strain to ethanolic extract. *Arzneim Forsch,* 1977;27:139.
[105] Glinnik AV, Gapanovich VYA. Antibacterial properties of propolis. *Zhurnal Ushnykh Nosovykhi Gorlovykh Bolezner,* 1981;4:75-76.
[106] Ibragimova AI, Pankratova NV. Combined antimicrobial effect of propolis and antibiotics on pathogenic staphylococci. *Sbornik Nauchnykh Trudov, Kazanskii Veterinarnyi Institute*, 1983:43-46.
[107] Meresta L, Meresta T. An attempt to use propolis extract in the treatment of mastitis of cows. *Medycyna Weterynaryjna,* 1985;41:489-492.
[108] Abdulsalam KS, Mohamed MI, El-Nawawy MA. Effect of propolis on some bacterial species. *Egyptian Journal of Phytopathology*, 1989;21:61-67.run.
[109] Castaldo S, Capasso F. Propolis, an old remedy used in modern medicine. *Fitoterapia*, 2002;73:S1-S6.
[110] Alencar SM, Oldoni TLC, Castro ML, Cabral ISR, Costa-Neto CM, Cury JA, Rosalen PL, Ikegakid M. Chemical composition and biological activity of a new type of Brazilian propolis: Red propolis. *Journal of Ethnopharmacology,* 2007;113:278-283.
[111] Burdock GA. Review of the biological properties and toxicity of bee propolis. *Food Chemical Toxicology,* 1998;36:347-363.
[112] Seidell V, Peyfoon E, Watson DG, Fearnley J. Comparative study of the antibacterial activity of propolis from different geographical and climatic zones. *Phytotherapy Research,* 2008; 22:1256-1263.
[113] Farnesi AP, Aquino-Ferreira R, De Jong D, Bastos JK, Soares AEE. Effects of stingless bee and honey bee propolis on four species of bacteria. *Genetics Molecular Research,* 2009;8:635-640.
[114] Cizmárik J, Trupl J. The effects of propolis on bacteria. *Pharmazie*, 1976;31:656-657.
[115] Shub TA, Kagramonova KA, Kivman GYA, Tikhonov AI, Gritsenko VI. Antimicrobial activity of propolis extracts. *Pharmaceutical Chemistry Journal*, 1978;11:1242-1424.
[116] Shub TA, Kagramanova KA, Voropaeva SD, Kivman GYA. Effect of propolis on strains of staphylococcus areus resistant to antibiotics. *Antibiotiki,* 1981;26:268-271.
[117] Krol W, Scheller S, Shani J, Pietsz G, Czuba Z. Synergistic effect of ethanolic extract of propolis and antibiotics on the growth of Staphylococcus aureus. *Arzneimittel Forschung-Drug Research,* 1993;43:607-609.
[118] Hegazi AG, El Hadyb F, Allah F. Chemical composition and antimicrobial activity of European propolis. *Zeitschrift für Naturforschung,* 2000;55:70-75.

[119] El-Fadaly H, El-Badrawy EEY. Flavonoids of propolis and their antibacterial activities. *Pakistan Journal of Biological Sciences*, 2001;21:204-207.

[120] Pepeljnjak S, Kosalec I. Galangin expresses bactericidal activity against multiple-resistant bacteria: MRSA, Enterococcus spp. and Pseudomonas aeruginosa. *FEMS Microbiology Lette*rs, 2004;240:111-116.

[121] Popova M, Bankova V, Naydensky Ch, Tsvetkova I, Kujumgiev A. Comparative study of the biological activity of propolis from different geographic origin: a statistical approach. *Macedonian Pharmaceutical Bulletin*, 2004; 50:9-14.

[122] Sforcin JM. Propolis and the immune system: a review. *Journal of Ethnopharmacology,* 2007;113:1-14.

[123] Júnior AF, Balestrin EC, Betoni JEC, RO Orsi, Cunha MLRS, Montelli AC. Propolis: anti-*Staphylococcus aureus* activity and synergism with antimicrobial drugs. *Memórias do Instituto Oswaldo Cruz, Rio de Janeiro*, 2005;100:563-566.

[124] Valdez GG, Hernandez NMR, Vera CM. Estudio comparativo de la acción antimicrobiana del propóleos con antibióticos y desinfectantes convencionales. *Ciencia y Técnica en la Agricultura. Apicultura*, 1985;1:23-36.

[125] Ikeno K, Ikeno T, Miyazawa C. Effects of propolis on dental caries in rats. *Caries Research*, 1991;25:347-351.

[126] Takaisi-Kikuni NB, Schilcher H. Electron microscopic and microcalorimetric investigations of the possible mechanism of the antibacterial action of propolis provenance. *Planta Medica*, 1994;60:222-227.

[127] Park YK, Koo MH, Abreu JAS, Ikegaki M, Cury JA, Rosalen PL. Antimicrobial activity of propolis on oral microorganisms. *Current Microbiology*, 1998;36:24-28.

[128] Bosio K, Avanzini C, D'Avolio A, Ozino O, Savoia D. In vitro activity of propolis against Streptococcus pyogenes. *Letters in Applied Microbiology*, 2000;31:174-177.

[129] Koo H, Rosalen PL, Cury JA, Park YK, Bowen WH. Effects of compounds found in propolis on Streptococcus mutans growth and on glucosiltransferase activity. *Antimicrobial Agents and Chemotherapy,* 2002;46:1302-1309.

[130] de Vargas AC, Loguercio AP, Witt NM, Costa MM, Silva MS, Viana LR. Atividade antimicrobiana "in vitro" de extrato alcoolico de propolis. *Ciência Rural Santa Maria,* 2004;1:159-163.

[131] Ugur A, Arslan T. An i*n vitro* study on antimicrobial activity of propolis from Mugla province of Turkey. *Journal of Medicinal Food*, 2004;7:90-94.

[132] Stepanović S, Antić N, Dakić I, Švabić-Vlahović M. *In vitro* antimicrobial activity of propolis and synergism between propolis and antimicrobial drugs. *Microbiological Research*, 2003;158:353-357.

[133] Wollenweber E, Hausen BM, Greenaway W. Phenolic constituents and sensitizing properties of propolis, poplar balsam and balsam of Peru. *Bulletin de Groupe Polyphenols,* 1990;15:112-120.

[134] Malimon GL, Shub TA, Kagramanova KA, Kivman GYA. Comparative study of alcoholic extracts of propolis from different geographic zones by spectrophotometric and antimicrobialaction. *Khimiko-farmatsevficheskii Zhural*,1980;14:114-117.

[135] Aga H, Shibuya T, Sugimoto T, Kurimoto M, Nakajima S. Isolation and identification of antimicrobial compounds in Brazilian Propolis. *Bioscience Biotechnology and Biochemistry*, 1994;58:945-946.

[136] Pepeljnjak S, Maysinger D, Jalsenjak I. Effect of propolis extract on some fungi. *Scientia Pharmacentica*, 1982;50:165-7.

[137] Pepeljnjak S, Jalsenjak I, Maysinger,D. Flavonoid content in propolis extracts and growth inhibition of Bacillus subtilis. *Pharmazie,* 1985;40:122-123.

[138] Trusheva B, Popova M, Bankova V, Simova S, Marcucci MC, Miorin PL, da Rocha Pasin F, Tsvetkova I. Bioactive constituents of Brazilian red propolis. *Evidence-based Complementary and Alternative Medicine,* 2006;3:249-254.

[139] Orsi RO, Sforcin JM, Rall VLM, Funari SRC, Barbosa L, Júnior FA.. Susceptibility profile of *Salmonella* against the antibacterial activity of propolis produced in two regions of Brazil. *Journal of Venomous Animals and Toxins including Tropical Diseases,* 2005;11:109-116.

[140] Silici S, Kutluca S. Chemical composition and antibacterial activity of propolis collected by three different races of honeybees in the same region. *Journal of Ethnopharmacology,* 2005;99:69-73.

[141] Banskota AH, Tezuka Y, Adnyana IK, Ishii E, Midorikawa K, Matsushige K, Kadota S. Hepatoprotective and anti- Helicobacter pylori activities of constituents from Brazilian propolis. *Phytomedicine.* 2001;8:16-23.[87] Boyanova L, Gergova G, Nikolov R, Derejian S, Lazarova E, Katsarov N, Mitov I, Krastev Z. Activity of Bulgarian propolis against Helicobacter pylori strains *in vitro* by agar-well diffusion, agar dilution and disc diffusion methods. *Journal of Medical Microbiology*, 2005;54:481-483.

[142] Lindenfelser LA. In vivo activity of propolis against *Bacillus larvae. Journal of Invertebrate Pathology*, 1968;12:129-131.

[143] Jozwik Z, Trytek J. The effect of propolis extracts containing flavonoid compounds on acid- resistant saprophytic bacilli. *Pszczelnicze Zeszyty Naukowe,*1985;29:47-65.

[144] Pereira AS, Seixas F, Neto F. Propolis: 100 anos de pesquisa e suas perspectivas futuras. *Química Nova*, 2002;25:321-326.

[145] Rojas Hernandez NM, Candelario M, Olivares E. Antimicrobial activity of propolis against representatives of the genus Mycobacterium. *Revista Biologia (Habana)*, 1993;7 :69-75.

[146] Koru O, Toksoy F, Acikel CH, Tunca YM, Baysallar M, Guclu AU, Akca E, Tuylu AO, Sorkun K, Tanyuksel M, Salih B. *In vitro* antimicrobial activity of propolis samples from different geographical origins against certain oral pathogens. *Anaerobe,* 2007;13:140-145.

[147] Santos FA, Bastos EMA, Uzeda M, Carvalho MAR, Farias LM, Moreira ESA, Braga FC. Antibacterial activity of Brazilian propolis and fractions against oral anaerobic bacteria. *Journal of Ethnopharmacology*, 2002;80:1-7.

[148] Simúth J, Trnovský J, Jeloková J. Inhibition of bacterial DNA-dependent RNA polymerases and restriction endonuclease by UV-absorbing components from propolis. *Pharmazie*, 1986;41:131-2.

[149] Mirzoeva OK, Grishanin RN, Colder PC. Antimicrobial action of propolis and some of its components: the effect on growth, membrane potential and motility of bacteria. *Microbiological Research*, 1997;52:239-246.

[150] Houghton PJ, Woldemariam TZ, Davey W, Baser A, Lau C, Quantitation of the pinocembrin content of propolis by densitometry and high performance liquid chromatography, *Phytochemical Analysis,* 1995;6:207-210.

[151] Afolayan AJ, Meyer JJM. The antimicrobial activity of 3,5,7-trihydroxyflavone isolated from the shoots of *Helichrysum aureonitens*. *Journal of Ethnopharmacology,* 1997;57:177-181.

[152] Bankova V, Christov R, Kujumgiev A, Marucci MC, Popov S. Chemical composition and antibacterial activity of Brazilian propolis, *Zeitschrift für Naturforschung*, 1995;50:167-172.

[153] White TC, Marr KA, Bowden RA. Clinical, cellular and molecular factors that contribute to antifungal drug resistance. *Clinical Microbiology Reviews*,1998;11:382-402.

[154] Ali I, Khan FG, Suri KA, Gupta BD, Satti NK, Dutt P, Afrin F, Qazi GN, Khan IA. In vitro antifungal activity of hydroxychavicol isolated from Piper betle L. *Annals of Clinical Microbiology and Antimicrobials*, 2010;9:7.

In: Beneficial Effects of Propolis on Human Health ... ISBN: 978-1- 62081-440-6
Editors: Tahira Farooqui and Akhlaq A. Farooqui 

*Chapter 11*

# PROPOLIS MEDIATED THERAPEUTIC POTENTIAL OF HEDTA AGAINST BERYLLIUM INDUCED TOXICOLOGICAL CONSEQUENCES

***Satendra Kumar Nirala[1,*], Monika Bhadauria[1], Sangeeta Shukla[1], Asha Mathur[2] and Ramesh Mathur[1]***
[1]School of Studies in Zoology, Jiwaji University, India
[2]Kamala Raja Autonomous Girls (P.G.) College, India

## ABSTRACT

Propolis (honeybee hive product; 200 mg/kg, po) mediated therapeutic potential of N-(2-hydroxy ethyl ethylene diamine triacetic acid) (HEDTA; 20 mg/kg, ip) was explored to encounter beryllium induced toxicological consequences in liver and kidney. Female albino rats were exposed to beryllium nitrate (1 mg/kg, ip) daily for 28 days followed by treatment with above mentioned therapeutic agents either individually or in combination for next 5 consecutive days. Exposure to beryllium increased its concentration in serum, liver and kidney and significantly altered drug metabolizing enzymes, lipid peroxidation and total proteins in liver microsomal fraction. Beryllium administration significantly altered lactate dehydrogenase, γ-glutamyl transpeptidase, bilirubin, creatinine and urea in serum. Activity of acid phosphatase, alkaline phosphatase, adenosine triphosphatase, glucose-6-phophatase and succinic dehydrogenase, triglycerides, cholesterol, protein contents, glycogen contents, lipid peroxidation and glutathione level were deviated in liver and kidney after beryllium intoxication. Severe alterations in histology and ultra morphology of liver and kidney proved its toxic consequences at cellular level. Individual treatment of propolis and HEDTA could reverse some of the studied parameters moderately towards control. Interestingly, combination of propolis and HEDTA reversed all the deviated variables more towards control possibly by additive or synergistic actions of two therapeutic agents at single or multiple target sites. Thus, it can be concluded that combination of propolis

* Address for correspondent author: Department of Zoology, Guru Ghasidas University, Bilaspur 495009, India, Mobile: +91-9406970472, Email: satendrak75@rediffmail.com.

and HEDTA provides excellent therapeutic potential in regulating beryllium induced hepatorenal dysfunction.

**Keywords:** Beryllium toxicity, propolis, HEDTA, hepatorenal ultramorphology, combined therapy

## INTRODUCTION

Propolis is an adhesive, resinous and balsamic material, which is collected by honey bees from sprouts, exudates of trees and other parts of the plants and is modified in the beehive by addition of salivated secretions and wax [1]. Honeybees employ it to smooth the internal walls, to seal holes in their honeycombs and protect the entrance of intruders. It has a long history of being used in folk medicine dating back to at least 300 BC [2]. More than 300 compounds of different functional groups and classes have been identified in propolis [3]; however, composition differs greatly due to variation in its geographical and botanical origin. The most important pharmacologically active constituents in propolis are flavonoids (flavones, flavonols, flavonones), phenolics, and aromatics [4]. Flavonoids are thought to account for much of the biological activity in propolis, including hepatoprotective [5-10], neuroprotective [11], antioxidant and antimicrobial [4], antiparasitic [12], anticancer [13], antidibetic [14], metal chelating [15-17] as well as adjuvant effects [18-20]. Chemical properties of propolis are not only beneficial to bees but also have general pharmacological value as a natural mixture. Thus, its diverse biological properties attracted us to think about its therapeutic potential against certain metal toxicities.

Exposure to toxic metals is inevitable because of wide distribution and extensive uses of metals in the era of industrialization and urbanization. Beryllium is second lightest metal, which has many desirable physico-chemical properties that make it useful in almost every modern industry like aerospace, defense, electronics, telecommunication and biomedical. People, working or living near beryllium related industries have the greatest risk for exposure to beryllium. A survey of previous literature with many clinical reports over last 20 years have incriminated beryllium as toxic metal with disease producing potentials, wherever improper industrial practices prevail [21,22]. Laboratory based experimental studies and industrial experiences have clearly established the toxic consequences of beryllium exposure in humans and experimental animals causing acute pneumonitis, contact dermatitis, hepatomegaly, spleenomegaly, bronchitis, pulmonary granulomatosis, chronic beryllium disease and cancer [23]. Changes in serum proteins and liver function, renal stones and osteosclerosis have also been found to be associated with chronic beryllium disease [24]. Beryllium inhibits a variety of enzymes, including alkaline phosphatase, phosphoglucomutase, $Na^{+}K^{+}$ ATPase [25] and DNA synthase [26] that results into serious physiological impairments.

Chelation therapy is one of the most effective approaches to detoxify beryllium toxicity but has certain limitations [27]. Treatment against metal poisonings is expensive with few chelators and may also impose untoward effects when administered at higher doses [28,29]. The HEDTA [N-(2-hydroxy ethyl ethylene diamine triacetic acid)] is a polyamino carboxylic acid, which contains three carboxylic, one hydroxyl and two amine groups. The therapeutic ability of HEDTA has successfully been tried in removing various toxic metal ions from biological systems like manganese [30], lead [31], beryllium [32] and aluminum [33] due to its multidentate polyfunctional chelating behaviour [34,35]. No marked changes in certain biochemical parameters were noticed after its *per se* administration in rats [36,37].

It is a need to develop a suitable companion formula with lesser side effects against beryllium poisoning. The activities of some compounds can be altered by their pharmacological intervention with other compounds. Thus, combined administration of chelators and therapeutically diverse natural products can achieve excellent protective effect against toxic manifestations by exerting beneficial effects through additive or synergistic actions at single or multiple target sites associated with a physiological process [38]. To validate this hypothesis, we evaluated therapeutic potential of relatively lower doses of HEDTA either individually or in combination with propolis to deal with beryllium induced toxicological consequences in liver and kidney.

## SCIENTIFIC APPROACH TO EVALUATE PROPOLIS

*Chemicals and animals:* Beryllium nitrate [$Be(NO_3)_2$] and HEDTA were procured from Sigma Aldrich Company, St Louis, MO, USA. Crude propolis was obtained generously from Prof. O.P. Agrawal, senior entomologist of School of Studies in Zoology, Jiwaji University, Gwalior. All the other chemicals used in the study were of analytical reagent grade and procured from reputed chemical companies.

Adult female Sprague-Dawely rats (10-12 weeks old) were taken as preferred model for beryllium toxicity. Animals were obtained from the departmental animal facility where they were housed under uniform husbandry conditions of light (14 h) and dark (10 h) with temperature ($25^{o} \pm 2^{o}$ C) and relative humidity (60-70%). Animals were fed on commercially available standard pelleted animal diet and drinking water *ad libitum*. Experimental protocols were approved by the Institutional Animal Ethics Committee.

*Preparation of doses, administration and study design:* Beryllium nitrate (1 mg/kg) was administered intraperitoneally (i.p.). Dose of HEDTA (20 mg/kg; i.p.) was prepared in normal saline; *p*H was adjusted to 7.4. Propolis extract was prepared as described previously [20] with the final yield of 65.38% (w/w). Its aqueous suspension (200 mg/kg) was prepared in gum acacia (2% w/v) and administered through gavage. Saline and 2% gum acacia suspension were used as vehicle and administered i.p. and p.o. respectively. Selection of doses of toxicant, therapeutic agents and duration of treatments were based on earlier work [34] as well as our previous studies [20,39,40]. Forty two animals were randomly assigned into seven groups of six each as following:

*Group 1:* received sodium nitrate (1 mg /kg, i.p.) once a day daily for 28 days followed by vehicle (i.p. and p.o. respectively) for 5 days and served as normal control.

*Group 2:* received vehicle for 28 days followed by HEDTA treatment along with suitable vehicle for 5 days and served as HEDTA *per se* group.

*Group 3:* received vehicle for 28 days followed by propolis treatment along with suitable vehicle for 5 days and served propolis as *per se* groups.

*Group 4:* received beryllium nitrate once a day daily for 28 days followed by vehicle as in group 1 for 5 days and served as experimental control.

*Group 5:* received toxicant as in group 2 and treated with HEDTA (i.p.) and vehicle (p.o.) for 5 consecutive days after toxicant administration.

*Group 6:* received toxicant as in group 2 and treated with vehicle (i.p.) and propolis (p.o.) for 5 consecutive days after toxicant administration.

*Group 7:* received toxicant as in group 2 and treated with HEDTA and propolis concomitantly for 5 consecutive days after toxicant administration.

After 24 h of the last administration, animals were euthanized under mild ether anesthesia. Blood was drawn by puncturing retro-orbital venous sinus to isolate serum. Liver and kidney were promptly excised, washed in chilled saline, blotted and processed for biochemical studies. Standard techniques were applied to determine various blood and tissue biochemical variables; beryllium mobilization as well as ultra structural observations as described previously [20, 40].

*Blood biochemical determination:* Serum was used to determine lactate dehydrogenase (LDH) [41]. Total bilirubin, creatinine, γ-glutamyl transpeptidase (γ-GT), albumin and urea were determined by commercially available diagnostic kits (Merck Specialities Pvt Ltd, India) as per manufacturer's instructions.

*Tissue biochemical determination:* Liver and kidney tissues were used to determine total proteins [42], glycogen [43], lipid peroxidation (LPO) [44], reduced glutathione (GSH) [45], triglycerides (TG) [46], total cholesterol [47], activities of acid phosphatase (ACPase) and alkaline phosphatase (ALPase) [48], adenosine triphosphatase (ATPase) [49], glucose-6-phosphatase (G-6-Pase) [50] and succinic dehydrogenase (SDH) [51].

*Microsomal fraction and drug metabolizing enzymes:* Microsomes were prepared by calcium precipitation method [52] for determination of microsomal protein and microsomal LPO. icrosomal drug metabolizing enzymes (MDME) of CYP1E1 cycle, i.e. aniline hydroxylase (AH) was assayed by measuring intensity of blue color conjugate of phenol and *p*-amino phenol [53].

Whereas amidopyrine-N-demethylase (AND) was determined by measuring formaldehyde formed [54] for the determination of CYP1A2 cycle.

*Beryllium mobilization:* Samples of serum, liver and kidney for beryllium mobilization study were prepared [40] and beryllium content was determined with atomic absorption spectrophotometer (Thermo Electron Corp., U.K.) at wavelength 235 nm [55].

*Transmission electron microscopy:* Small pieces of 1 $mm^3$ of liver and kidney were fixed in Karnovsky's fixative at 4°C for 18 h followed by washing with PBS. Post fixation was carried out with osmium tetraoxide (1%) followed by dehydration in acetone series. Subsequently, samples were embedded in epoxy resin and polymerised at 70°C for 20 h. Ultrathin sections were cut on Reichert Jung Ultracut-E microtome. The sections were placed on uncoated grids and stained with uranyl acetate and lead citrate, then examined under FEI Philips Morgagni 268D transmission electron microscope [56].

*Statistical analyses:* Results are presented as mean ± SEM of 6 animals used in each group. Statistical significance was determined by one-way analysis of variance ($P \leq 0.05$) followed by student's t test ($P \leq 0.01$ and $P \leq 0.05$) for comparison between two groups [57]. Tukey's honestly significant difference *post hoc* test was used for comparison among groups of individual and combined treatments ($P \leq 0.05$).

## SCIENTIFIC EVIDENCES FOR THERAPEUTIC PROSPECTIVE OF PROPOLIS

Figure 1 (A-F) represents the consequences of various treatments on blood biochemical variables. *Per se* treatment of HEDTA and propolis did not alter any of these variables significantly. Beryllium administration provoked the leakage of LDH and γ-GT, hence, increased their level into the circulation significantly ($P \leq 0.01$). Individual administration of HEDTA and propolis as well as their combination reversed both variables significantly towards control ($P \leq 0.01$). Tukey's HSD *post hoc* test revealed significant reversal in these parameters by combined therapy of HEDTA and propolis in comparison to monotherapy ($P \leq 0.05$). Significant fall was observed in serum albumin and urea ($P \leq 0.01$), whereas serum bilirubin and creatinine were significantly increased ($P \leq 0.01$) after beryllium intoxication. Monotherapy and combined therapy of HEDTA and propolis showed significant improvement in serum urea ($P \leq 0.01$). Individual treatment of HEDTA reversed serum albumin ($P \leq 0.05$), whereas monotherapy of propolis did not ameliorate serum albumin. Combined therapy reversed albumin towards control significant at 1% level of probability. Serum bilirubin and creatinine were down regulated significantly after individual and combined administration of HEDTA and propolis ($P \leq 0.01$). Tukey's HSD *post hoc* test indicated significant reversal of bilirubin, albumin and urea by combined therapy of HEDTA and propolis in comparison to monotherapy ($P \leq 0.05$). The percent protection apparently established the fact that combined therapy of HEDTA and propolis exerted more beneficial effects in modulating serological endpoints towards control and showed its merit over monotherapy by providing more than 70% protection in these parameters. Figure 2 (A-D) demonstrates beryllium induced alterations in hepatic microsomal fraction and influence of different treatments on them. *Per se* administration of therapeutic agents did not affect these parameters appreciably.

Significant fall in the activity of AH and AND and microsomal protein content ($P \leq 0.01$), whereas significant increase in microsomal LPO ($P \leq 0.01$) were observed after beryllium administration. Monotherapy of HEDTA and propolis could protect the alterations of microsomal enzymes significantly ($P \leq 0.05$) except the AH activity, which was not reversed with propolis treatment. However, combined treatment of HEDTA and propolis was found to be more effective than monotherapy on the basis of percent protection. Therapy of HEDTA, propolis and their combination inhibited LPO in microsomal fraction ($P \leq 0.01$), whereas microsomal proteins were significantly enhanced towards control only with combined treatment ($P \leq 0.01$). Tukey's HSD *post hoc* test indicated that combined therapy of HEDTA and propolis was significantly effective to inhibit microsomal LPO in comparison to monotherapy ($P \leq 0.05$). Exposure to beryllium intensified hepatorenal LPO, whereas diminished GSH level significantly ($P \leq 0.01$) indicating severe oxidative stress in liver and kidney (Figure 3; A-D).

Monotherapy and combined therapy of HEDTA and propolis significantly inhibited LPO towards control ($P \leq 0.01$). Monotherapy of HEDTA and propolis were not able to improve hepatic GSH; however, combined treatment restored it significantly towards control ($P \leq 0.01$).Individual treatment of propolis recovered renal GSH towards control ($P \leq 0.05$), whereas combined therapy of HEDTA and propolis up regulated GSH production more profoundly ($P \leq 0.01$) and found to be more beneficial in suppressing beryllium induced oxidative stress. Tukey's HSD *post hoc* test revealed significant inhibition in LPO in liver and kidney by combined therapy of HEDTA and propolis in comparison to monotherapy ($P \leq 0.05$).

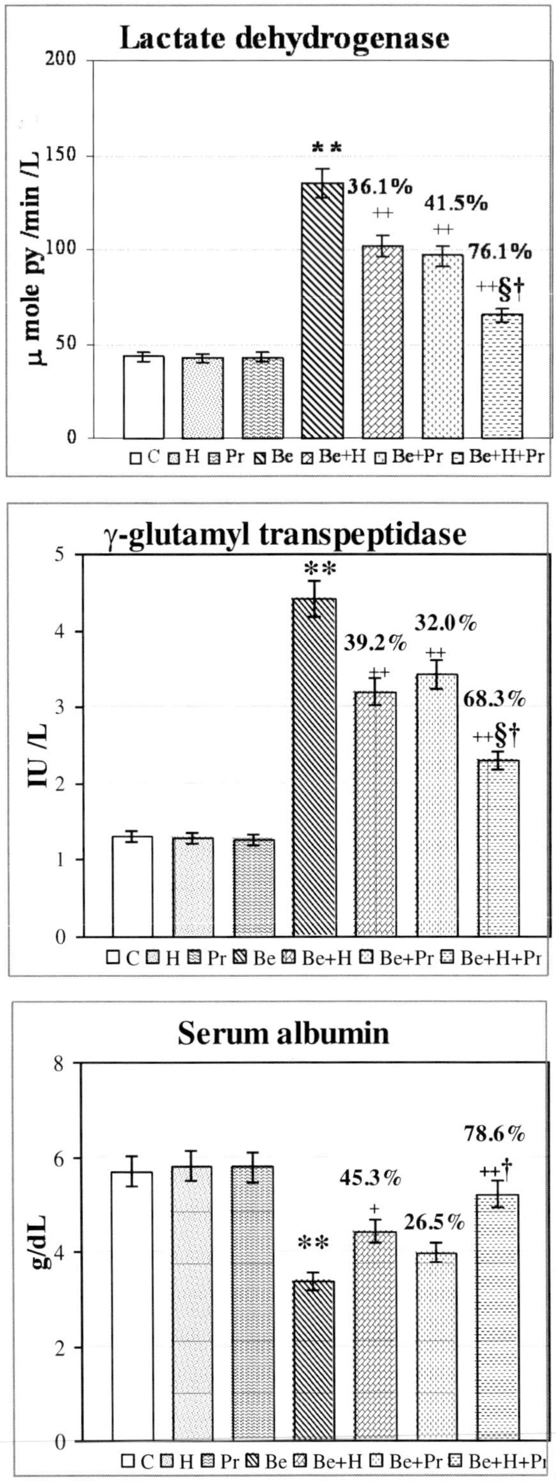


(a)

(b)

(c)

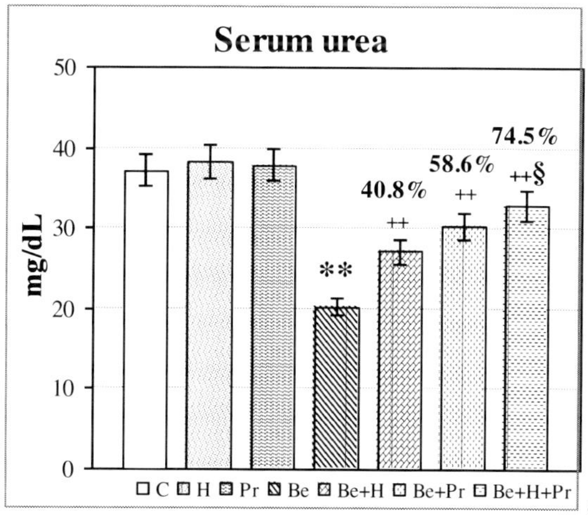


(d)

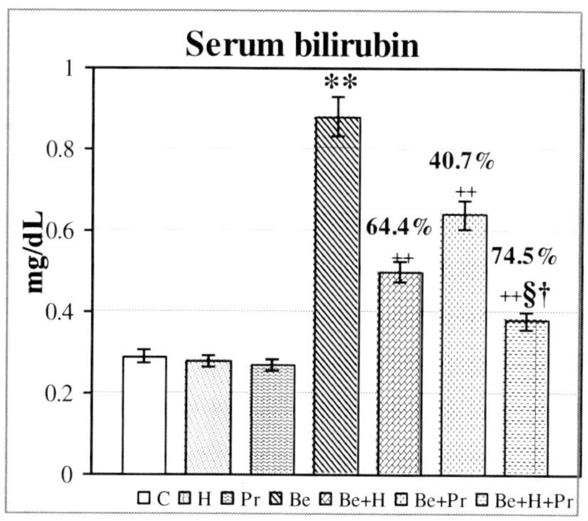


(e)

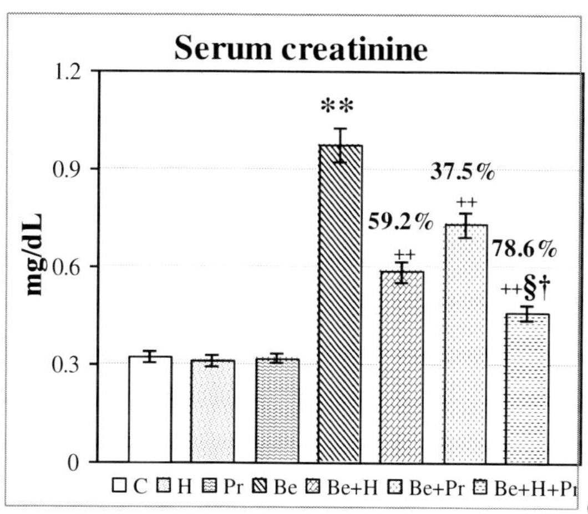


(f)

Figure.1. (A-F).

Beryllium administration significantly diminished the activities of G-6-Pase and SDH with subsequent decrease in glycogen store in liver and kidney ($P \leq 0.01$) (Table 1). Mono therapy of HEDTA significantly recovered renal G-6-Pase as well as hepatorenal SDH and glycogen. Individual treatment of propolis recovered all the variables significantly except hepatic glycogen store.

Co-administration of HEDTA and propolis recovered all these variables more profoundly rather than monotherapy at 1 % level of probability.

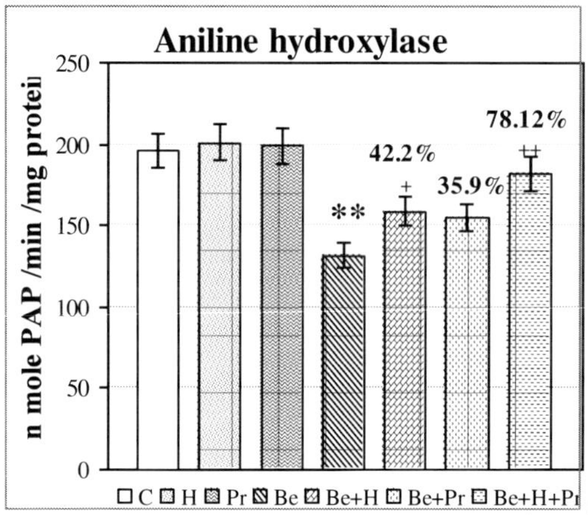


(a)

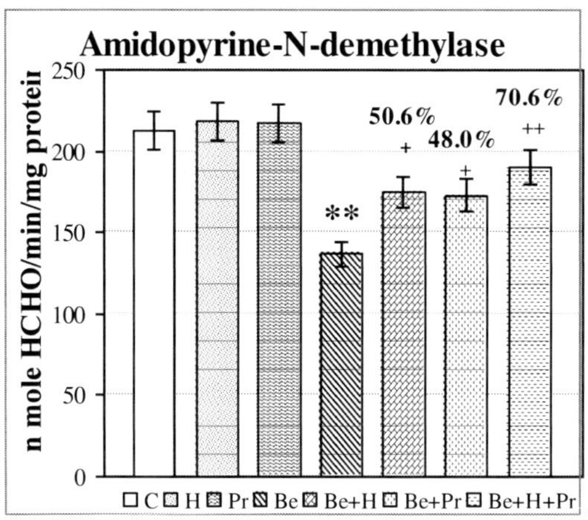


(b)

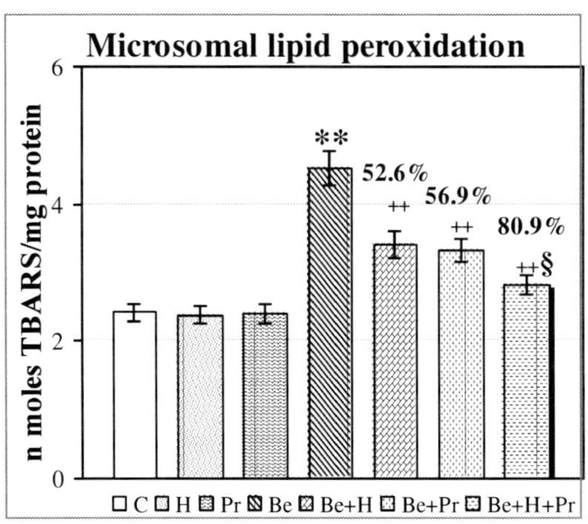


(c)

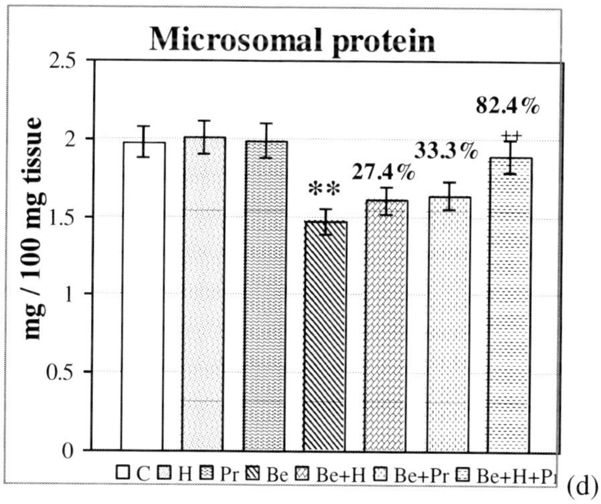


Figure.2. (A-D).

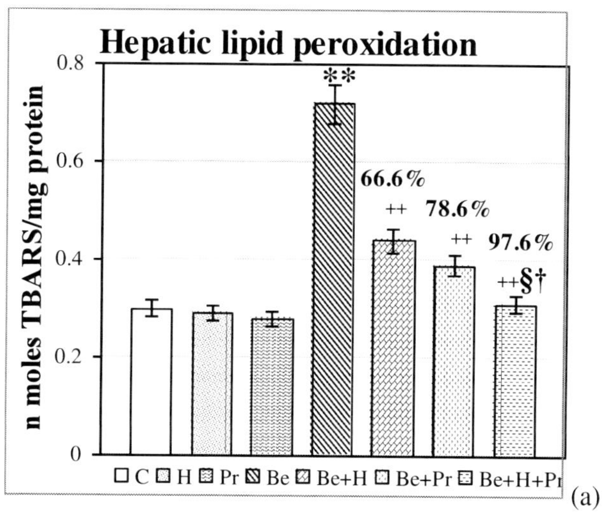


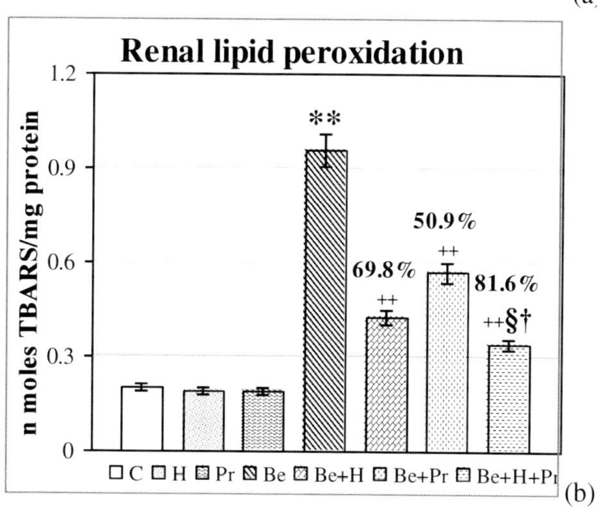


Figure 3. (Continued)

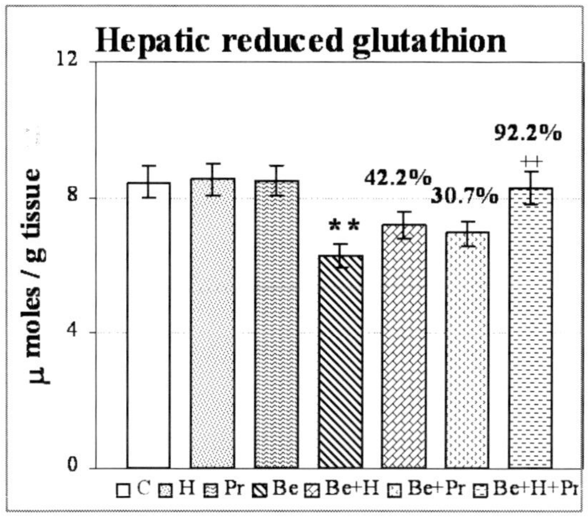


(c)

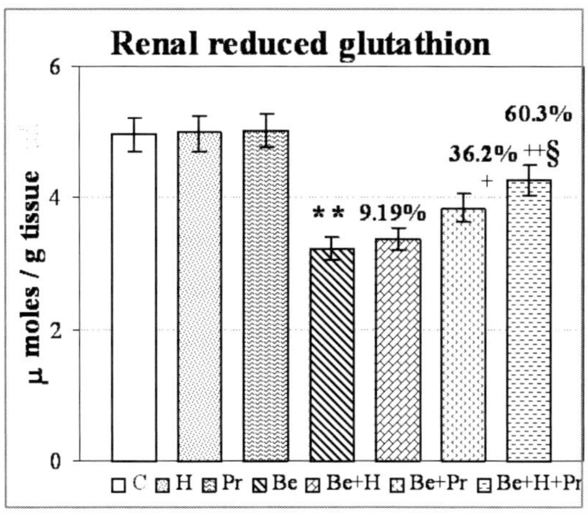


(d)

Figure 3. (A-D).

Tukey's HSD *post hoc* test showed significant reversal in G-6-Pase and SDH by combined therapy in comparison to monotherapy ($P \leq 0.05$). *Per se* treatment of HEDTA and propolis caused no significant changes in the values of these variables.

Beryllium intoxication inhibited the activities of renal ATPase and hepatorenal ALPase ($P \leq 0.01$); however, hepatic ATPase was diminished significantly at 5% level of probability (Table 2). Activity of ACPase was significantly increased after beryllium toxicity in liver only ($P \leq 0.01$). Monotherapy of HEDTA did not activate hepatorenal ATPase and ALPase significantly, whereas renal ATPase and renal ALPase were replenished with individual treatment of propolis ($P \leq 0.05$).

Combined treatment of HEDTA and propolis significantly up regulated the activities of renal ATPase ($P \leq 0.05$) and hepatorenal ALPase ($P \leq 0.01$). Individual administration of HEDTA and propolis down regulated the activity of hepatic ACPase significantly ($P \leq 0.05$). Co-administration of HEDTA and propolis did not show significant reversal in renal ACPase while hepatic ACPase was down regulated significantly ($P \leq 0.01$). Tukey's HSD *post hoc* test reflected significant reversal of hepatorenal ALPase by combined therapy in comparison to monotherapy of HEDTA and propolis ($P \leq 0.05$).

**Table 1. HEDTA and propolis against beryllium induced deviation in G-6-Pase, SDH and glycogen content**

| Treatments | G-6-Pase (mg Pi/ 100mg/ min) | | SDH ($K_3Fe(CN)_6$ reduced/ min /mg protein) | | Glycogen (mg /100 g) | |
|---|---|---|---|---|---|---|
| | Hepatic | Renal | Hepatic | Renal | Hepatic | Renal |
| Control | 7.26 ± 0.40 | 3.89 ± 0.21 | 46.3 ± 2.55 | 38.1 ± 2.10 | 2810 ± 155 | 88.8 ± 4.90 |
| H *per se* | 7.28 ± 0.41 | 3.95 ± 0.22 | 49.1 ± 2.71 | 39.3 ± 2.17 | 2882 ± 159 | 92.8 ± 5.13 |
| Pr *per se* | 7.31 ± 0.41 | 3.97 ± 0.22 | 48.5 ± 2.68 | 38.5 ± 2.12 | 2847 ± 157 | 91.7 ± 5.06 |
| Be | 2.96 ± 0.16** | 1.69 ± 0.09** | 20.9 ± 1.15** | 22.3 ± 1.23** | 1928 ± 106** | 41.9 ± 2.31** |
| Be + H | 3.41 ± 0.18 | 2.24 ± 0.12$^{++}$ | 31.8 ± 1.75$^{++}$ | 28.5 ± 1.57$^{+}$ | 2360 ± 130$^{+}$ | 64.8 ± 3.58$^{++}$ |
| ***% Protection*** | ***10.46%*** | ***25.00%*** | ***42.91%*** | ***39.24%*** | ***48.99%*** | ***48.83%*** |
| Be + Pr | 3.96 ± 0.21$^{++}$ | 2.06 ± 0.11$^{+}$ | 30.3 ± 1.67$^{++}$ | 26.2 ± 1.44$^{+}$ | 2268 ± 125 | 66.4 ± 3.67$^{++}$ |
| ***% Protection*** | ***23.25%*** | ***16.81%*** | ***37.00%*** | ***24.68%*** | ***38.55%*** | ***52.24%*** |
| Be + H + Pr | 5.24 ± 0.28$^{++}$§† | 3.50 ± 0.19$^{++}$§† | 43.5 ± 2.40$^{++}$§† | 32.6 ± 1.80$^{++}$† | 2752 ± 152$^{++}$† | 71.6 ± 3.95$^{++}$ |
| ***% Protection*** | ***53.02%*** | ***82.27%*** | ***88.97%*** | ***65.18%*** | ***93.42%*** | ***63.33%*** |
| F variance | 46.6$^{\Psi}$ | 39.1$^{\Psi}$ | 29.5$^{\Psi}$ | 16.6$^{\Psi}$ | 8.00$^{\Psi}$ | 27.4$^{\Psi}$ |

F variance at 5 % level, $^{\Psi}$significant for ANOVA, **significant Be vs control at $P \leq 0.01$; $^{+}$significant treatments vs Be at $P \leq 0.05$; $^{++}$significant treatments vs Be at $P \leq 0.01$.

§ Significant difference Be+H+Pr vs Be+H, †significant difference Be+H+Pr vs Be+Pr for Tukey's HSD *post hoc* test ($P \leq 0.05$).

Abbreviations: Be=beryllium; H=HEDTA; Pr=propolis; G-6-Pase=glucose-6-phosphatase; SDH=succinic dehydrogenase.

**Table 2. HEDTA along with propolis against altered enzymatic variables after beryllium exposure**

| Treatments | Adenosine triphosphatase (mg Pi/ 100 g/ min) | | Acid phosphatase (mg Pi/ 100 g/ h) | | Alkaline phosphatase (mg Pi/ 100 g/ h) | |
|---|---|---|---|---|---|---|
| | Hepatic | Renal | Hepatic | Renal | Hepatic | Renal |
| Control | 1992 ± 110 | 2465 ± 136 | 243 ± 13.4 | 284 ± 15.7 | 74.1 ± 4.09 | 2645 ± 146 |
| H *per se* | 2010 ± 111 | 2510 ± 138 | 248 ± 13.7 | 289 ± 15.9 | 76.2 ± 4.21 | 2682 ± 148 |
| Pr *per se* | 1999 ± 110 | 2527 ± 139 | 244 ± 13.5 | 287 ± 15.8 | 77.2 ± 4.26 | 2679 ± 148 |
| Be | 1648 ± 91* | 1772 ± 97** | 339 ± 18.7** | 337 ± 18.6 | 52.7 ± 2.91** | 1767 ± 97** |
| Be + H | 1892 ± 104 | 2082 ± 115 | 271 ± 14.9$^{+}$ | 312 ± 17.2 | 58.3 ± 3.22 | 2025 ± 111 |
| ***% Protection*** | ***70.93%*** | ***44.73%*** | ***70.83%*** | ***47.17%*** | ***26.17%*** | ***29.38%*** |
| Be + Pr | 1859 ± 102 | 2124 ± 117$^{+}$ | 284 ± 15.6$^{+}$ | 304 ± 16.8 | 62.5 ± 3.45 | 2230 ± 123$^{+}$ |
| ***% Protection*** | ***61.33%*** | ***50.79%*** | ***57.29%*** | ***62.26%*** | ***45.79%*** | ***52.73%*** |
| Be + H + Pr | 1957 ± 108 | 2378 ± 131$^{++}$ | 256 ± 14.1$^{++}$ | 287 ± 15.9 | 73.2 ± 4.04$^{++}$§ | 2644 ± 146$^{++}$§ |
| ***% Protection*** | ***89.82%*** | ***87.44%*** | ***86.46%*** | ***94.33%*** | ***95.79%*** | ***99.88%*** |
| F variance | 1.76$^{ns}$ | 6.01$^{\Psi}$ | 6.66$^{\Psi}$ | 1.62$^{ns}$ | 8.04$^{\Psi}$ | 9.54$^{\Psi}$ |

F variance at 5 % level, $^{\Psi}$significant for ANOVA, * significant Be vs control at $P \leq 0.05$; ** significant Be vs control at $P \leq 0.01$.

$^{+}$ significant treatments vs Be at $P \leq 0.05$; $^{++}$ significant treatments vs Be at $P \leq 0.01$.

§ Significant difference Be+H+Pr vs Be+H for Tukey's HSD *post hoc* test ($P \leq 0.05$).

Abbreviations: Be=beryllium; H=HEDTA; Pr=propolis.

**Table 3. Effects of combined therapy on triglycerides, cholesterol and total protein content after beryllium toxicity**

| Treatments | Triglycerides (mg/ 100 mg) | | Total cholesterol (mg/ 100 mg) | | Total protein (mg/ 100 mg) | |
|---|---|---|---|---|---|---|
| | Hepatic | Renal | Hepatic | Renal | Hepatic | Renal |
| Control | 13.2 ± 0.72 | 10.8 ± 0.59 | 0.15 ± 0.008 | 0.129 ± 0.007 | 15.9 ± 0.87 | 14.3 ± 0.79 |
| H *per se* | 13.1 ± 0.72 | 10.6 ± 0.58 | 0.148 ± 0.008 | 0.128 ± 0.007 | 16.1 ± 0.89 | 14.8 ± 0.82 |
| Pr *per se* | 13.0 ± 0.71 | 10.7 ± 0.59 | 0.142 ± 0.007 | 0.125 ± 0.006 | 15.9 ± 0.88 | 14.7 ± 0.81 |
| Be | 31.2 ± 1.70** | 28.4 ± 1.56** | 0.264 ± 0.014** | 0.229 ± 0.012** | 12.3 ± 0.67** | 8.95 ± 0.49** |
| Be + H | 27.4 ± 1.51 | 22.2 ± 1.22$^{+}$ | 0.182 ± 0.010$^{++}$ | 0.194 ± 0.010 | 14.3 ± 0.79 | 11.2 ± 0.61$^{+}$ |
| ***% Protection*** | ***21.11%*** | ***35.23%*** | ***71.93%*** | ***35.00%*** | ***55.55%*** | ***42.05%*** |
| Be + Pr | 23.3 ± 1.28$^{++}$ | 21.7 ± 1.19$^{++}$ | 0.187 ± 0.010$^{++}$ | 0.186 ± 0.010$^{+}$ | 13.9 ± 0.76 | 12.2 ± 0.67$^{++}$ |
| ***% Protection*** | ***43.88%*** | ***38.07%*** | ***67.54%*** | ***43.00%*** | ***44.44%*** | ***60.75%*** |
| Be + H + Pr | 22.3 ± 1.23$^{++}$§ | 20.8 ± 1.14$^{++}$ | 0.154 ± 0.008$^{++}$† | 0.159 ± 0.008$^{++}$§ | 15.1 ± 0.83$^{+}$ | 13.8 ± 0.76$^{++}$§ |
| ***% Protection*** | ***49.44%*** | ***43.18%*** | ***96.49%*** | ***70.00%*** | ***77.77%*** | ***90.65%*** |
| F variance | 47.1$^{\Psi}$ | 55.2$^{\Psi}$ | 22.3$^{\Psi}$ | 21.9$^{\Psi}$ | 3.41$^{\Psi}$ | 11.1$^{\Psi}$ |

F variance at 5 % level, $^{\Psi}$significant for ANOVA, ** significant Be vs control at P≤0.01; $^{+}$significant treatments vs Be at P≤0.05; $^{++}$significant treatments vs Be at P≤0.01.

§ Significant difference Be+H+Pr vs Be+H, † significant difference Be+H+Pr vs Be+Pr for Tukey's HSD *post hoc* test (P≤0.05).

Abbreviations: Be=beryllium; H=HEDTA; Pr=propolis.

Significant enhance in total triglyceride and total cholesterol contents, whereas significant fall in total protein contents were observed after induction of beryllium toxicity (*P*≤0.01) (Table 3). *Per se* treatment of therapeutic agents did not show any adverse effect on these variables. Individual treatment of HEDTA significantly decreased only renal triglyceride (*P*≤0.05) and hepatic cholesterol contents (*P*≤0.01). Monotherapy of propolis significantly decreased hepatorenal triglyceride and cholesterol contents (*P*≤0.01) except renal cholesterol, which was declined significantly at 5% level of probability.

Co-administration of HEDTA and propolis decreased triglyceride and total cholesterol content in both the organs (*P*≤0.01). Monotherapy of HEDTA and propolis did not reveal any significant reversal in hepatic total protein contents, whereas they enhanced renal protein content significantly at 5 and 1% level of probability respectively. Combined therapy of HEDTA and propolis significantly improved total protein contents of liver (*P*≤0.05) and kidney (*P*≤0.01) and showed more profound therapeutic effects on the basis of percent protection.

Tukey's HSD *post hoc* test found that combined therapy of HEDTA and propolis in comparison to monotherapy was significantly effective (*P*≤0.05) in reversal of hepatic triglyceride, renal protein and hepatorenal cholesterol contents.

Table 4 represents the influence of therapeutic agents on mobilization of beryllium in different tissues. Beryllium concentration was found to be increased significantly in serum, liver and kidney after its administration for 28 days (*P*≤0.01).

Monotherapy of HEDTA reduced beryllium concentration in liver and kidney (*P*≤0.01), whereas individual treatment of propolis was able to reduce beryllium concentration moderately in serum and kidney (*P*≤0.05). Combined treatment of HEDTA and propolis exerted more pronounced effects in reducing beryllium burden in these tissues (*P*≤0.01).

Tukey's HSD *post hoc* test found significant difference in beryllium mobilization in all the tissues by combined therapy in comparison to monotherapy ($P \leq 0.05$).

**Table 4. Beryllium mobilization after treatment of HEDTA, propolis and their combination**

| Treatments | Beryllium mobilization | | |
|---|---|---|---|
| | Serum (µg/100ml) | Hepatic (µg/100mg) | Renal (µg/100mg) |
| Control | 0.39 ± 0.02 | 0.55 ± 0.03 | 0.78 ± 0.04 |
| H *per se* | 0.38 ± 0.02 | 0.55 ± 0.03 | 0.77 ± 0.04 |
| Pr *per se* | 0.39 ± 0.02 | 0.56 ± 0.03 | 0.78 ± 0.04 |
| Be | 14.8 ± 0.81** | 46.2 ± 2.55** | 13.7 ± 0.75** |
| Be + H | 12.7 ± 0.70 | 30.9 ± 1.70$^{++}$ | 9.72 ± 0.53$^{++}$ |
| ***% Protection*** | ***14.57%*** | ***33.51%*** | ***30.80%*** |
| Be + Pr | 12.1 ± 0.66$^{+}$ | 40.2 ± 2.22 | 11.1 ± 0.61$^{+}$ |
| ***% Protection*** | ***18.73%*** | ***13.14%*** | ***20.12%*** |
| Be + H + Pr | 4.96 ± 0.27$^{++}$§† | 17.2 ± 0.95$^{++}$§† | 5.20 ± 0.28$^{++}$§† |
| ***% Protection*** | ***68.28%*** | ***63.52%*** | ***65.78%*** |
| F ratio | 210$^{\Psi}$ | 215$^{\Psi}$ | 191$^{\Psi}$ |

F variance at 5 % level, ψsignificant for ANOVA.
** significant Be vs control at $P \leq 0.01$.
$^{+}$ Significant treatments vs Be at $P \leq 0.05$; $^{++}$significant treatments vs Be at $P \leq 0.01$.
§ Significant difference Be+H+Pr vs Be+H, †significant difference Be+H+Pr vs Be+Pr for Tukey's HSD post hoc test ($P \leq 0.05$).
Abbreviations: Be=beryllium; H=HEDTA; Pr=propolis.

Beryllium administration for 28 days caused severe damage in histology of liver and kidney, which was recovered profoundly by combined therapy of HEDTA and propolis (data not shown). Beryllium induced ultra morphological alterations were prominently reversed after co-administration of HEDTA and propolis. Figure 4A depicts electron micrograph of hepatocyte of control liver with nucleus having intact nuclear envelop, extensive endoplasmic reticulum, plenty of mitochondria and rosettes of glycogen granules in granular cytoplasm. Figure 4B demonstrates beryllium induced hepatocellular damage with deformed nucleus, degenerated nuclear envelop, irregular nucleolus and heterochromatin, less prominent mitochondria and endoplasmic reticulum, scanty of glycogen granules and high cytoplasmic vacuolation due to degeneration of cellular organelles.

Figure 4C illustrates the micrograph of recovered hepatic ultrastructure after combined effects of HEDTA and propolis that shows well formed and increased number of mitochondria, conspicuously extensive endoplasmic reticulum and rosettes of glycogen in the cytoplasm.

Figure 5A illustrates the ultrastructure of the glomerulus of control kidney. The filtration apparatus of glomerulus in kidney cortex comprises glomerular capillary and adjacent podocytes, where the foot processes of the podocytes rest on the basal lamina surrounding the capillary endothelium and together the three form a filtration apparatus.

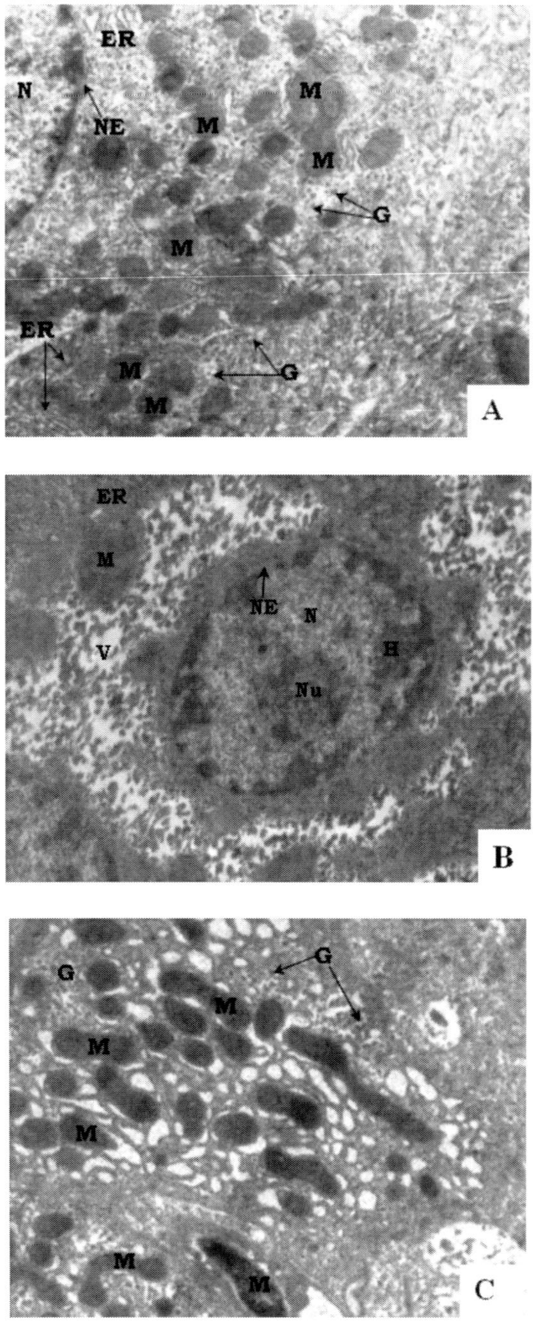


Figure.4. (A-C).

Electron dense glomerular basement membrane was of uniform thickening. Podocytes were normal in appearance with several epithelial foot processes arranged on lamina lucida externa.

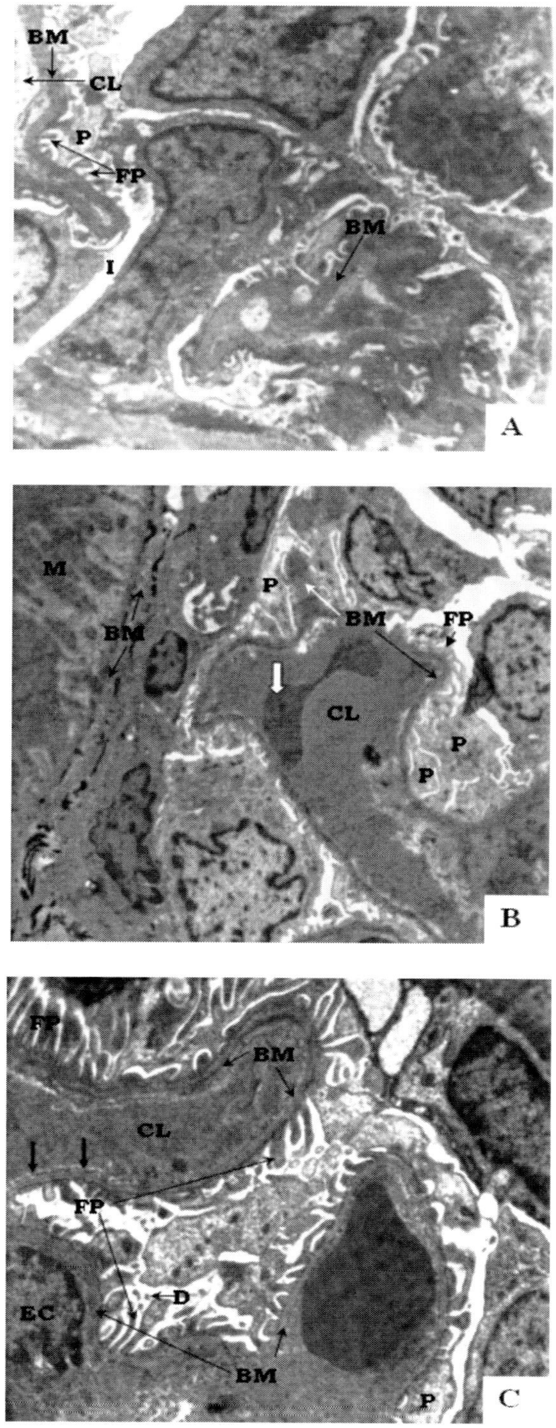


Figure.5. (A-C).

Fenestrated endothelial cells were normal in appearance. Figure 5B exhibits beryllium induced ultra structural alterations in glomerulus of kidney. The glomerular basement membrane was thinner than control but was unusually thickened and tortuous at places. The podocytes were enlarged; foot processes were less in number, deteriorated and fused at places. The interstitium was widened due to shrinkage of constituent cells, whereas membrane detritus was present in interstitium. Capillary lumen was filled with some electron dense material. Mitochondria were not in their normal appearance and their arrangement was disturbed with the degeneration of basement membrane. Figure 5C reveals electron micrograph of the glomerulus capillary and its adjacent podocytes in the glomerulus after combined therapy, which was more similar to the control kidney indicating the reversal of the cellular changes. The capillary lumen was obviously surrounded by uniform fenestrated glomerular basement membrane with uniformly presented podocytes and foot processes. The interstitium was normal in appearance; however, few podocytes were still enlarged.

## Anticipation for Beneficial Role of Propolis

Propolis mediated therapeutic potential of HEDTA was explored to attenuate beryllium induced hepatorenal toxicity considering important biochemical endpoints. Use of chelating agents against metal toxicity facilitates to decrease concentration of toxic metal ions in tissues to the levels that would be unable to induce toxic manifestations. Beryllium accumulation is supposed to increase reactive oxygen species (ROS) [58,59], which injure microsomes, lysosomes, endoplasmic reticulum, plasma membrane and growth receptors that lead to structural and functional impairments [60]. Peroxidative cellular damage and lack of metabolic regulations increased the level of triglyceride and cholesterol contents in liver and kidney due to beryllium intoxication. Although these organs possess an antioxidant defense system that scavenges ROS, the capacity of this system might be overwhelmed during toxic circumstances. (Mechanism of beryllium induced toxicity has been summarized in figure 6). Combination of HEDTA and propolis more profoundly reduced beryllium accumulation in various tissues probably as a result of their chelating action. Polyaminocarboxylic acids are used as effective therapeutic agents in removing toxic metals from biological systems due to their multidentate polyfunctional chelating ability [36,61]. In fact, the chelating efficacy of HEDTA mainly resides in the hydroxyl, carboxyl and amine groups present in it. Beryllium ion may covalently bind after replacing the proton from its carboxylic group and coordinate with nitrogen of amine group as occurs in its congener EDTA. Polyphenolic compounds behave as ROS scavengers, metal chelators and enzyme modulators [59,62] and may play a major role in enhancing cellular antioxidant defense. Being a complex mixture of more than 300 compounds, including phenolics, organic acids and their derivatives; propolis acted as a $Be^{2+}$chelator [15,16]. Propolis is reported to increase bioavailability of certain drugs [63] so it is plausible that propolis might also increase the bioavailability of HEDTA, which in turn sequestered much amount of beryllium ions from the tissues. The capacity of propolis to pass through the membrane and to accumulate in both hydrophilic and hydrophobic environments might also facilitate to scavenge free radicals [64]. Combined treatment reduced the degradation rate of hepatocytes and erythrocytes due to antioxidant action of the flavonoids found in propolis [65,66], which consequently reduced bilirubin level. Combined treatment of propolis and HEDTA improved albumin and protein as a result of intracellular glutathione regulated cellular protein turnover [67]. The cellular recovery was also evident by ultra structural observations.

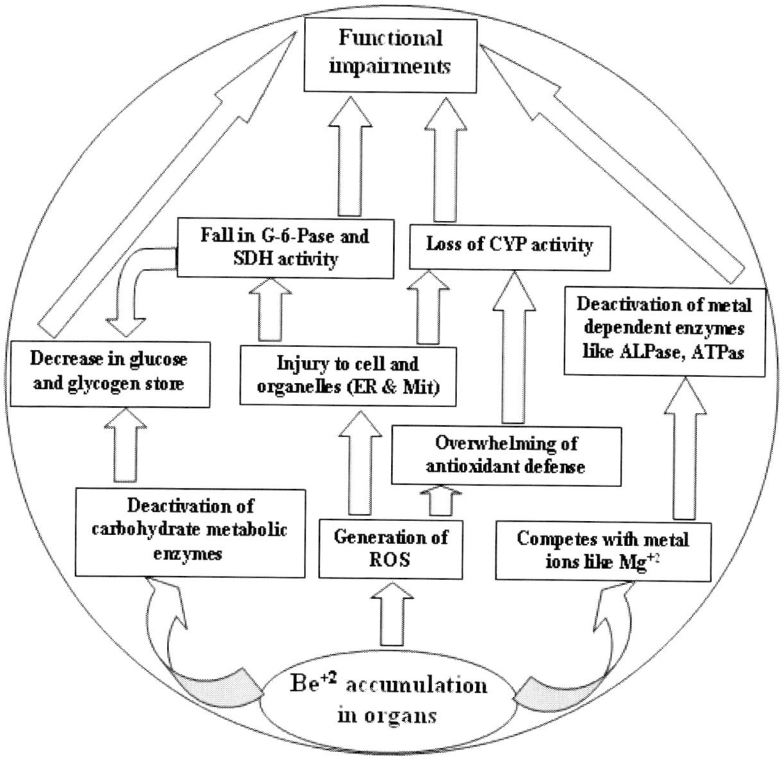


Figure 6. Mechanism of beryllium induced toxicity.

Liver is one of the principal target organs for toxicological action of beryllium [68]. Induction of LDH reflected liver injury associated with necrosis, whereas γ-GT pointed to hepatic cholestasis [69]. Decreased serum urea reflected destruction in the deammination ability of liver due to beryllium intoxication, whereas increased serum creatinine pointed to functional impairment and damage in kidney. Cellular damage and diminishment in glycogenesis due to inactivation of carbohydrate metabolic enzymes after beryllium poisoning [70] declined hepatorenal glycogen. HEDTA diminished beryllium burden in various tissues and acted as an indirect antioxidant by removing beryllium ions from the site [27] as well as phenolic compounds present in propolis extract might protect these marker enzymes by diminishing cellular damage [20], which was also well persuaded by histological and ultra structural observations and proved the merit of combined therapy over monotherapy. Elevated hepatorenal ACPase indicated injurious effects of beryllium on lysosomes [68], which are responsible for increased cellular autophagy, cell death and certain physiological and pathological conditions [71]. Reduction in the release of this enzyme after co-treatment of HEDTA and propolis reflected conspicuous protection of liver and kidney against beryllium toxicity. The ALPase, ATPase and G-6-Pase are membrane bound enzymes and decreased activities of these enzymes [72] corroborated membrane lipid alterations due to toxic consequences of beryllium exposure. Beryllium ions are notorious to inhibit these enzymes by combining their phosphate groups [73]. Displacement of $Mg^{2+}$ by $Be^{2+}$ also results in blocking of phosphatase causing depletion in these enzymes for *in vivo* beryllium toxicity [74]. Decreased beryllium burden in tissues after combined chelation therapy by HEDTA and propolis revived these enzymes. Propolis is a rich source of essential elements, including $Zn^{2+}$, $Mg^{2+}$, $Cu^{2+}$, $Fe^{2+}$, $Mn^{2+}$, $Ni^{2+}$, $Ca^{2+}$ etc. [75], which might also be responsible to reactivate these enzymes by providing optimum trace elements. Propolis is also supposed to be helpful in absorption and utilization of various minerals due to the presence of organic acid derivatives in it, which in turn improved physiological functions by regulating the ion dependent enzymatic activities [76].

Fall in SDH activity after beryllium exposure reflected mitochondrial impairment and inhibition in tricarboxylic acid cycle [77], which would impair the energy supply and subsequently led to cellular degeneration. Ultra structural observations evidently demonstrated degeneration and loss of mitochondria in hepatocytes and renal tubules after exposure to beryllium. Reactivation of SDH and structural improvement in mitochondria evidently proved better therapeutic effects of combination therapy rather than montherapy.

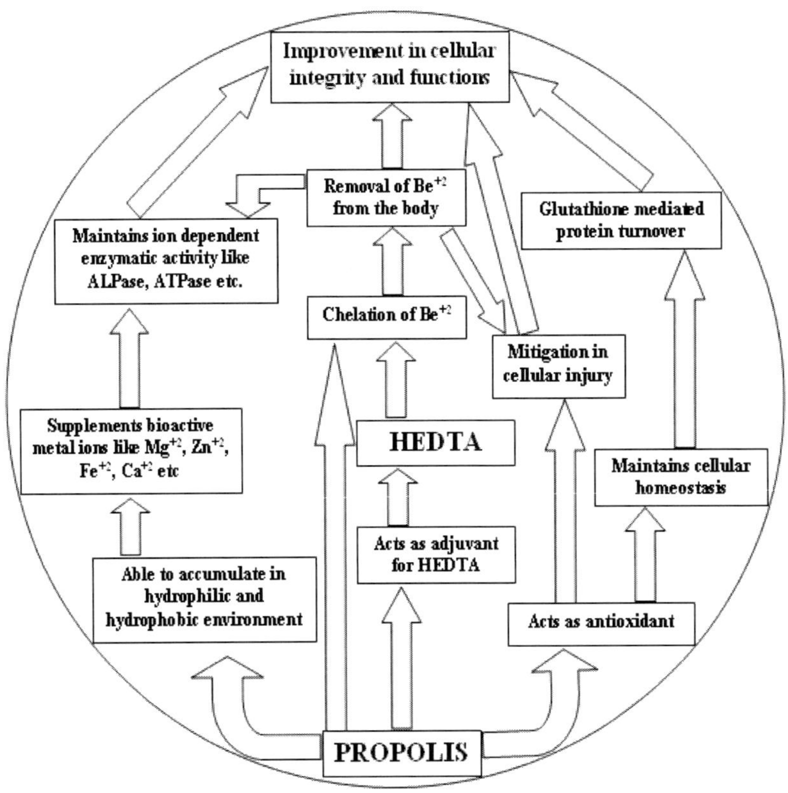


Figure 7. An over all action of propolis and HEDTA in reducing beryllium induced toxicity.

CYP450s belong to a multigenic superfamily involved in the metabolism of endogenous and exogenous compounds [78] and CYP2E1 enzymes are specifically implicated in the metabolism of several compounds [79]. Beryllium inhibits some form of cytochrome P450 specially those are responsible for hydroxylation of substances and inhibits protein and many enzymes, including drug metabolizing enzymes [80]. Thus, beryllium ions might attack on microsomal membranes and destructed microsomal protein and drug metabolizing enzymes i.e., AH and AND by inducing LPO, which were reversed after combined therapy. Several flavonoids and phenolic compounds present in propolis might be capable to encounter beryllium induced microsomal LPO through their combined actions to recover sub cellular architecture and functional integrity of cells that eventually rejuvenated AH and AND activities. (Figure 7 represents an over all action of propolis and HEDTA in reducing beryllium induced toxicity).

Propolis is relatively nontoxic [81,82] and is reported to increase the therapeutic index of a variety of drugs by increasing their bioavailability [63,20]. The dose of HEDTA, used in the experiment was relatively lower and far from any toxic effects [37]. It was assumed that several flavonoids present in propolis might enhance the bioavailability of HEDTA to enhance its subsequent effectiveness by influencing its absorption, transport and entry into cells [83]. It can be concluded that propolis mediated action of HEDTA provides excellent therapeutic potential in regulating beryllium induced hepatorenal dysfunction and propolis could be considered as complementary medicine along with chelation therapy in management of beryllium intoxication.

## ACKNOWLEDGMENTS

Authors are thankful to All India Institute of Medical Sciences, New Delhi for EM facility. Indian Council of Medical Research (45/3/2004/PHA/BMS) and University Grants Commission (F-3/70/2001, SR-II.) are gratefully acknowledged for financial assistance.

## REFERENCES

[1] Ahn MR, Kunimasa K, Ohta T, Kumazawa S, Kamihira M, Kaji K, Uto Y, Hori H, Nagasawa H, Nakayama T. Suppression of tumor-induced angiogenesis by Brazilian propolis: Major component artepillin C inhibits in vitro tube formation and endothelial cell proliferation. *Cancer Letters,* 2007;252:235–243.

[2] Arkhipova OG, Demokidova NK. Effect of phosphoorganic complexons on the activity of alkaline phosphatase in beryllium poisoning *Farmakol Toksikol,* (Russian) 1967;30:352-356.

[3] ATSDR (Agency for Toxic Substances and Disease Registry) Toxicological profile for beryllium. Atlanta, Georgia, ATSDR, US department of health and human services, Public Health Service, September 2002.

[4] Baginski ES, Foa PP, Zak B, Glucose -6-phosphate. *In*: Bergmeyer HU editor, *Methods in Enzymatic analysis,* 2$^{nd}$ Edn; New York: Verlag Chemie Weinheiem, Academy press Inc.,: 1974, 876-880.

[5] Bankova VS, Castro SL, Marcucci MC. Propolis: recent advances in chemistry and plant origin. *Apidologie,* 2000;31:3-15.

[6] Bhadauria M, Nirala SK, Shukla S. Duration dependent hepatoprotective effect of propolis extract against carbon tetrachloride induced acute damage in rats. *Advances in Therapy,* 2007;24:1134-1143.

[7] Bhadauria M, Nirala SK, Shukla S. Hepatoprotective efficacy of propolis extract: A biochemical and histopathological approach. *Iranian Journal of Pharmacology and Therapeutics,* 2007;6:145-154.

[8] Bhadauria M, Nirala SK, Shukla S. Multiple treatment of propolis extract ameliorates carbon tetrachloride induced liver injury in rats. *Food and Chemical Toxicology,* 2008;46:2703-2712.

[9] Bhadauria M, Nirala SK, Shukla S. Propolis protects CYP2E1 enzymatic activities and oxidative stress induced by carbon tetrachloride. *Molecular and Cellular Biochemistry,* 2007;302:215-224.

[10] Bhadauria M, Nirala SK. Reversal of acetaminophen induced sub chronic hepatorenal injury by propolis extract in rats. *Environmental Toxicology and Pharmacology,* 2009; 27:17-25.

[11] Bokowski DL. Rapid determination of beryllium by direct reading spectrophotometer. *American Industrial Hygienic Association Journal,* 1968;29:474-481.

[12] Bosque MA, Domingo JL, Corbella J. Assessment of the developmental toxicity of deferoxamine in mice. *Archives of Toxicology,* 1995;69:467-471.

[13] Boukhalfa H, Lewis JG, Crumbliss AL. Beryllium (II) binding to ATP and ADP: Potentiometric determination of thermodynamic constants and implications for *in vivo* toxicity. *Biometals,* 2004;17:105-109.

[14] Brehe JE, Burch HB. Enzymatic assay for glutathione. *Analytical Biochemistry,* 1976;74:189-197.

[15] Burdock GA. Review of the biological properties and toxicity of bee propolis (Propolis). *Food and Chemical Toxicology,* 1998;36:347-368.

[16] Cantilena LR, Klassen CD. Comparison of effectiveness of several chelators after single administration on the toxicity, excretion and distribution of cadmium. *Toxicology and Applied Pharmacology,* 1981;58:452-460.

[17] Catarina FPT, Wilson JY, Luiziana FS, Tereza TO, Seizi O. Inhibitory effects of beryllium chloride on rat liver microsomal enzymes. *Toxicology,* 1990;61;293-301.

[18] Cochin J, Axelrod J. Biochemical Pharmacological changes in the rats following chronic administration of morphine nalorphine and normorphine. *Journal of Pharmacology and Experimental Therapeutics,* 1959;125:105-110.

[19] Cunha IBDS, Salomao K, Shimizu M, Bankova VS, Custodio AR, De Castro S L, Marcuccie MC. Antitrypanosomal activity of Brazilian propolis from *Apis mellifera. Chemical and Pharmceutical Bulletin,* 2004;52:602-604.

[20] Demasi M, Davies KJ. Proteasome inhibitors induce intracellular protein aggreagation and cell death by an oxygen dependent mechanism. *FEBS Lett,* 2003;542:89-94.

[21] Dobrowolski JW, Tomaszewski R, Druzga M, Zawodny Z. Herb-honeys with pollens as natural sources of deficient and biologically essential elements *In*: Said M, Rahman MA, D'Silva LA editors Elements in health and diseases, Karachi, Pakistan: Hamdard University Press, 1987, 63-73.

[22] Dobrowolski JW, Vohora SB, Sharma K, Shah SA, Naqvi SA, Dandiya PC. Antibacterial, antifungal, antiamoebic, anti-inflammatory, and antipyretic studies on propolis bee products. *Journal of Ethnopharmacology,* 1991;35:77-82.

[23] Fischer G, Cleff MB, Dummer LA, Paulino N, Paulino AS, Vilela CO, Campos FS, Storch T, Vargas GD, Hubner SO, Vidor T. Adjuvant effect of green propolis on

humoral immune response of bovines immunized with bovine herpes virus type 5. *Veterinary Immunology and Immunopathology,* 2007;116:79-84.

[24] Fiske CH, Subbarow Y. The colorimetric determination of phosphatase. *Journal of Biological Chemistry,* 1925;66:375-400.

[25] Flora SJS, Mehta A, Satsangi K, Kannan GM, Gupta M. Aluminum induced oxidative stress in rat brain: response to combined administration of citric acid and HEDTA. *Comparative Biochemistry and Biophysics Part C,* 2003;134:319-328.

[26] Franchini M, Veneri D. Iron-chelation therapy: an update. *Hematology Journal,* 2004;5:287-292.

[27] Friberg L. Edathamil calcium disodium in cadmium poisoning; a study of the excretion, distribution, and toxicity of cadmium in animals. *A M A Archives of Industrial Health,* 1956;13:18-23.

[28] Fulianga HU, Hepburnb HR, Xuana H, Chenc M, Dayad S, Radloffe SE. Effects of propolis on blood glucose, blood lipid and free radicals in rats with diabetes mellitus. *Pharmacological Research,* 2005;51:147-152.

[29] Geckil H, ates B, Durmaz G, Erdogan S, Yilmaz I. Antioxidant, free radical scavenging and metal chelating characteristic of propolis. *American Journal of Biochemistry and Biotechnology,* 2005;1:27-21.

[30] Ghisalberti E. Propolis: a review. *Bee World,* 1979; 60 (2): 59-84

[31] Haro A, Lopez-Aliaga I, Lisbona F, Barrionuevo M, Alferez MJM, Campos MS. Beneficial effect of pollen and/or propolis on the metabolism of iron, calcium, phosphorus, and magnesium in rats with nutritional ferropenic anemia. *Journal of Agriculture and Food Chemistry,* 2000;48:5715-5722.

[32] Hayat A, Arif M. Principles and techniques of electron microscopy. Biological application. New York, Van Nostrard Reinhold Company, 1970.

[33] Hema-Iswarya S, Doble M. Potential synergism of natural products in the treatment of cancer. *Phytotherapy Research,* 2006;20:239-249.

[34] Holtzman NA. Medical and ethical issue in genetic screening-an academic view. *Environmental Health Perspective,* 1996;104:987-990.

[35] Jaiswal AK, Venugopal R, Mucha J, Carothers AM, Grunberger D. Caffeic acid phenethyl ester stimulates human antioxidant response element-mediated expression of the NAD(P)H: Quinone oxidoreductase (NQO1) gene. *Cancer Research,* 1997;57:440-446.

[36] Kato R, Gillette JR. Effect of starvation on NADPH- dependent enzymes in liver microsomes of male and female rats. *Journal of Pharmacology and Experimental Therapeutics,* 1965;150:279-284.

[37] Kepcija D, Dimitrijevic M, Stojanovic M. Une investigation sur les proprie´te´s antioxidants de la propolis *Acta. Vet.,* (Belgrado) 1981;31:181-184.

[38] Khayyal MT, el-Ghazaly MA, el-Khatib AS, Hatem AM, de Vries PJ, el-Shafei S, Khattab MM. A clinical pharmacological study of the potential beneficial effects of a propolis food product as an adjuvant in asthmatic patients. *Fundamental and Clinical Pharmacology,* 2003;17: 93-102.

[39] Leonard SS, Harris GK, Shi X. Metal induced oxidative stress and signal transduction. Free radicals as mediators of alcohol toxicity. *Free Radical Biology of Medicine,* 2004;37:1921-1942.

[40] Lowry OH, Rosenbrough NJ, Farr AL, Randall RJ. Protein measurement with Folin's phenol reagent. *Journal of Biological Chemistry,* 1951;193:265-275.
[41] Mainigi KD, Bresnick E. Inhibition of deoxythymidine kinase by beryllium. *Biochemical Pharmacology,* 1969;18:2003-2007.
[42] Martin JA, Blanco MD, Olmo R, Gomezy C, Teijon JM. Acute administration of beryllium in Rats: Renal, hepatic and haematologic effects and implications of the plasmatic lysozyme levels. *Ecotoxicology and Environmental Restoration,* 2000;3:42-46.
[43] Mathur R, Nirala SK, Mathur A. Comparative effectiveness of $CaNa_3$DTPA and Tiron along with α-tocopherol against beryllium induced biochemical alterations in rats. *Indian Journal of Experimental Biology,* 2004;42:570-574.
[44] Mathur S, Flora SJS, Mathur R, Das Gupta S. Mobilization and distribution of beryllium over the course of chelation therapy with some polyaminocarboxylic acids in rats. *Human and Experimental Toxicology,* 1993;12:19-24.
[45] Mathur S, Flora SJS, Mathur R, DasGupta S. Mobilization and distribution of beryllium over the course of chelation therapy with some polyaminocarboxylic acids in rats. *Human and Experimental Toxicology,* 1993;12:19-24.
[46] Mehta A, Flora SJS. Possible role of metal redistribution, hepatotoxicity and oxidative stress in chelating agents induced hepatic and renal metallothionein in rats. *Food and Chemical Toxicology,* 2001;39:1029-1038.
[47] Moskaug JO, Carlsen H, Myhrstad MCW, Blomhoff R. Polyphenols and glutathione synthesis regulation. *American Journal of Clinical Nutrition,* 2005;81:277S-283S.
[48] Mukhina ST. Effect of magnesium on oxidative processes in rat liver and lung homogenates as a result of experimental beryllium intoxication. *Gig Tr Proj Zabol,* (Russian) 1967;11:43-46.
[49] Nelson DR, Koymans L, Kamataki T, Stegeman JJ, Feyereisen R, Waxman DJ, Waterman MR, Gotoh O, Coon MJ, Estabrook RW, Gunsalus IC, Nebert DW. P450 superfamily: update on new sequences, gene mapping, accession numbers and nomenclature. *Pharmacogenetics,* 1996;6:1-42.
[50] Neri BP, Frings CS. Improved method for determination for triglycerides in serum. *Clinical Chemistry,* 1973;19:1201-1202.
[51] Nirala SK, Bhadauria M, Mathur R, Mathur A. Amelioration of beryllium induced alterations in hepatorenal biochemistry and ultramorphology by co-administration of tiferron and adjuvants. *Journal of Biomedical Sciences,* 2007;14:331-345.
[52] Nirala SK, Bhadauria M, Mathur R, Mathur A. Influence of α-tocopherol, propolis and piperine on therapeutic potential of tiferron against beryllium induced toxic manifestations. *Journal of Applied Toxicology,* 2008;28:44-54.
[53] Nirala SK, Bhadauria M, Shukla S, Agrawal OP, Mathur A, Li PQ, Mathur R. Pharmacological intervention of tiferron and propolis to alleviate beryllium-induced hepatorenal toxicity. *Fundamental and Clinical Pharmacology,* 2008;*22*:403-415.
[54] Nirala SK, Bhadauria M. Propolis reverses acetaminophen induced hepatorenal biochemical and histopathological alterations. *Archives of Pharmacal Research,* 2008; 31:451-461.
[55] Nirala SK, Bhadauria M. Synergistic effects of ferritin and propolis in modulation of beryllium induced toxicogenic alterations. *Food and Chemical Toxicology,* 2008;46:3069–3079.

[56] Nirala SK, Mathur R, Mathur A. Amelioration of beryllium induced biochemical alterations by combined treatment of propolis and chelator. *Journal of Ecophysiology and Occupational Health,* 2004;4:45-54.

[57] Nostro A, Cellini L, Di Bartolomeo S, Cannatelli MA, Di Campli E, Procopio F, Grande R, Marzio L, Alonzo V. Effects of combining extracts (from propolis or Zingiber officinale) with clarithromycin on *Helicobacter pylori. Phytotherapy Research,* 2006;20:187-190.

[58] Novikoff AB. The cell *In*: Brachet J, Mirsky AE editors, Lysosomes and related particles Vol. 2, New York: Academic Press: 1961, 432.

[59] Pietta P, Simonetti P, Gordana C, Brusamolino A, Morazzoni P, Bombardelli E. Relationship between rate and extent of cathechin absorption and plasma antioxidant status. *Biochemical and Molecular Biology International,* 1998;46:895-903.

[60] Pucci L, Chirulli V, Marini S, Lucchesi D, Penno G, Gervasi PG, Prato SD, Longob V. Expression and activity of CYP2E1 in circulating lymphocytes are not altered in diabetic individuals. *Pharmacology Research,* 2005;51:561-565.

[61] Rodriguez-Garay EA. Cholestasis: human disease and experimental animal models. *Annals of Hepatology,* 2003;2:150-158.

[62] Schenkman JB, Cinti DL. Prepareation of microsomes from calcium. *Methods of Enzymology,* 1978;52:83-89.

[63] Seifter S, Dayton S, Novic B, Muintwyler E. The estimation of glycogen with anthrone reagent. *Archives of Biochemistry,* 1950;25:191-200.

[64] Seth PK, Tangri KK. Biochemical effects of newer salicylic acid congeners. *Journal of Pharmacy and Pharmacology,* 1966;18:831-833.

[65] Sharma SK, Krishna Murti CR. Production of lipid peroxides by brain. *Journal of Neurochemistry,* 1968;15:147-149.

[66] Shimazawa M, Chikamatsu S, Morimoto N, Mishima S, Nagai H, Hara H. Neuroprotection by Brazilian Green Propolis against *In vitro and In vivo* Ischemic Neuronal Damage. *Evidence Based Complementary and Alternative Medicine,* 2005;2:201-207.

[67] Simoes LM, Gregorio LE, Da Silva Filho AA, de-Souza ML, Azzolini AE, Bastos JK, Lucisano-Valim YM. Effect of Brazilian Propolis on the production of reactive oxygen species by stimulated neutrophils. *Journal of Ethnopharmacology,* 2004;94:59-65.

[68] Slater EC, Bonner WD. The effect of fluoride on the succinic oxidase system. *Biochemistry Journal,* 1952;82:185-191.

[69] Snedecor GW, Cochran WG. Statistical Method, 8$^{th}$ Edition, Ames. Iowa, Iowa State University Press:1994, 217-236.

[70] Stange AW, Furman FJ, Hillmas DE. Rocky flats beryllium health surveillance. *Environmental Health Perspective,* 1996;104:981-986.

[71] Sun F, Hayami S, Haruna S, Ogiri Y, Tanaka K, Yamada Y, Ikeda K, Yamaha H, Sujimoto H, Kaeai N, Kojo S. *In vivo* antioxidative activity of propolis evaluated by the interaction with vitamin C and E and the level of lipid hydroperoxides in rats. *Journal of Agricultural Food Chemistry*, 2000;48:1462-1465.

[72] Tandon SK, Behari JR, Singh S. Chelation in metal intoxication. XIII. Polyamino carboxylic acids as chelators in lead poisoning. *Bulletin of Environmental Contamination and Toxicology,* 1983;30:552-558.

[73] Tandon SK, Khandelwal S. Chelation in metal intoxication X: Influence of different polyaminocarboxylic acids and thiol chelators in the excretion and tissue distribution of $Mn^{54}$ in rat. *Research and Communication in Chemistry Pathology Pharmacology,* 1982;36:337-340.

[74] Tandon SK, Mathur AK. Chelation in metal intoxication, III. Lowering of Nickel content in poisoned rat organs. *Acta Pharmacology Toxicology,*1976;38:401-408.

[75] Tepper LB. Beryllium. *CRC Critical Reviews in Toxicology* 1972;1:235-259.

[76] Thomas M, Aldridge WN. The inhibition of enzymes by beryllium *Biochemical Journal,* 1966; 98: 94-99.

[77] Uzel A, Sorkun K, Oncag O, Cogulu D, Gencay O, Salih B. Chemical compositions and antimicrobial activities of four different Anatolian propolis samples. *Microbiological Research,* 2005;160:189-195.

[78] WHO (World Health Organization) Environmental Health Criteria: 106 'Beryllium'. International programme on Chemical Safety. World Health Organization, Geneva, 1990.

[79] Witschi HP, Aldridge WN. Uptake, Distribution and binding of beryllium to organelles of the rat liver. *Cell and Biochemistry Journal,* 1968;106:811-820.

[80] Witschi HP. Effects of beryllium on deoxyribonucleic acid synthesizing enzymes in regenerating liver cell. *Biochemistry Journal,* 1970;120:623-634.

[81] Wroblewski F, La Due JS. Lactic dehydrogenase activity in blood. *Proceedings of Social and Experimental Biology and Medicine,* 1955;90:210-213.

[82] Zhao JQ, Du GZ, Xiong YC, Wen YF, Bhadauria M, Nirala SK. Gallic acid in combination with piperine attenuates beryllium induced hepatocellular dysfunction and oxidative stress in rodent. *Archives of Pharmcal Research,* 2007;30:1575-1583.

[83] Zlatkis A, Zak B, Boyle AJ. A new method for direct determination of serum cholesterol. *Journal of Lab Clincal Medicine,* 1953;41:486-492.

In: Beneficial Effects of Propolis on Human Health ... ISBN: 978-1- 62081-440-6
Editors: Tahira Farooqui and Akhlaq A. Farooqui 

*Chapter 12*

# A Sticky Problem: Unraveling the Health Benefits of Polyphenols in Propolis

***E. Paul Cherniack***
Geriatrics Institute, Division of Gerontology and Geriatric Medicine, Department of Medicine, University of Miami Miller School of Medicine, and the Bruce W. Carter Veterans Affairs Medical Center, Miami, FL, US

## Abstract

The complex mixture of substances that comprises propolis includes multiple polyphenols. Many of these polyphenols are believed to have health benefits. These substances include phenolic acid esters, flavones, flavonones, chalcones, dihydrochalcones, phenolic acids, and aliphatic acids,

The most common constituents are phenolic acid esters, particular caffeic acid. Caffeic acid has been studied in vitro for its anti-carcinogenic, anti-microbial, anti-viral, and anti-inflammatory properties.

Another well studied polyphenol that can be found in propolis is resveratrol. Resveratrol has multiple potential benefits including treatment of cognitive disorders, cancer, metabolic syndrome, osteoporosis, and aging. Resveratrol increased the lifespan of several invertebrate and one vertebrate species, Clinical trials of the use of resveratrol in dementia, glucose and lipid metabolism disorders are currently underway.

Quercetin is a constituent with many potential effects on health. Quercetin in vitro has anti-inflammatory, anti-tumor, and neuroprotective effects. In animal models it enhances lifespan and treats metabolic syndrome.

Kaempferol is a polyphenol with medicinal activity found in propolis that has been the topic of in vitro and epidemiological studies. Kaempferol is an anti-inflammatory agent with antimicrobial, anti-tumor, neuroprotective, and cardioprotective properties.

Other polyphenols include chrysin, pinocembrin, myricetin, and rutin, which have anticarcinogenic activity and beneficial effects on lipids.

A major question that remains in the application of these polyphenols is there bioavailability. Since they are quickly and highly metabolized in the liver and intestine, delivery at sufficient concentrations to elicit health benefits will be a challenge.

In this chapter the health-enhancing properties of multiple polyphenols will be reviewed, including studies in which propolis was the actual source of the polyphenol used in the investigation.

**Keywords:** Propolis, polyphenol. resveratrol. quercetin, caffeic acid, kaempferol

## INTRODUCTION

Among the plethora of substances present in propolis are a class of molecules known as polyphenols, whose health benefits are the source of increasing study. Characterized by the presence of multiple phenol rings, these substances are the focus of intense investigation for their role as antinflammatory, antineoplastic, antimicrobial, anti-aging, and neuroprotective agents.In several investigations, the polyphenol content of propolis was analyzed [1]. Propolis contains many polyphenols including resveratrol, quercetin, chrysin, myricetin, kaempferol, rutin, and caffeic acid [1]. In this chapter, the health of effects of these polyphenols will be analyzed, including studies in which propolis was the source of the polyphenol.

## RESVERATROL

Resveratrol is probably the most-well studied of all of these polyphenols. Resveratrol has been investigated for multiple possible health enhancing-effects, such as prolonging lifespan, reducing heart disease and metabolic syndrome, inhibiting carcinogenesis, and treating cognitive dysfunction [2-4].

Resveraterol has been touted as an anti-aging substance due to effect on the lifespan of certain species. The lifespan of the yeast *S. cervevisiae* grown in a 10 μM solution of resveratrol was 70% longer than yeast grown in culture media without the polyphenol [5]. A concentration of 100 μM prolonged the lifespan of the flatworm *C. elegans* by 20% and the fruit fly *Drosophila melanogaster* by 29% [6]. However, the lifespans of human fibroblasts and mice did were not augmented by resveratrol [7, 8].

Resveratrol may alter lifespan by acting upon nutrient-sensing genes that regulate cellular growth, such as AKT and P13k [2]. It may also activate genes called sirtuins, that deacetylate histones, fostering gene integrity when DNA is disrupted, although there is some controversy as to whether resveratrol actually stimulates sirtins [2]. Sirtuins, in turn, activate AMP-mediated kinase, an important gene in mitochondrial synthesis and energy regulations [2].

There are other mechanisms by which resveratrol may retard the aging process in multicellular organisms. Resveratrol has anti-inflammatory activity and mitochondrial-enhancing activity [2]. Resveratrol counteracts inflammation through inhibition of angioensin-II, LDL oxidation, and platelet clustering [2].

An important anti-inflammatory action of resveratrol may be its effect on adipocytes. Resveratrol suppresses an important gene in adipocyte function, peroxisome proliferator-activated receptor (PPARγ), reducing levels of PPARγ protein [9]. This causes a loss of insulin sensitivity and glucose intake by adipocytes and prevents adipocyte development from precursor cells [10]. Resveratrol also inhibits adipoctye maturation by its effect on mitochondrial genes, such as sirtuins [10]. Sirtuins stimulate transcriptional coactivator peroxisome proliferator-activated receptor gamma coactivator 1-alpha (PGC-1α). PGC-1α regulates mitochondrial synthesis and oxidizes fatty acids [10]. Resveratrol also prevents accretion of lipids with rat lipocytes [10]. When rat adipocytes were incubated in 10-100μM resveratrol, lipolysis resulted [11]. The release of proinflammatory cytokines from adipocytes, such as tumor necrosis factor alpha (TNF-α), interleukin-6 (IL-6), IL-8, monocyte chemoattractant protein 1 (MCP-1), extracellular receptor-activated kinase (ERK), COX-2, vascular endothelial growth factor (VEGF), NF-kappaB(NF-κB), plasminogen activator inhibitor (PAI-1), and adiponectin is averted by resveratrol [3, 10].

A study was performed in which mice were fed either a normal or a high-fat diet together with or without 400mg/kg/day resveratrol for 15 weeks [12]. Resveratrol prevented weight gain and loss of endurance of grip strength, ability to hang onto a rotating rod, and maze tests induced by a high-fat diet. Mitochondria from the muscle biopsies of resveratrol-treated mice were larger and more active than mitochondria from control mice. There was an increased activation of mitochondrial genes in mice fed the polyphenol. Resveratrol-treated mice did not lose aerobic and oxidative capacity that mice fed a high-fat diet without resveratrol did.

Mice on a high-fat diet also live shorter lives. However, mice that consumed an added 22.4mg/kg/day of resveratrol lived as long as normal mice [7].

Zucker rats, a rodent model of metabolic syndrome, were treated with either 10mg/kg resveratrol or a placebo [13]. The resveratrol-treated rats had a better lipid profile, and a lower glucose and blood pressure than control animals. Zucker rats who ingested 15mg/kg resveratrol had less fatty liver disease than control rats [14]. Normal rats fed a high-fat diet in addition to resveratrol added to water for 30 days had improved insulin in glucose control than rats not treated with resveratrol [15]. Diabetic rats that consumed resveratrol also noted better glucose and insulin levels, improved concentration of carbohydrate metabolism regulation enzymes, and lower concentrations of proinflammatory cytokines [16-19].

Other mammals have improved lipid metabolism on resveratrol ingestion. Pigs who consumed 100mg/kg/d over seven weeks also had a lower weight, lipid profile, and blood pressure than placebo pigs [20]. Lemurs who consumed 200mg/kg/d resveratrol for one month had a greater metabolic rate and a lower seasonal weight gain [21].

While few human trials of resveratrol have been performed to test the beneficial effects of resveratrol in humans, resveratrol has been postulated to be, at least, in part, responsible for the "French paradox" [22]. In France, there is a lower than expected incidence of cardiovascular disease given the high-fat content of the diet [23]. This low incidence of disease has been associated with wine consumption, and resveratrol, a component of red wine, has been postulated to be responsible [23]. Although cardioprotection has not been proven in humans, resveratrol has lowered blood pressure in hypertensive rats, and reduced experimental infarct size [24]. Macrophages from humans grown in resveratrol had fewer lipoproteins, and were less permeable to cholesterol transport than those grown without resveratrol [25]. When participants of another investigation took 100mg/d for a month and a half and had blood macrophages cultured, the macrophages showed evidence of downregulation of proinflammatory cytokine genes [26]. Several human trials of the effects of resveratrol on glucose and lipid regulation in humans are underway [27, 28]. In one, currently taking place at the Albert Einstein College of Medicine, thirty subjects ages 50-80 with impaired glucose tolerance will ingest 2g of resveratrol a day for a month and a half [27]. At the University of Maastricht in the Netherlands, fifty individuals ages 45 to 70 will take 150mg of resveratrol for a month or a placebo, and the effects on apolipoprotein A-1 and HDL will be analyzed [29].

Another beneficial effect of resveratrol on adipocytes is the induction of apoptosis. This induction may occur through the stress activated protein(SAP)/MAPK cell pathway which includes p38, ERK and JNK kinases [3]. In turn, stress activated protein kinase-1 (MSK) is induced [30].

The ability of resveratrol to induce apoptosis may extend to other cell types and result in other potential positive health outcomes. Resveratrol has been found to have an anticarcinogenic effect. In hepatic cancer cells, resveratrol had multiple actions. At lower doses, it prevented DNA synthesis, and at higher doses, caused cells to undergo apoptosis [31]. Resveratrol placed on the skin of mice in addition to a carcinogen prevented the development of skin cancer [32]. Resveratrol caused apoptosis in cultured pancreatic cell lines [33]. In cancer cells, resveratrol may act upon additional signaling pathways. Resveratrol causes tumor apoptosis through the Fas receptor, phosphoinositol 3 kinase/Akt,, Wnt, and NF-κB as well as the sirtuin pathways [34]. Prostate cancer cell lines were also suppressed by resveratrol, and the polyphenol prevented the malignant histological transformation of breast cancer cells [35, 36].

Reduction of inflammatory cytokines through adipocyte apoptosis may also suggest a neuroprotective role for resveratrol. This has been tested in several animal models of experimentally-induced dementia. In pathologic studies, neonatal rats receiving head trauma that were pretreated with resveratrol retained greater numbers of neurons than those that did not receive resveratrol.[37] Mice that were given agents causing neuronal loss had less injury with concomitant resveratrol administration [38]. In one investigation, dementia was induced in rats by pretreatment with streptozocin [39]. Rodents that also were given resveratrol performed better than streptozocin-treated control rats on maze tests of acquisition of knowledge.

Human trials are underway to determine the cognitive effects of resveratrol. At the University of Florida, healthy elderly subjects age 65 or older are being randomized to take either a placebo, 300mg, or 1000mg daily doses of resveratrol for three months, during which they are being assessed for cognitive performance on several neuropsychological tests and physical performance. Three other studies have also been undertaken on effects of resveratrol on cognition, and one other is currently in progress, the results of which have not been published yet [40-43].

## QUERCETIN

Quercetin, like resveratrol, has anti-aging, anti-carcinogenic, and anti-inflammatory effects[44-46]. When the roundworm *C. elegans* was cultured in 200μM quercetin, its lifespan was prolonged by 15% [47, 48]. The polyphenol reduced the invasiveness of human breast cancer cells *in vitro*.[49] Quercetin thwarted the growth of cultured lung cancer cells.[50]

Quercetin administered *in vitro* to colon cancer cells downregulated Ras, an important regulatory protein[51]. Quercetin has demonstrated anti-inflammatory effects on multiple cell types. In one investigation, quercetin suppressed certain genes encoding the proinflammatory cytokines IL1β, IL-6, IL-8, and MCP-1 in TNF-α treated adipocytes as much if not more so than resveratol [52]. Mice fed a high-fat diet with quercetin 0.8g/kg/d had lower concentrations of IL-1α, IL-4, and interferon-γ than animals that did not ingest quercetin [53].

Quercetin has been studied for its anti-atherogenic effects. Zucker rats were given 2-10/mg/kg quercetin for two and a half months or a placebo [54]. The rats who consumed quercetin had a lower systolic blood pressure, free fatty acids, cholesterol, and triglycerides than those who did not. The rats who took quercetin also had a lower serum nitrous oxide, and lower adipose tissue TNF-α levels.

In a human quercetin trial, 172 participants, some of whom were hypertensive, ages 25-65, took 150mg/d quercetin or a placebo for a month and a half [55]. In hypertensive individuals, there was a mean reduction of systolic blood pressure by 2.9mmHg. Participants who ingested quercetin had a mean lower oxidized LDL, but also a lower HDL. There was no change in the serum inflammatory markers C-reactive protein and TNF-α. Monocytes from the sera of health individuals was incubated in vitro with different concentrations of quercetin and a macrophage stimulatory substrate [56]. Quercetin caused a dose-dependent inhibition of monocyte TNF-α production.

Quercetin has also been tested for a neuroprotective effect. Rats with ethanol- induced brain injury were given 10-50mg/kg/d quercetin for a month [57]. Quercetin improved the cognitive test performance of these rats.

## Caffeic Acid

Caffeic acid is a polyphenol found in propolis that has been studied for its antineoplastic activity. Caffeic acid phenylethyl ester (CAPE) is a form of caffeic acid that can be synthesized from propolis and has been tested against several different types of tumors *in vitro* [58]. CAPE reduced the tumor cell volume in ascites from tumors implanted into the peritoneums of mice [59]. When five melanoma tumor cell lines were grafted into mice, CAPE successfully suppressed their growth [60]. The growth of a rat glioma cell line was inhibited *in vitro*, and xenografts and neoplastic growth factors were suppressed by CAPE[61]. Propolis-derived CAPE was tested *in vitro* in mice against breast cancer *in vitro* and in xenografts to live mice.[58] CAPE suppressed tumor growth *in vitro*, and reduced expression by the xenograft of the angiogenesis-promoting factor vascular endothelial growth factor (VEGF). CAPE also suppressed breast cancer stem cell growth[62]. CAPE was cytotoxic to a human gastric cancer cell line *in vitro* [63]. Gastric cancer may be promulgated by chronic *Helicobacter pylori* infection, with concomitant proinflammatory cytokine release of NF-κB, IL1β, IL-6, and MMP-9 [64]. CAPE reduced the proinflammatory cytokine release when *H. pylori* was cultured with gastric cancer cells and *in vivo* in the stomachs of *H. pylori*-infected Mongolian gerbils [63, 65]. CAPE has also induced apoptosis of cells in human pancreatic and cervical cancer cell lines.[66, 67] The polyphenol also retarded the growth of human neurofibromatosis tumor xenografts to mice [68].

The ability of CAPE to modulate cytokine levels suggests potential roles in the treatment of atherosclerosis and infection. CAPE prevented the replication of vascular smooth muscle cells via p38 and MAPK intracellular signaling pathways [69]. However, there are no reported currently funded trials of CAPE use in humans.

## Chrysin

Chrysin is another polyphenol with health-enhancing properties. It was isolated from Brazilian and Chinese propolis as an anti-allergenic component that prevents the degranulation of rat mast cells in response to antigen stimulation[70]. Chrysin prevented inhibited proinflammatory cytokine and histamine release from mast cells in mice and alleviated cutaneous allergic reactions in experimentally-induced allergic reactions [71]. Chrysin protected cultured human keratinocytes from ultraviolet radiation-induced damage.[72] Applied to mouse skin, it caused no adverse effects. Chyrsin may have neuroprotective properties; the polyphenol averted experimentally-induced apoptosis in human neuroblastoma cells [73].

Chrysin also has antineoplastic effects. The polyphenol downregulates NF-κB, activating TNF-α to induce apoptosis in cancer cells [74]. Chrysin induced apoptosis in vitro in human colon cancer, hepatoma, nasopharyngeal, leukemia, cervical, glioma, thyroid, prostate, lung, and breast cancer cell lines [75-77]. There are no reported funded human trials underway of chyrsin use.

## Kaempferol

Kaempferol is a polyphenol that has anti-inflammatory properties, reducing cellular nitric cyclooxygenase and nitric oxide synthetase[78]. Kaempferol reduces proinflammatory cytokine release in human macrophages [79]. Calineurin, an important immune regulatory enzyme in T cells, is inhibited by kaempferol [80]. The polyphenol has displayed a neuroprotective effect; lowering amyloid beta peptide levels in rat pheochromocytoma cells [81]. Despite its anti-inflammatory effect, kaempferol was able to synergize with antibiotics to enhancing killing of the bacteria *Staphlococcus aureus*, possibility due to its ability to bind to bacterial membrane proteins [82].Kaempferol, like chrysin, has been able to induce neoplastic cells to undergo apoptosis *in vitro*. The polyphenol induced apoptosis in human oral squamous, breast, pancreatic, colon, glioma, ovarian carcinoma cells *in vitro* [83-89].

## Rutin

Rutin is another polyphenol with anti-inflammatory and antineoplastic properties. Rutin reduced the lifespan of human leukemic stem cells and colon cancer cell lines *in vitro* and prevented leukemia proliferation in rodent xenografts [90-92]. Non-steroidal anti-inflammatory drug-induced ulcers were prevented in rats by the administration of rutin [93].

The polyphenol has beneficial effects on lipid and glucose metabolism. Rutin reduced production of the carbohydrate metabolizing enzyme maltase and serum glucose levels when it was fed by gavage to rats.[94] Inflammatory nitric oxide synthetase gene expression was reduced by rutin [95]. Diabetic rats that ingested rutin for a month and a half had improved lipid oxidation product and fasting glucose levels [96]. Rutin altered levels of glucose-metabolizing enzymes in these rats and improved pancreatic histology [97]. Rutin also reduced the lipid content of hepatocytes *in vitro*.[98] The polyphenol lowered total LDL cholesterol levels in rats.[99]

## Myrcetin

Myrcetin has anticarginogenic, metabolic, and neuroprotective effects. The polyphenol is believed to retard cancer cell growth through the MEK 1 pathway or alteration of intracellular redox reactions [100-102]. Myricetin shielded murine and human skin from the adverse effects of ultraviolet radiation [103, 104]. Myricetin also prevented or reduced tumor size in experimental animal models of colon cancer and retarded the growth of colon cancer cells *in vitro* [105, 106].

The polyphenol caused the apoptosis of pancreatic cancer cells *in vitro* [107]. Human glioma cells were rendered more susceptible to apoptosis *in vitro* by myricetin [108]. Myricetin altered insulin signaling and reduces insulin resistance in rodents [109, 110]. The polyphenol averted neurotoxicity in a human *in vitro* experimental cell line [111, 112].

## Pinocembrin

Pinocembebrin is a polyphenol that has been evaluated for a possible role in the treatment of cancer and neurological disorders. The polyphenol caused mitochondrial apoptosis in colon carcinoma cells *in vitro* [113]. Rats given pinocembrin after experimentally-induced ischemia had improved brain histology [114-116]. Pinocembrin averted toxicity to neurons created by glutamate administration [117].

## Bioavailability of Polyphenols

One of the challenges to the use of polyphenols is limited bioavailability [2, 4]. When ingested, the availability of many is at most ten percent [118]. The pharmacokinetics of resveratrol and quercetin have been outlined in a limited number of human studies [119]. When polyphenols, such as resveratrol and quercetin are ingested, they are readily metabolized through conjugation in the intestine and the liver [119, 120]. In one of the few pharmokinetic trials on other polyphenols found in propolis, in a rodent study, pinocembrin also achieved a poor bioavailability [121].

However, the metabolites of polyphenols might also have biological activity, although this has not been well characterized [119]. Preliminary studies of resveratrol metabolites have identified variation in concentrations among different tissues, and some anti-neoplastic activity, albeit not as strong as the parent substance [122]. In nature, polyphenols are often not found in isolation, but in combination in plant products, which bees collect to create propolis. Whether the presence of a polyphenol in a propolis mixture alters the bioavailability of individual polyphenols is also not known.

## CONCLUSION

There has been a proliferation over the past few decades of scientific publications about polyphenols, reflecting an increasing interest in their health effects. In the past decade, the number of articles about resveratrol alone has grown by more than eightfold [123]. Despite this wealth of new knowledge about polyphenols, none has yet become an established preventative measure or treatment for any health disorder. Given the limited bioavailability and fact that naturally, these substances occur not singly, but in mixtures with other substances, the optimal method of obtaining the health benefits of polyphenol may be as compounds [2, 4, 123].

Propolis is one such polyphenol-containing compound. Newer studies of its polyphenol content show its varied nature; additional propolis polyphenols have been identified, such as epicatechin, and chlorgenic acid [124]. In a recent propolis trial, when a cervical cancer cell line was treated with propolis *in vitro*, the antineoplastic effects were not dependent on the concentration any given polyphenol, which suggested that synergistic effects between components might account for the activity of propolis rather than the amount of any given polyphenol.[125] Future studies of propolis should determine the utility of propolis-derived polyphenols, and the relative contribution of polyphenols to the health benefits of propolis.

## REFERENCES

[1] Abdel-Raheem IT. Gastroprotective effect of rutin against indomethacin-induced ulcers in rats. *Basic Clin. Pharmacol. Toxicol.*, 2010;107:742-50.

[2] Araujo JR, Goncalves P, Martel F. Chemopreventive effect of dietary polyphenols in colorectal cancer cell lines. *Nutr. Res.*, 2011;31:77-87.

[3] Bae Y, Lee S, Kim SH. Chrysin suppresses mast cell-mediated allergic inflammation: Involvement of calcium, caspase-1 and nuclear factor-kappaB. *Toxicol. Appl. Pharmacol.*, 2011;254:56-64.

[4] Baile CA, Yang JY, Rayalam S, Hartzell DL, Lai CY, Andersen C, Della-Fera MA. Effect of resveratrol on fat mobilization. *Ann. NY Acad. Sci.*, 2011;1215:40-7.

[5] Barbaric M, Miskovic K, Bojic M, Loncar MB, Smolcic-Bubalo A, Debeljak Z, Medic-Saric M. Chemical composition of the ethanolic propolis extracts and its effect on HeLa cells. *J. Ethnopharmacol.*, 2011;135:772-8.

[6] Baur JA, Pearson KJ, Price NL, Jamieson HA, Lerin C, Kalra A, Prabhu VV, Allard JS, Lopez-Lluch G, Lewis K, Pistell PJ, Poosala S, Becker KG, Boss O, Gwinn D, Wang M, Ramaswamy S, Fishbein KW, Spencer RG, Lakatta EG, Le Couteur D, Shaw RJ, Navas P, Puigserver P, Ingram DK, de Cabo R, Sinclair DA. Resveratrol improves health and survival of mice on a high-calorie diet. *Nature*, 2006;444:337-42.

[7] Berrougui H, Grenier G, Loued S, Drouin G, Khalil A. A new insight into resveratrol as an atheroprotective compound: inhibition of lipid peroxidation and enhancement of cholesterol efflux. *Atherosclerosis*, 2009;207:420-7.

[8] Bischoff SC. Quercetin: potentials in the prevention and therapy of disease. *Curr. Opin. Clin. Nutr. Metab. Care*, 2008;11:733-40.

[9] Boots AW, Haenen GR, Bast A. Health effects of quercetin: from antioxidant to nutraceutical. *Eur. J. Pharmacol.*, 2008;585:325-37.

[10] Boots AW, Wilms LC, Swennen EL, Kleinjans JC, Bast A, Haenen GR. In vitro and ex vivo anti-inflammatory activity of quercetin in healthy volunteers. *Nutrition*, 2008;24:703-10.

[11] Bourogaa E, Bertrand J, Despeaux M, Jarraya R, Fabre N, Payrastre L, Demur C, Fournie JJ, Damak M, Feki AE, Racaud-Sultan C. Hammada scoparia flavonoids and rutin kill adherent and chemoresistant leukemic cells. *Leuk. Res.*, 2011;35:1093-101.

[12] Chang WC, Hsieh CH, Hsiao MW, Lin WC, Hung YC, Ye JC. Caffeic acid induces apoptosis in human cervical cancer cells through the mitochondrial pathway. *Taiwan. J. Obstet. Gynecol.*, 2011;49:419-24.

[13] Chen MJ, Chang WH, Lin CC, Liu CY, Wang TE, Chu CH, Shih SC, Chen YJ. Caffeic acid phenethyl ester induces apoptosis of human pancreatic cancer cells involving caspase and mitochondrial dysfunction. *Pancreatology*, 2008;8:566-76.

[14] Cherniack EP. Polyphenols: planting the seeds of treatment for the metabolic syndrome.Cherniack EP. The potential influence of plant polyphenols on the aging process. *Forsch. Komplementmed.*, 2010;17:181-7.

[15] Choi EJ, Ahn WS. Kaempferol induced the apoptosis via cell cycle arrest in human breast cancer MDA-MB-453 cells. *Nutr. Res. Pract.*, 2008;2:322-5.

[16] Chuang CC, Martinez K, Xie G, Kennedy A, Bumrungpert A, Overman A, Jia W, McIntosh MK. Quercetin is equally or more effective than resveratrol in attenuating tumor necrosis factor-{alpha}-mediated inflammation and insulin resistance in primary human adipocytes. *Am. J. Clin. Nutr.*, 2010;92:1511-21.

[17] Csaki C, Keshishzadeh N, Fischer K, Shakibaei M. Regulation of inflammation signalling by resveratrol in human chondrocytes in vitro. *Biochem. Pharmacol.*, 2008;75:677-87.

[18] Dal-Pan A, Blanc S, Aujard F. Resveratrol suppresses body mass gain in a seasonal non-human primate model of obesity. *BMC Physiol.*, 2010;10:11.

[19] Dandona, P., Mohanty, P., Ghanim, H., Marumganti, A., Sia, C., Abuaysheh, S., Rajeswari, J. Resveratrol Suppresses Pro-Inflammatory Genes Causing Insulin Resistance. The Endocrine Society's 90th Annual Meeting. San Francisco, CA, 2008.

[20] Demestre M, Messerli SM, Celli N, Shahhossini M, Kluwe L, Mautner V, Maruta H. CAPE (caffeic acid phenethyl ester)-based propolis extract (Bio 30) suppresses the growth of human neurofibromatosis (NF) tumor xenografts in mice. *Phytother. Res.*, 2009;23:226-30.

[21] DeToma AS, Choi JS, Braymer JJ, Lim MH. Myricetin: a naturally occurring regulator of metal-induced amyloid-beta aggregation and neurotoxicity. *Chembiochem*, 2011;12:1198-201.

[22] Egert S, Bosy-Westphal A, Seiberl J, Kurbitz C, Settler U, Plachta-Danielzik S, Wagner AE, Frank J, Schrezenmeir J, Rimbach G, Wolffram S, Muller MJ. Quercetin reduces systolic blood pressure and plasma oxidised low-density lipoprotein concentrations in overweight subjects with a high-cardiovascular disease risk phenotype: a double-blinded, placebo-controlled cross-over study. *Br. J. Nutr.*, 2009;102:1065-74.

[23] El-Refaei MF, El-Naa MM. Inhibitory effect of caffeic acid phenethyl ester on mice bearing tumor involving angiostatic and apoptotic activities. *Chem. Biol. Interact.*, 2010;186:152-6.

[24] Erdogan S, Ates B, Durmaz G, Yilmaz I, Seckin T. Pressurized liquid extraction of phenolic compounds from Anatolia propolis and their radical scavenging capacities. *Food Chem. Toxicol.*, 2011;49:1592-7.

[25] Falcao-Silva VS, Silva DA, Souza Mde F, Siqueira-Junior JP. Modulation of drug resistance in Staphylococcus aureus by a kaempferol glycoside from Herissantia tiubae (Malvaceae). *Phytother. Res.*, 2009;23:1367-70.

[26] Floyd ZE, Wang ZQ, Kilroy G, Cefalu WT. Modulation of peroxisome proliferator-activated receptor gamma stability and transcriptional activity in adipocytes by resveratrol. *Metabolism*, 2008;57:S32-8.

[27] Fontana Pereira D, Cazarolli LH, Lavado C, Mengatto V, Figueiredo MS, Guedes A, Pizzolatti MG, Silva FR. Effects of flavonoids on alpha-glucosidase activity: Potential targets for glucose homeostasis. *Nutrition*, 2011.

[28] Gao M, Liu R, Zhu SY, Du GH. Acute neurovascular unit protective action of pinocembrin against permanent cerebral ischemia in rats. *J. Asian. Nat. Prod. Res.*, 2008;10:551-8.

[29] Gao M, Zhang WC, Liu QS, Hu JJ, Liu GT, Du GH. Pinocembrin prevents glutamate-induced apoptosis in SH-SY5Y neuronal cells via decrease of bax/bcl-2 ratio. *Eur. J. Pharmacol.*, 2008;591:73-9.

[30] Goldberg DM, Yan J, Soleas GJ. Absorption of three wine-related polyphenols in three different matrices by healthy subjects. *Clin. Biochem.*, 2003;36:79-87.

[31] Gomez-Zorita S, Fernandez-Quintela A, Macarulla MT, Aguirre L, Hijona E, Bujanda L, Milagro F, Martinez JA, Portillo MP. Resveratrol attenuates steatosis in obese Zucker rats by decreasing fatty acid availability and reducing oxidative stress. *Br. J. Nutr.*, 2011:1-9.

[32] H, Rankin GO, Li Z, Depriest L, Chen YC. Kaempferol induces apoptosis in ovarian cancer cells through activating p53 in the intrinsic pathway. *Food Chem.*, 2011;128:513-9.

[33] Howitz KT, Bitterman KJ, Cohen HY, Lamming DW, Lavu S, Wood JG, Zipkin RE, Chung P, Kisielewski A, Zhang LL, Scherer B, Sinclair DA. Small molecule activators of sirtuins extend Saccharomyces cerevisiae lifespan. *Nature*, 2003;425:191-6.

[34] Hu M. Commentary: bioavailability of flavonoids and polyphenols: call to arms. *Mol. Pharm.*, 2007;4:803-6.

[35] Huang CH, Jan RL, Kuo CH, Chu YT, Wang WL, Lee MS, Chen HN, Hung CH. Natural flavone kaempferol suppresses chemokines expression in human monocyte THP-1 cells through MAPK pathways. *J. Food Sci.*, 2010;75:H254-9.

[36] Huang JH, Huang CC, Fang JY, Yang C, Chan CM, Wu NL, Kang SW, Hung CF. Protective effects of myricetin against ultraviolet-B-induced damage in human keratinocytes. *Toxicol. In Vitro,* 2010;24:21-8.

[37] Izuta H, Shimazawa M, Tazawa S, Araki Y, Mishima S, Hara H. Protective effects of Chinese propolis and its component, chrysin, against neuronal cell death via inhibition of mitochondrial apoptosis pathway in SH-SY5Y cells. *J. Agric. Food Chem.*, 2008;56:8944-53.

[38] Jang M, Cai L, Udeani GO, Slowing KV, Thomas CF, Beecher CW, Fong HH, Farnsworth NR, Kinghorn AD, Mehta RG, Moon RC, Pezzuto JM. Cancer chemopreventive activity of resveratrol, a natural product derived from grapes. *Science*, 1997;275:218-20.

[39] Jeong JC, Kim MS, Kim TH, Kim YK. Kaempferol induces cell death through ERK and Akt-dependent down-regulation of XIAP and survivin in human glioma cells. *Neurochem. Res.*, 2009;34:991-1001.

[40] Jung SK, Lee KW, Kim HY, Oh MH, Byun S, Lim SH, Heo YS, Kang NJ, Bode AM, Dong Z, Lee HJ. Myricetin suppresses UVB-induced wrinkle formation and MMP-9 expression by inhibiting Raf. *Biochem. Pharmacol.*, 2010;79:1455-61.

[41] Kamalakkannan N, Prince PS. Antihyperglycaemic and antioxidant effect of rutin, a polyphenolic flavonoid, in streptozotocin-induced diabetic wistar rats. Basic *Clin. Pharmacol. Toxicol.*, 2006;98:97-103.

[42] Kang JW, Kim JH, Song K, Kim SH, Yoon JH, Kim KS. Kaempferol and quercetin, components of Ginkgo biloba extract (EGb 761), induce caspase-3-dependent apoptosis in oral cavity cancer cells. *Phytother. Res.*, 2010;24 Suppl 1:S77-82.

[43] Kang NJ, Jung SK, Lee KW, Lee HJ. Myricetin is a potent chemopreventive phytochemical in skin carcinogenesis. *Ann. NY Acad. Sci.*, 2011;1229:124-32.

[44] Kelly GS. Quercetin. Monograph. *Altern. Med. Rev.*, 2011;16:172-94.

[45] Khoo BY, Chua SL, Balaram P. Apoptotic effects of chrysin in human cancer cell lines. *Int. J. Mol. Sci.*, 2010;11:2188-99.

[46] Kim BW, Lee ER, Min HM, Jeong HS, Ahn JY, Kim JH, Choi HY, Choi H, Kim EY, Park SP, Cho SG. Sustained ERK activation is involved in the kaempferol-induced apoptosis of breast cancer cells and is more evident under 3-D culture condition. *Cancer Biol. Ther.*, 2008;7:1080-9.

[47] Kim JK, Choi SJ, Cho HY, Hwang HJ, Kim YJ, Lim ST, Kim CJ, Kim HK, Peterson S, Shin DH. Protective effects of kaempferol (3,4',5,7-tetrahydroxyflavone) against amyloid beta peptide (Abeta)-induced neurotoxicity in ICR mice. *Biosci. Biotechnol. Biochem.*, 2010;74:397-401.

[48] Kudugunti SK, Vad NM, Ekogbo E, Moridani MY. Efficacy of caffeic acid phenethyl ester (CAPE) in skin B16-F0 melanoma tumor bearing C57BL/6 mice. *Invest. New Drugs*, 2011;29:52-62.

[49] Kumar MA, Nair M, Hema PS, Mohan J, Santhoshkumar TR. Pinocembrin triggers Bax-dependent mitochondrial apoptosis in colon cancer cells. *Mol. Carcinog.*, 2007;46:231-41.

[50] Lagouge M, Argmann C, Gerhart-Hines Z, Meziane H, Lerin C, Daussin F, Messadeq N, Milne J, Lambert P, Elliott P, Geny B, Laakso M, Puigserver P, Auwerx J. Resveratrol improves mitochondrial function and protects against metabolic disease by activating SIRT1 and PGC-1alpha. *Cell*, 2006;127:1109-22.

[51] Lea MA, Ibeh C, Deutsch JK, Hamid I, desBordes C. Inhibition of growth and induction of alkaline phosphatase in colon cancer cells by flavonols and flavonol glycosides. *Anticancer. Res.*, 2010;30:3629-35.

[52] Lee KW, Kang NJ, Rogozin EA, Kim HG, Cho YY, Bode AM, Lee HJ, Surh YJ, Bowden GT, Dong Z. Myricetin is a novel natural inhibitor of neoplastic cell transformation and MEK1. *Carcinogenesis*, 2007;28:1918-27.

[53] Lekli I, Ray D, Das DK. Longevity nutrients resveratrol, wines and grapes. *Genes. Nutr.*, 2010;5.

[54] Li W, Du B, Wang T, Wang S, Zhang J. Kaempferol induces apoptosis in human HCT116 colon cancer cells via the Ataxia-Telangiectasia Mutated-p53 pathway with

the involvement of p53 Upregulated Modulator of Apoptosis. *Chem. Biol. Interact.*, 2009;177:121-7.

[55] Li X, Huang Q, Ong CN, Yang XF, Shen HM. Chrysin sensitizes tumor necrosis factor-alpha-induced apoptosis in human tumor cells via suppression of nuclear factor-kappaB. *Cancer Lett.*, 2010;293:109-16.

[56] Li X, Wang JN, Huang JM, Xiong XK, Chen MF, Ong CN, Shen HM, Yang XF. Chrysin promotes tumor necrosis factor (TNF)-related apoptosis-inducing ligand (TRAIL) induced apoptosis in human cancer cell lines. *Toxicol. In Vitro,* 2010;25:630-5.

[57] Lin CW, Hou WC, Shen SC, Juan SH, Ko CH, Wang LM, Chen YC. Quercetin inhibition of tumor invasion via suppressing PKC delta/ERK/AP-1-dependent matrix metalloproteinase-9 activation in breast carcinoma cells. *Carcinogenesis*, 2008;29:1807-15.

[58] Lin JP, Yang JS, Lin JJ, Lai KC, Lu HF, Ma CY, Sai-Chuen Wu R, Wu KC, Chueh FS, Gibson Wood W, Chung JG. Rutin inhibits human leukemia tumor growth in a murine xenograft model *in vivo. Environ. Toxicol*. 2011.

[59] Lin WL, Liang WH, Lee YJ, Chuang SK, Tseng TH. Antitumor progression potential of caffeic acid phenethyl ester involving p75(NTR) in C6 glioma cells. *Chem. Biol. Interact.*, 2010;188:607-15.

[60] Liu IM, Tzeng TF, Liou SS, Lan TW. Myricetin, a naturally occurring flavonol, ameliorates insulin resistance induced by a high-fructose diet in rats. *Life Sci.*, 2007;81:1479-88.

[61] Lotfy M. Biological activity of bee propolis in health and disease. *Asian Pac. J. Cancer Prev.*, 2006;7:22-31.

[62] Lu J, Papp LV, Fang J, Rodriguez-Nieto S, Zhivotovsky B, Holmgren A. Inhibition of Mammalian thioredoxin reductase by some flavonoids: implications for myricetin and quercetin anticancer activity. *Cancer Res.*, 2006;66:4410-8.

[63] Mahat MY, Kulkarni NM, Vishwakarma SL, Khan FR, Thippeswamy BS, Hebballi V, Adhyapak AA, Benade VS, Ashfaque SM, Tubachi S, Patil BM. Modulation of the cyclooxygenase pathway via inhibition of nitric oxide production contributes to the anti-inflammatory activity of kaempferol. *Eur. J. Pharmacol.*, 2010;642:169-76.

[64] Meng F, Liu R, Gao M, Wang Y, Yu X, Xuan Z, Sun J, Yang F, Wu C, Du G. Pinocembrin attenuates blood-brain barrier injury induced by global cerebral ischemia-reperfusion in rats. *Brain Res.*, 2011;1391:93-101.

[65] Metzner J, Bekemeier H, Schneidewind EM, Wenzel U. [Pharmacokinetic studies of the propolis constituent pinocembrin in the rat (author's transl)]. *Pharmazie*, 1979;34:185-7.

[66] Molina-Jimenez MF, Sanchez-Reus MI, Cascales M, Andres D, Benedi J. Effect of fraxetin on antioxidant defense and stress proteins in human neuroblastoma cell model of rotenone neurotoxicity. Comparative study with myricetin and N-acetylcysteine. *Toxicol. Appl. Pharmacol.*, 2005;209:214-25.

[67] Morimoto M, Takagi Y, Higashi N, Suzuki T. Orally Administrated Rutin Inhibits the Gene Expression of Th2 Cytokines in the Gut and Lung in Aged Mice. *J. Vet. Med. Sci.*, 2011.

[68] Nakamura R, Watanabe K, Oka K, Ohta S, Mishima S, Teshima R. Effects of propolis from different areas on mast cell degranulation and identification of the effective components in propolis. *Int. Immunopharmacol.*, 2010;10:1107-12.

[69] Ndiaye M, Kumar R, Ahmad N. Resveratrol in cancer management: where are we and where we go from here? *Ann. NY Acad. Sci.*, 2011;1215:144-9.

[70] Nguyen TT, Tran E, Nguyen TH, Do PT, Huynh TH, Huynh H. The role of activated MEK-ERK pathway in quercetin-induced growth inhibition and apoptosis in A549 lung cancer cells. *Carcinogenesis*, 2004;25:647-59.

[71] Nirmala P, Ramanathan M. Effect of myricetin on 1,2 dimethylhydrazine induced rat colon carcinogenesis. *J. Exp. Ther. Oncol.*, 2011;9:101-8.

[72] Omene CO, Wu J, Frenkel K. Caffeic Acid Phenethyl Ester (CAPE) derived from propolis, a honeybee product, inhibits growth of breast cancer stem cells. Invest. New Drugs 2011.

[73] Palsamy P, Sivakumar S, Subramanian S. Resveratrol attenuates hyperglycemia-mediated oxidative stress, proinflammatory cytokines and protects hepatocytes ultrastructure in streptozotocin-nicotinamide-induced experimental diabetic rats. *Chem. Biol. Interact.*, 186:200-10.

[74] Palsamy P, Subramanian S. Ameliorative potential of resveratrol on proinflammatory cytokines, hyperglycemia mediated oxidative stress, and pancreatic beta-cell dysfunction in streptozotocin-nicotinamide-induced diabetic rats. *J. Cell Physiol.*,;224:423-32.

[75] Palsamy P, Subramanian S. Modulatory effects of resveratrol on attenuating the key enzymes activities of carbohydrate metabolism in streptozotocin-nicotinamide-induced diabetic rats. *Chem. Biol. Interact.*, 2009;179:356-62.

[76] Palsamy P, Subramanian S. Resveratrol, a natural phytoalexin, normalizes hyperglycemia in streptozotocin-nicotinamide induced experimental diabetic rats. *Biomed. Pharmacother.*, 2008;62:598-605.

[77] Pezzuto JM. The phenomenon of resveratrol: redefining the virtues of promiscuity. *Ann. NY Acad. Sci.*, 2011;1215:123-30.

[78] Phan T, Yu XM, Kunnimalaiyaan M, Chen H. Antiproliferative Effect of Chrysin on Anaplastic Thyroid Cancer. *J. Surg. Res.*, 2011. Epub ahead of print May 17.

[79] Phillips PA, Sangwan V, Borja-Cacho D, Dudeja V, Vickers SM, Saluja AK. Myricetin induces pancreatic cancer cell death via the induction of apoptosis and inhibition of the phosphatidylinositol 3-kinase (PI3K) signaling pathway. *Cancer Lett.*, 2011;308:181-8.

[80] Pietsch K, Saul N, Menzel R, Sturzenbaum SR, Steinberg CE. Quercetin mediated lifespan extension in Caenorhabditis elegans is modulated by age-1, daf-2, sek-1 and unc-43. *Biogerontology*, 2008.

[81] Psahoulia FH, Moumtzi S, Roberts ML, Sasazuki T, Shirasawa S, Pintzas A. Quercetin mediates preferential degradation of oncogenic Ras and causes autophagy in Ha-RAS-transformed human colon cells. *Carcinogenesis*, 2007;28:1021-31.

[82] Ribeiro U, Jr., Safatle-Ribeiro AV. Caffeic acid phenethyl ester (CAPE) may be a promising adjuvant treatment in gastric cancer. *J. Clin. Gastroenterol.*, 2007;41:871-3.

[83] Rivera L, Moron R, Sanchez M, Zarzuelo A, Galisteo M. Quercetin ameliorates metabolic syndrome and improves the inflammatory status in obese Zucker rats. *Obesity (Silver Spring)* 2008;16:2081-7.

[84] Rivera L, Moron R, Zarzuelo A, Galisteo M. Long-term resveratrol administration reduces metabolic disturbances and lowers blood pressure in obese Zucker rats. *Biochem. Pharmacol.*, 2009;77:1053-63.

[85] Robich MP, Chu LM, Chaudray M, Nezafat R, Han Y, Clements RT, Laham RJ, Manning WJ, Coady MA, Sellke FW. Anti-angiogenic effect of high-dose resveratrol in a swine model of metabolic syndrome. *Surgery*, 2010;148:453-62.

[86] Rocha KK, Souza GA, Ebaid GX, Seiva FR, Cataneo AC, Novelli EL. Resveratrol toxicity: effects on risk factors for atherosclerosis and hepatic oxidative stress in standard and high-fat diets. *Food Chem. Toxicol.*, 2009;47:1362-7.

[87] Roos TU, Heiss EH, Schwaiberger AV, Schachner D, Sroka IM, Oberan T, Vollmar AM, Dirsch VM. Caffeic acid phenethyl ester inhibits PDGF-induced proliferation of vascular smooth muscle cells via activation of p38 MAPK, HIF-1alpha, and heme oxygenase-1. *J. Nat. Prod.*, 2011;74:352-6.

[88] running head: plant polyphenols and the metabolic syndrome. *Nutrition*, 2011;27:617-23.

[89] Sakata Y, Zhuang H, Kwansa H, Koehler RC, Dore S. Resveratrol protects against experimental stroke: Putative neuroprotective role of heme oxygenase 1. Exp Neurol.

[90] Saul N, Pietsch K, Menzel R, Steinberg CE. Quercetin-mediated longevity in Caenorhabditis elegans: Is DAF-16 involved? *Mech. Ageing Dev.*, 2008;129:611-3.

[91] Seeni A, Takahashi S, Takeshita K, Tang M, Sugiura S, Sato SY, Shirai T. Suppression of prostate cancer growth by resveratrol in the transgenic rat for adenocarcinoma of prostate (TRAP) model. *Asian Pac. J. Cancer Prev.*, 2008;9:7-14.

[92] Shakibaei M, Harikumar KB, Aggarwal BB. Resveratrol addiction: to die or not to die. *Mol. Nutr. Food Res.*, 2009;53:115-28.

[93] Sharma M, Gupta YK. Chronic treatment with trans resveratrol prevents intracerebroventricular streptozotocin induced cognitive impairment and oxidative stress in rats. *Life Sci.*, 2002;71:2489-98.

[94] Shi LL, Chen BN, Gao M, Zhang HA, Li YJ, Wang L, Du GH. The characteristics of therapeutic effect of pinocembrin in transient global brain ischemia/reperfusion rats. *Life Sci.*, 2011;88:521-8.

[95] Shukla Y, Singh R. Resveratrol and cellular mechanisms of cancer prevention. *Ann. NY Acad. Sci.*, 2011;1215:1-8.

[96] Siegelin MD, Gaiser T, Habel A, Siegelin Y. Myricetin sensitizes malignant glioma cells to TRAIL-mediated apoptosis by down-regulation of the short isoform of FLIP and bcl-2. *Cancer Lett.*, 2009;283:230-8.

[97] Singh A, Naidu PS, Kulkarni SK. Reversal of aging and chronic ethanol-induced cognitive dysfunction by quercetin a bioflavonoid. *Free Radic. Res.*, 2003;37:1245-52.

[98] Smoliga JM, Baur JA, Hausenblas HA. Resveratrol and health - A comprehensive review of human clinical trials. *Mol. Nutr. Food Res.*, 2011;55:1129-41.

[99] Sonmez U, Sonmez A, Erbil G, Tekmen I, Baykara B. Neuroprotective effects of resveratrol against traumatic brain injury in immature rats. *Neurosci. Lett.*, 2007;420:133-7.

[100] Stanley Mainzen Prince P, Kamalakkannan N. Rutin improves glucose homeostasis in streptozotocin diabetic tissues by altering glycolytic and gluconeogenic enzymes. *J. Biochem. Mol. Toxicol.*, 2006;20:96-102.

[101] Stefani M, Markus MA, Lin RC, Pinese M, Dawes IW, Morris BJ. The effect of resveratrol on a cell model of human aging. *Ann. NY Acad. Sci.*, 2007;1114:407-18.

[102] Stewart LK, Soileau JL, Ribnicky D, Wang ZQ, Raskin I, Poulev A, Majewski M, Cefalu WT, Gettys TW. Quercetin transiently increases energy expenditure but persistently decreases circulating markers of inflammation in C57BL/6J mice fed a high-fat diet. *Metabolism*, 2008;57:S39-46.

[103] Szkudelska K, Nogowski L, Szkudelski T. Resveratrol, a naturally occurring diphenolic compound, affects lipogenesis, lipolysis and the antilipolytic action of insulin in isolated rat adipocytes. *J. Steroid. Biochem. Mol. Biol.*, 2009;113:17-24.

[104] Toyoda T, Tsukamoto T, Takasu S, Shi L, Hirano N, Ban H, Kumagai T, Tatematsu M. Anti-inflammatory effects of caffeic acid phenethyl ester (CAPE), a nuclear factor-kappaB inhibitor, on Helicobacter pylori-induced gastritis in Mongolian gerbils. *Int. J. Cancer,* 2009;125:1786-95.

[105] Tzeng TF, Liou SS, Liu IM. Myricetin Ameliorates Defective Post-Receptor Insulin Signaling via beta-Endorphin Signaling in the Skeletal Muscles of Fructose-Fed Rats. *Evid. Based Complement Alternat. Med.,* 2011;2011:150752.

[106] U.S. National Institute of Health, ClinicalTrials.gov. Effects of Dietary Interventions on the Brain in Mild Cognitive Impairment (MCI). Availableat: http://www.clinicaltrials. gov/ct2/show/NCT01 219244? term= resveratrolandrank=30 Acessed August 16, 2011.

[107] U.S. National Institute of Health, ClinicalTrials.gov. Long-term Investigation of Resveratrol in Obesity (LIRMOI). Available at: http://www.clinicaltrials. gov/ct2/show/NCT01412645?term=resveratrolandrank=8 Acessed August 16, 2011.

[108] U.S. National Institute of Health, ClinicalTrials.gov. Pilot Study of Resveratrol in Older Adults With Impaired Glucose Tolerance (RSV). Available at: http://www. clinicaltrials.gov/ct2/show/NCT01375959? term=resveratrolandrank=9 Acessed August 16, 2011.

[109] U.S. National Institute of Health, ClinicalTrials.gov. Resveratrol and Serum Apo A-I. Available at: http://www.clinicaltrials. gov/ct2/show/NCT01 364961?term= resveratrolandrank=11 Acessed August 16, 2011.

[110] U.S. National Institute of Health, ClinicalTrials.gov. The Effects of Resveratrol Supplementation on Measurements of Health and Human Performance (MUresv). Available at: http://www.clinicaltrials.gov/ct2 /show/NCT01244360?term= resveratrolandrank=10 Acessed August 16, 2011.

[111] U.S. National Institutes of Health, ClinicalTrials.gov. Pilot Study of the Effects of Resveratrol Supplement in Mild-to-Moderate Alzheimer's Disease. Accessed May 12, 2010. Available at: http://www.clinicaltrials. gov/ct2/show/NCT00743743? term= cognition+resveratrolandrank=1 Acessed.

[112] U.S. National Institutes of Health, ClinicalTrials.gov. Randomized Trial of a Nutritional Supplement in Alzheimer's Disease. Accessed May 3, 2010. Available at: http://www.clinicaltrials.gov/ct2/show /NCT00678431?term=mount+sinai+ resveratro landrank=1 Acessed.

[113] Vang O, Ahmad N, Baile CA, Baur JA, Brown K, Csiszar A, Das DK, Delmas D, Gottfried C, Lin HY, Ma QY, Mukhopadhyay P, Nalini N, Pezzuto JM, Richard T, Shukla Y, Surh YJ, Szekeres T, Szkudelski T, Walle T, Wu JM. What is new for an old molecule? Systematic review and recommendations on the use of resveratrol. *PLoS One,* 2011;6:e19881.

[114] Vergara D, Valente CM, Tinelli A, Siciliano C, Lorusso V, Acierno R, Giovinazzo G, Santino A, Storelli C, Maffia M. Resveratrol inhibits the epidermal growth factor-induced epithelial mesenchymal transition in MCF-7 cells. *Cancer Lett.,* 2011;310:1-8.

[115] Vidavalur R, Otani H, Singal PK, Maulik N. Significance of wine and resveratrol in cardiovascular disease: French paradox revisited. Exp Clin Cardiol 2006;11:217-25.

[116] Wang H, Zhou CL, Lei H, Zhang SD, Zheng J, Wei Q. Kaempferol: a new immunosuppressant of calcineurin. *IUBMB Life,* 2008;60:549-54.

[117] Wood JG, Rogina B, Lavu S, Howitz K, Helfand SL, Tatar M, Sinclair D. Sirtuin activators mimic caloric restriction and delay ageing in metazoans. *Nature,* 2004;430:686-9.

[118] Wu CH, Lin MC, Wang HC, Yang MY, Jou MJ, Wang CJ. Rutin inhibits oleic acid induced lipid accumulation via reducing lipogenesis and oxidative stress in hepatocarcinoma cells. *J. Food Sci.,* 2011;76:T65-72.

[119] Wu CS, Chen MF, Lee IL, Tung SY. Predictive role of nuclear factor-kappaB activity in gastric cancer: a promising adjuvant approach with caffeic acid phenethyl ester. *J. Clin. Gastroenterol.,* 2007;41:894-900.

[120] Wu J, Omene C, Karkoszka J, Bosland M, Eckard J, Klein CB, Frenkel K. Caffeic acid phenethyl ester (CAPE), derived from a honeybee product propolis, exhibits a diversity of anti-tumor effects in pre-clinical models of human breast cancer. *Cancer Lett.,* 2011;308:43-53.

[121] Wu NL, Fang JY, Chen M, Wu CJ, Huang CC, Hung CF. Chrysin Protects Epidermal Keratinocytes from UVA- and UVB-Induced Damage. *J. Agric. Food. Chem.,* 2011.

[122] Zhang Y, Chen AY, Li M, Chen C, Yao Q. Ginkgo biloba extract kaempferol inhibits cell proliferation and induces apoptosis in pancreatic cancer cells. *J. Surg. Res.,* 2008;148:17-23.

[123] Zhou JH, Cheng HY, Yu ZQ, He DW, Pan Z, Yang DT. Resveratrol induces apoptosis in pancreatic cancer cells. *Chin. Med. J.,* (Engl) 2011;124:1695-9.

[124] Zhou R, Fukui M, Choi HJ, Zhu BT. Induction of a reversible, non-cytotoxic S-phase delay by resveratrol: implications for a mechanism of lifespan prolongation and cancer protection. *Br. J. Pharmacol.,* 2009;158:462-74.

[125] Ziaee A, Zamansoltani F, Nassiri-Asl M, Abbasi E. Effects of rutin on lipid profile in hypercholesterolaemic rats. *Basic Clin. Pharmacol. Toxicol.,* 2009;104:253-8.

In: Beneficial Effects of Propolis on Human Health ... ISBN: 978-1- 62081-440-6
Editors: Tahira Farooqui and Akhlaq A.Farooqui 

*Chapter 13*

# COMPARISON OF PROPOLIS AND HONEY USING STANDARDIZED METHODS

***Raúl C. Peña*[*] *and Gloria Montenegro***
Departamento Ciencias Vegetales, Facultad de Agronomía e Ingeniería Forestal de la Universidad Católica de Chile, Campus San Joaquín, Macul, Santiago, Chile

## ABSTRACT

Propolis has remarkable chemical variability; hundreds of its chemical compounds have been characterized, but systematic studies on geographical variability are needed, even when various authors have already described many types of propolis based on physicochemical features as a means of standardization. The bibliography of the past ten years focused on physicochemical methods, although it underlined the difficulty that a variable product regarding plant source and geographic origin presents, of which there is no reference on pollen assessment: palynological profiles. A decade of bibliographical sources on chemical characterization of crude materials was reviewed and completed on propolis and honey within the results of this chapter. It can be concluded from the results and review that an array of morphological, palynological, physicochemical and sensory methods is the best way for solving the problems that standardization of complex matrices for propolis or honey demands. This chapter describes a sequence of protocols for microscopy, sensory (instrumental or panels), quantification analyses; chromatographic quantification features like microscopy and sensory; and qualitative and quantitative methods, including thin layer chromatography (TLC), high pressure liquid chromatography (HPLC), in addition to spectral analysis associated (MS or NMR). Standardization of commercial products whose accurate geographic origin is unknown represents an additional challenge.

[*] E-mail address: penarc@gmail.com. Corresponding author.

# 1. INTRODUCTION

Several physicochemical and biological methods, particularly palynological and microscopic, have been developed to classify propolis. This study evaluates the analytical knowledge gained from ensuring the quality of honey, from which useful lessons can be learned to apply on the characterization of propolis. Although the development of chromatographic methods, related to spectral analysis, has sought to replace melissopalynology, this method is still recommended in national pharmacopoeias.

## 1.1. Botany, Phytochemistry and Pharmacological Topics

Propolis is a resin whose composition depends on the location, floral pattern, phenology of plant sources and types of forage species [1, 2, 3, 4, 5]. Some authors described *Tetragonisca* as very constant forage, while *Apis* is dependent on the crop region. *Jataí* (*T. angustula*) is distributed from Mexico to Argentina, discounting the Andes, Caatinga, and parts of the Amazon. Velikova et al. [6] concluded that only the propolis from *A. mellifera* contained prenylated p-coumaric acids typical of Brazil, but lacks Meliponinae products. According to Miorin et al. [7], *T. angustula* propolis contained mainly 3.5-diprenyl-4-hydroxycinnamic acid, 3-prenyl-4-hydroxycinnamic acid, 2.2-dimethyl-8-prenyl-2H-1-benzopyran-6-propenoic acid and the derivative 1 of cinnamic acid. Sawaya et al. [8] reported that *Tetragonisca* prefered species of *Schinus terebinthifolius* as a source of resins. Silici and Kutluca [9] found higher antibacterial activity in the propolis of *A. mellifera caucasica*, compared to *A. m. anatolica* or *A. m. carnica.*

*Frieseomelitta* Meliponinae, a Brazilian endemic, builds its nests in rotting logs, its workers carry resins in basket-like structures; the resin is used to glue the pollen to the corbicula [10]. Morgan studied three *Frieseomelitta* species (*silvestris, languida* and *varia*), finding differences among their volatile compounds. He also found differences between the waxes of honey bee and *Melipona bicolor* [11]. In general, the Meliponinae wax composition is simpler than the wax of Apis.

European, American and extratropical area propolis are based on resins of several *Populus* species. In Brazil, green propolis, originally from the Amazon and El Cerrado, has a distinctive composition [12, 13].

Zhang et al. [14] have underlined the skills and visual plasticity in the honey bee to reject locations and depleted harvest sites, and also, that probably a set of visual, external but not aromatic stimuli are considered by this forage [15]. The aromatic stimuli are the most difficult to establish for purposes of standardization and quality control [16].

Already at the beginning of the last decade, Bankova [17] was aware that the key to recognizing propolis was the source plant, the classification was then an analytical approach based on plant source [18]. Bankova [17] recommended three parameters for poplar propolis characterization: flavones and total flavonols, flavanones and total dihydroflavonol, and phenolic content [19]. Similarly, Chang et al. [20] proposed to determine the total flavonoid content with a 2.4-dinitrophenylhydrazine reaction as well as reactions with aluminum chloride.

**Table 1. Propolis compounds of different provenances**

| | | | | | | | | | | | | | | | | | | | | | | | | | | | | |
|---|---|---|---|---|---|---|---|---|---|---|---|---|---|---|---|---|---|---|---|---|---|---|---|---|---|---|---|---|
| caffeic acid | 1 | 1 | 0 | 0 | 0 | 0 | 0 | 0 | 0 | 1 | 0 | 0 | 0 | 1 | 1 | 1 | 1 | 0 | 0 | 0 | 1 | 0 | 0 | 0 | 0 | 0 | 1 | 0 |
| coumaric acid | 1 | 1 | 0 | 0 | 0 | 0 | 0 | 0 | 0 | 1 | 0 | 0 | 0 | 1 | 1 | 0 | 1 | 0 | 0 | 0 | 1 | 0 | 0 | 0 | 0 | 0 | 0 | 0 |
| vanillin | 1 | 0 | 0 | 0 | 0 | 0 | 0 | 0 | 0 | 0 | 0 | 0 | 1 | 0 | 0 | 0 | 0 | 0 | 0 | 0 | 0 | 0 | 0 | 0 | 0 | 0 | 1 | 0 |
| methyl caffeate | 1 | 0 | 0 | 0 | 0 | 0 | 0 | 0 | 0 | 0 | 0 | 0 | 0 | 0 | 0 | 0 | 0 | 0 | 0 | 0 | 0 | 0 | 0 | 0 | 0 | 0 | 0 | 0 |
| ferulic acid | 1 | 0 | 0 | 0 | 0 | 0 | 1 | 0 | 0 | 1 | 0 | 0 | 0 | 0 | 0 | 0 | 0 | 0 | 0 | 0 | 1 | 0 | 0 | 0 | 0 | 0 | 0 | 0 |
| ferulic acid methyl ester | 1 | 0 | 0 | 0 | 0 | 0 | 0 | 0 | 0 | 0 | 0 | 0 | 0 | 0 | 0 | 0 | 0 | 0 | 0 | 0 | 0 | 0 | 0 | 0 | 0 | 0 | 0 | 0 |
| luteolin | 1 | 0 | 0 | 0 | 0 | 0 | 0 | 0 | 0 | 0 | 0 | 0 | 0 | 0 | 0 | 0 | 0 | 0 | 0 | 0 | 0 | 0 | 0 | 0 | 0 | 0 | 0 | 0 |
| quercetin | 1 | 1 | 0 | 0 | 0 | 0 | 0 | 0 | 0 | 0 | 0 | 0 | 0 | 0 | 0 | 0 | 0 | 0 | 0 | 0 | 0 | 0 | 0 | 1 | 0 | 0 | 0 | 0 |
| sakuranetin | 1 | 0 | 0 | 0 | 0 | 0 | 0 | 0 | 0 | 0 | 0 | 0 | 0 | 0 | 0 | 0 | 0 | 0 | 0 | 0 | 0 | 0 | 0 | 0 | 0 | 0 | 0 | 0 |
| methyl quercetin | 1 | 0 | 0 | 0 | 0 | 0 | 0 | 0 | 0 | 0 | 0 | 0 | 0 | 0 | 0 | 0 | 0 | 0 | 0 | 0 | 0 | 0 | 0 | 0 | 0 | 0 | 0 | 0 |
| cinnamic acid | 1 | 0 | 0 | 0 | 0 | 0 | 0 | 0 | 0 | 0 | 0 | 0 | 0 | 0 | 0 | 0 | 0 | 0 | 0 | 0 | 0 | 0 | 0 | 0 | 0 | 0 | 0 | 0 |
| tectochry1n | 1 | 0 | 0 | 0 | 0 | 0 | 1 | 0 | 0 | 0 | 0 | 0 | 0 | 1 | 1 | 0 | 0 | 0 | 0 | 0 | 1 | 0 | 0 | 0 | 0 | 0 | 0 | 0 |
| apigenin | 1 | 1 | 0 | 0 | 0 | 0 | 0 | 0 | 0 | 0 | 0 | 0 | 0 | 0 | 0 | 0 | 0 | 0 | 0 | 0 | 0 | 0 | 0 | 0 | 0 | 0 | 0 | 0 |
| naringenin | 1 | 0 | 1 | 1 | 1 | 0 | 0 | 0 | 0 | 0 | 0 | 0 | 0 | 0 | 0 | 0 | 0 | 0 | 0 | 0 | 0 | 0 | 0 | 0 | 0 | 0 | 0 | 0 |
| pinobanksin | 1 | 0 | 0 | 0 | 0 | 0 | 1 | 0 | 0 | 0 | 0 | 0 | 0 | 0 | 0 | 0 | 0 | 1 | 0 | 0 | 0 | 0 | 0 | 0 | 0 | 0 | 1 | 0 |
| kaempferol | 1 | 1 | 0 | 0 | 0 | 0 | 0 | 0 | 0 | 0 | 0 | 0 | 0 | 1 | 1 | 0 | 0 | 0 | 0 | 0 | 0 | 0 | 0 | 0 | 0 | 0 | 0 | 0 |
| kaempferide | 1 | 0 | 0 | 0 | 0 | 0 | 0 | 0 | 0 | 0 | 0 | 0 | 0 | 0 | 0 | 0 | 0 | 0 | 0 | 0 | 0 | 0 | 0 | 0 | 0 | 0 | 0 | 0 |
| bis-methylated quercetin | 1 | 0 | 0 | 0 | 0 | 0 | 0 | 0 | 0 | 0 | 0 | 0 | 0 | 0 | 0 | 0 | 0 | 0 | 0 | 0 | 0 | 0 | 0 | 0 | 0 | 0 | 0 | 0 |
| acacetin | 1 | 0 | 0 | 0 | 0 | 0 | 0 | 0 | 0 | 0 | 0 | 0 | 0 | 0 | 0 | 0 | 0 | 0 | 0 | 0 | 0 | 0 | 0 | 0 | 0 | 0 | 0 | 0 |
| hesperetin | 1 | 0 | 0 | 0 | 0 | 0 | 0 | 0 | 0 | 0 | 0 | 0 | 0 | 0 | 0 | 0 | 0 | 0 | 0 | 0 | 0 | 0 | 0 | 0 | 0 | 0 | 0 | 0 |
| prenyl caffeate | 1 | 0 | 0 | 0 | 0 | 0 | 0 | 0 | 0 | 0 | 0 | 0 | 0 | 0 | 0 | 0 | 0 | 0 | 0 | 0 | 0 | 0 | 0 | 0 | 0 | 0 | 0 | 0 |
| chrysin | 1 | 1 | 0 | 0 | 0 | 1 | 1 | 0 | 0 | 0 | 0 | 0 | 0 | 1 | 1 | 0 | 1 | 0 | 0 | 0 | 0 | 0 | 0 | 0 | 0 | 0 | 1 | 0 |
| pinocembrin | 1 | 1 | 0 | 0 | 1 | 1 | 0 | 0 | 0 | 0 | 0 | 0 | 0 | 1 | 1 | 0 | 1 | 1 | 0 | 0 | 0 | 0 | 0 | 1 | 0 | 0 | 0 | 1 |
| galangin | 1 | 1 | 0 | 0 | 0 | 1 | 0 | 0 | 0 | 0 | 0 | 0 | 0 | 1 | 1 | 0 | 1 | 0 | 0 | 0 | 0 | 0 | 0 | 1 | 0 | 0 | 1 | 0 |
| caffeic acid phenylethyl ester | 1 | 0 | 0 | 0 | 0 | 1 | 0 | 0 | 0 | 0 | 0 | 0 | 0 | 0 | 0 | 1 | 1 | 0 | 0 | 0 | 0 | 0 | 0 | 1 | 0 | 0 | 0 | 0 |
| pinobanksin-3-acetate | 1 | 0 | 0 | 0 | 0 | 0 | 0 | 0 | 0 | 0 | 0 | 0 | 0 | 1 | 1 | 0 | 0 | 1 | 0 | 0 | 0 | 0 | 0 | 0 | 0 | 0 | 0 | 0 |
| isopenthyl ferulate | 1 | 0 | 0 | 0 | 0 | 0 | 0 | 0 | 0 | 0 | 0 | 0 | 0 | 0 | 0 | 0 | 0 | 0 | 0 | 0 | 0 | 0 | 0 | 0 | 0 | 0 | 0 | 0 |
| pinobanksin-3-propionate | 1 | 0 | 0 | 0 | 0 | 0 | 0 | 0 | 0 | 0 | 0 | 0 | 0 | 0 | 0 | 0 | 0 | 0 | 0 | 0 | 0 | 0 | 0 | 0 | 0 | 0 | 0 | 0 |
| clerodane diterpenoid I | 1 | 0 | 0 | 0 | 0 | 0 | 0 | 0 | 0 | 0 | 0 | 0 | 0 | 0 | 0 | 0 | 0 | 0 | 0 | 0 | 0 | 0 | 0 | 0 | 0 | 0 | 0 | 0 |
| clerodane diterpenoid II | 1 | 0 | 0 | 0 | 0 | 0 | 0 | 0 | 0 | 0 | 0 | 0 | 0 | 0 | 0 | 0 | 0 | 0 | 0 | 0 | 0 | 0 | 0 | 0 | 0 | 0 | 0 | 0 |
| palmitic acid | 1 | 0 | 0 | 0 | 0 | 0 | 0 | 0 | 0 | 0 | 0 | 0 | 0 | 0 | 0 | 0 | 0 | 0 | 0 | 0 | 0 | 0 | 0 | 0 | 0 | 0 | 0 | 0 |
| isosakuranetin | 0 | 0 | 0 | 0 | 0 | 0 | 1 | 0 | 0 | 0 | 0 | 0 | 0 | 0 | 0 | 0 | 0 | 0 | 0 | 0 | 0 | 0 | 0 | 0 | 1 | 0 | 0 | 0 |
| benzoic acid | 0 | 1 | 0 | 0 | 0 | 0 | 1 | 0 | 0 | 0 | 0 | 0 | 0 | 0 | 0 | 0 | 0 | 0 | 0 | 0 | 0 | 0 | 0 | 0 | 0 | 0 | 1 | 0 |
| viscidone | 0 | 0 | 0 | 0 | 0 | 0 | 0 | 1 | 0 | 0 | 0 | 0 | 1 | 0 | 0 | 0 | 0 | 0 | 0 | 0 | 0 | 0 | 0 | 0 | 0 | 0 | 0 | 0 |
| bornyl-p-benzoate | 0 | 0 | 0 | 0 | 0 | 0 | 0 | 0 | 1 | 0 | 0 | 0 | 0 | 0 | 0 | 0 | 0 | 0 | 0 | 0 | 0 | 0 | 0 | 0 | 0 | 0 | 0 | 0 |
| ferutinol p-hydroxybenzoate | 0 | 0 | 0 | 0 | 0 | 0 | 0 | 0 | 1 | 0 | 0 | 0 | 0 | 0 | 0 | 0 | 0 | 0 | 0 | 0 | 0 | 0 | 0 | 0 | 0 | 0 | 0 | 0 |
| bornyl-p-vanillate | 0 | 0 | 0 | 0 | 0 | 0 | 0 | 0 | 1 | 0 | 0 | 0 | 0 | 0 | 0 | 0 | 0 | 0 | 0 | 0 | 0 | 0 | 0 | 0 | 0 | 0 | 0 | 0 |
| rosmarinic ACID | 0 | 0 | 0 | 0 | 0 | 0 | 0 | 0 | 0 | 1 | 0 | 0 | 0 | 0 | 0 | 0 | 0 | 0 | 0 | 0 | 0 | 0 | 0 | 0 | 0 | 0 | 0 | 0 |
| rutin | 0 | 0 | 0 | 0 | 0 | 0 | 0 | 0 | 0 | 0 | 0 | 0 | 0 | 0 | 0 | 0 | 0 | 1 | 0 | 0 | 0 | 0 | 0 | 0 | 0 | 0 | 0 | 0 |
| liquiritegenin | 0 | 0 | 0 | 0 | 0 | 0 | 0 | 0 | 0 | 0 | 0 | 0 | 0 | 0 | 0 | 0 | 0 | 1 | 0 | 0 | 0 | 0 | 0 | 0 | 0 | 0 | 0 | 0 |
| daidzein | 0 | 0 | 0 | 0 | 0 | 0 | 0 | 0 | 0 | 0 | 0 | 0 | 0 | 0 | 0 | 0 | 0 | 1 | 0 | 0 | 0 | 0 | 0 | 0 | 0 | 0 | 0 | 0 |
| dalbergin | 0 | 0 | 0 | 0 | 0 | 0 | 0 | 0 | 0 | 0 | 0 | 0 | 0 | 0 | 0 | 0 | 0 | 1 | 0 | 0 | 0 | 0 | 0 | 0 | 0 | 0 | 0 | 0 |
| isoliquiretigenin | 0 | 0 | 0 | 0 | 0 | 0 | 0 | 0 | 0 | 0 | 0 | 0 | 0 | 0 | 0 | 0 | 0 | 1 | 0 | 0 | 0 | 0 | 0 | 0 | 0 | 0 | 0 | 0 |
| formononetin | 0 | 0 | 0 | 0 | 0 | 0 | 0 | 0 | 0 | 0 | 0 | 0 | 0 | 0 | 0 | 0 | 0 | 1 | 0 | 0 | 0 | 0 | 0 | 0 | 0 | 0 | 0 | 0 |
| biochanin A | 0 | 0 | 0 | 0 | 0 | 0 | 0 | 0 | 0 | 0 | 0 | 0 | 0 | 0 | 0 | 0 | 0 | 1 | 0 | 0 | 0 | 0 | 0 | 0 | 0 | 0 | 0 | 0 |
| isonympheol B | 0 | 0 | 0 | 0 | 0 | 0 | 0 | 0 | 0 | 0 | 0 | 0 | 0 | 0 | 0 | 0 | 0 | 0 | 1 | 0 | 0 | 0 | 0 | 0 | 0 | 0 | 0 | 0 |
| nymphaeol A | 0 | 0 | 0 | 0 | 0 | 0 | 0 | 0 | 0 | 0 | 0 | 0 | 0 | 0 | 0 | 0 | 0 | 0 | 1 | 0 | 0 | 0 | 0 | 0 | 0 | 0 | 0 | 0 |
| nymphaeol C | 0 | 0 | 0 | 0 | 0 | 0 | 0 | 0 | 0 | 0 | 0 | 0 | 0 | 0 | 0 | 0 | 0 | 0 | 1 | 0 | 0 | 0 | 0 | 0 | 0 | 0 | 0 | 0 |
| medicarpin | 0 | 0 | 0 | 0 | 0 | 0 | 0 | 0 | 0 | 0 | 0 | 0 | 0 | 0 | 0 | 0 | 0 | 0 | 0 | 1 | 0 | 0 | 0 | 0 | 0 | 0 | 0 | 0 |
| (S)-vestitol | 0 | 0 | 0 | 0 | 0 | 0 | 0 | 0 | 0 | 0 | 0 | 0 | 0 | 0 | 0 | 0 | 0 | 0 | 0 | 1 | 0 | 0 | 0 | 0 | 0 | 0 | 0 | 0 |
| 3,4,2',3' tetrahydrochalcone | 0 | 0 | 0 | 0 | 0 | 0 | 0 | 0 | 0 | 0 | 0 | 0 | 0 | 0 | 0 | 0 | 0 | 0 | 0 | 1 | 0 | 0 | 0 | 0 | 0 | 0 | 0 | 0 |
| cis asarone | 0 | 0 | 0 | 0 | 0 | 0 | 0 | 0 | 0 | 0 | 0 | 0 | 0 | 0 | 0 | 0 | 0 | 0 | 0 | 1 | 0 | 0 | 0 | 0 | 0 | 0 | 0 | 0 |
| methoxy eugenol | 0 | 0 | 0 | 0 | 0 | 0 | 0 | 0 | 0 | 0 | 0 | 0 | 0 | 0 | 0 | 0 | 0 | 0 | 0 | 1 | 0 | 0 | 0 | 0 | 0 | 0 | 0 | 0 |
| narigenin-8-C-hexo1de | 0 | 0 | 0 | 0 | 0 | 0 | 0 | 0 | 0 | 0 | 0 | 0 | 0 | 0 | 0 | 0 | 0 | 0 | 0 | 1 | 0 | 0 | 0 | 0 | 0 | 0 | 0 | 0 |
| (3*S*)-7-*O*-methylvestitol | 0 | 0 | 0 | 0 | 0 | 0 | 0 | 0 | 0 | 0 | 0 | 0 | 0 | 0 | 0 | 0 | 0 | 0 | 0 | 0 | 0 | 0 | 0 | 0 | 0 | 0 | 0 | 0 |
| gallic ac | 0 | 1 | 0 | 0 | 0 | 0 | 0 | 0 | 0 | 0 | 0 | 0 | 0 | 0 | 0 | 0 | 0 | 0 | 0 | 0 | 0 | 0 | 0 | 0 | 0 | 0 | 0 | 0 |
| ellagic ac | 0 | 1 | 0 | 0 | 0 | 0 | 0 | 0 | 0 | 0 | 0 | 0 | 0 | 0 | 0 | 0 | 0 | 0 | 0 | 0 | 0 | 0 | 0 | 0 | 0 | 0 | 0 | 0 |
| 4 OH 3 Meox benzoic | 0 | 1 | 0 | 0 | 0 | 0 | 0 | 0 | 0 | 0 | 0 | 0 | 0 | 0 | 0 | 0 | 0 | 0 | 0 | 0 | 0 | 0 | 0 | 0 | 0 | 0 | 0 | 0 |
| pinobanksin 5 methyl-ether | 0 | 0 | 0 | 0 | 0 | 0 | 0 | 0 | 0 | 0 | 0 | 0 | 0 | 0 | 0 | 0 | 0 | 0 | 0 | 0 | 1 | 0 | 0 | 0 | 0 | 0 | 0 | 0 |
| Cynnamylideneacetic acid | 0 | 0 | 0 | 0 | 0 | 0 | 0 | 0 | 0 | 0 | 0 | 0 | 0 | 1 | 1 | 0 | 0 | 0 | 0 | 0 | 0 | 0 | 0 | 0 | 0 | 0 | 0 | 0 |
| dimethylallylcaffeic acid | 0 | 0 | 0 | 0 | 0 | 0 | 0 | 0 | 0 | 0 | 0 | 0 | 0 | 0 | 0 | 0 | 0 | 0 | 0 | 0 | 0 | 0 | 0 | 0 | 1 | 0 | 0 | 0 |
| 3,5-diprenyl-4-hydroxycinnamic | 0 | 0 | 0 | 0 | 0 | 0 | 0 | 0 | 0 | 0 | 0 | 0 | 0 | 0 | 0 | 0 | 0 | 0 | 0 | 0 | 0 | 0 | 0 | 0 | 0 | 1 | 0 | 0 |
| 3-Prenyl-4-hydroxycinnamic acid | 0 | 0 | 0 | 0 | 0 | 0 | 0 | 0 | 0 | 0 | 0 | 0 | 0 | 0 | 0 | 0 | 0 | 0 | 0 | 0 | 0 | 0 | 0 | 0 | 0 | 0 | 1 | 0 |
| 7-Hydroxyflavanone | 0 | 0 | 0 | 0 | 0 | 0 | 0 | 0 | 0 | 0 | 0 | 0 | 0 | 0 | 0 | 0 | 0 | 0 | 0 | 0 | 0 | 0 | 0 | 0 | 0 | 0 | 0 | 1 |
| Mucronulatol | 0 | 0 | 0 | 0 | 0 | 0 | 0 | 0 | 0 | 0 | 0 | 0 | 0 | 0 | 0 | 0 | 0 | 0 | 0 | 0 | 0 | 0 | 0 | 0 | 0 | 0 | 0 | 1 |
| arizonicanolA | 0 | 0 | 0 | 0 | 0 | 0 | 0 | 0 | 0 | 0 | 0 | 0 | 0 | 0 | 0 | 0 | 0 | 0 | 0 | 0 | 0 | 0 | 0 | 0 | 0 | 0 | 0 | 1 |
| Vestitol | 0 | 0 | 0 | 0 | 0 | 0 | 0 | 0 | 0 | 0 | 0 | 0 | 0 | 0 | 0 | 0 | 0 | 0 | 0 | 0 | 0 | 0 | 0 | 0 | 0 | 0 | 0 | 1 |
| melilotocarpanA | 0 | 0 | 0 | 0 | 0 | 0 | 0 | 0 | 0 | 0 | 0 | 0 | 0 | 0 | 0 | 0 | 0 | 0 | 0 | 0 | 0 | 0 | 0 | 0 | 0 | 0 | 0 | 1 |
| melilotocarpanD | 0 | 0 | 0 | 0 | 0 | 0 | 0 | 0 | 0 | 0 | 0 | 0 | 0 | 0 | 0 | 0 | 0 | 0 | 0 | 0 | 0 | 0 | 0 | 0 | 0 | 0 | 0 | 1 |
| salicylic acid | 0 | 1 | 0 | 0 | 0 | 0 | 0 | 0 | 0 | 0 | 0 | 0 | 0 | 0 | 0 | 0 | 0 | 0 | 0 | 0 | 0 | 0 | 0 | 0 | 0 | 0 | 0 | 0 |
| | 1 | 2 | 3 | 4 | 5 | 6 | 7 | 8 | 9 | 10 | 11 | 12 | 13 | 14 | 15 | 16 | 17 | 18 | 19 | 20 | 21 | 22 | 23 | 24 | 25 | 26 | 27 | 28 |

Argentine: 2, 3; Azerbaijan: 4; Brazil: 13, 18, 20, 25, 26, 27; Chile: 8, 24; China: 6, 15, 17; Croatia: 21; Irak: 1; Iran 9; Italy: 5; Japan: 19, 22, 23; Korea: 14, 16; Lituania: 10; Mexico: 28; Polonia: 11; Riga: 12.

A number of methods have been used in the analysis of propolis, for example, via capillary electrophoresis, identifying twelve flavonoids such as pinocembrin, acacetine, chrysin, rutin, catechin, naringenin, galangin, luteolin, myricetin, kaempferol, quercetin, two phenolic acids, cinnamic and caffeic, and revesratrol stilbene [21]. A good correlation between CZE and HPLC was observed [22].

The first chromatographic methods were based on the European perspective of compositions with similar characteristics to that of *Populus*. Popova et al. [19] insisted that the method of Salatino [23] lacks the gallic acid control substance, taking into account that this is a minor compound in propolis. A mixture of flavonol and flavanone is recommended in the propolis that *Populus* is presumed to be the source plant. Pinocembrin and galangin had a recovery of 86%. Although when comparing to HPLC, this method may have flaws, the spectrophotometric methods are useful for routine analysis due to their simplicity, reproducibility and acceptable accuracy.

Park et al. [24] distinguished 12 types of propolis from Brazil, five from the South of the country designated as group 3, one from the Southeast called 12, and six from the North called Group 6. By comparing the spectra, the authors concluded that the resin comes from *Hypsis divaricata.*

Isla et al. [25] found similarities between the north of Argentina propolis and those from southern Brazil. Daugsch et al. [26] attributed to *Dalberghia*, the color of red propolis, also correlated the profile of propolis with the compounds found in such legume [27] (Table 1). Trusheva et al. [28] described the plant *Clusia* as the source of the red color in the propolis from Brazil, which is also reported for Cuban red propolis. Teixera et al. [29] confirmed the Kumasawa et al. results [30] with respect to the origin of *Baccharis dracunculifolia*-based green propolis; while these authors got the morphological characteristics by direct observation, Teixeira et al. [29] obtained values of corbicular content through Africanized honeybees.

In the late 90's, Valcic et al. [31] developed a microscopic technique for the analysis of propolis residues, pollen grains and also both morphological and vegetative debris, including trichomes and stomatal apparatus remains, describing *Baccharis* as source of resin for Chilean propolis. Through morphological remnants, *B. linearis* and other species of Chilean matorral, as *Lithraea Kageneckia* and *Trevoa*, could be traced.

Not significant phytochemical-morphoanatomical correlation was obtained, this may be due to Chilean propolis also contains Salicaceae pollen of the genus *Salix* and eucalyptus, with a predominance of pollen from eucalyptus between July and October. In Chile, the maximum production of propolis occurs between August and September [32].

Salatino et al. [33] described that conifers and aspen trees, found in temperate areas, are more significant in those propolis, while in tropical areas, only *Baccharis* is a resource for propolis production. There are similarities between European and Argentinean samples [34], probably due to a much interfered agroecosystem in the New World by European settlers, who inserted their trees. Lignans seemed to be not geographically restricted to the Canary Islands, Chile and Kenya.

The distribution of benzophenone is not useful either as they are present in two different climates, Venezuelan and Chilean Mediterranean [35, 36]. Prenylated benzophenones have been identified in red propolis from *Clusia*, obtained from Cuban sites, corresponding to the same vegetal source (Clusia species) than Venezuelan products [17].

Unlike some genres with traceable geographic distribution through chemotaxonomy, *Baccharis* or *Populus* are not taxonomical descriptive [37, 38, 39] (Figure 1). Isosakuranetin and two ursolic acid derivatives can be identified as antibiotics, present in propolis and in *B. dracunculifolia* extracts [40].

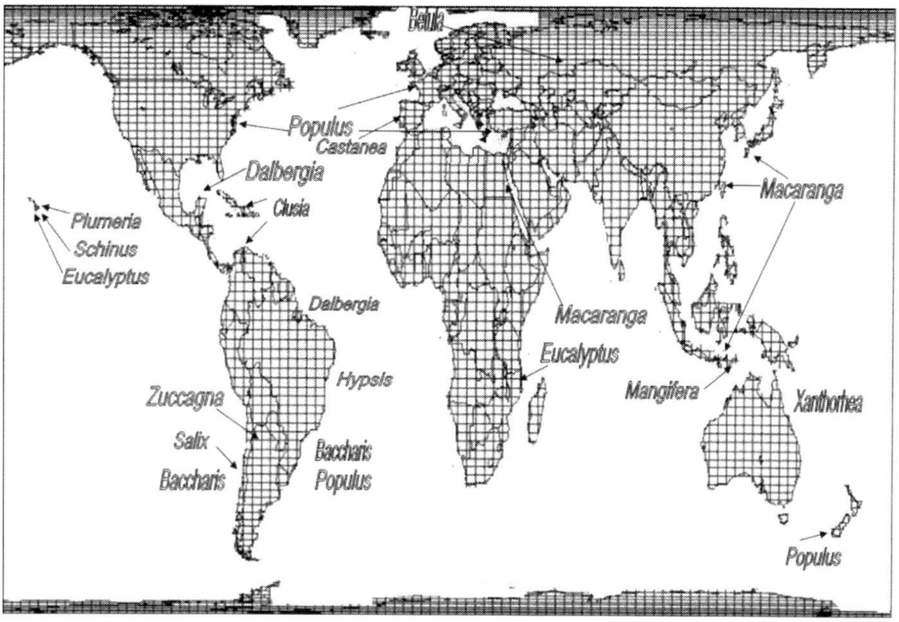


Figure 1. Genres source of resins for the foraging of *Apis mellifera* honeybee.

Fujimoto et al. [41] distinguished a Brazil-type and a *Populus*-type propolis. Marcucci et al. [42] distinguished at least three types of Brazilian propolis. *T. angustula* obtained resins from *Schinus terebinthifolius* (known locally as *aroeira vermelha*), and although the composition of propolis from *A. mellifera* in the South and Southeast of Brazil varies considerably, three well defined types can be obtained using HPLC and ESI (-)-MS sampling, as a result of different plant sources and geographical origins.

Moreira et al. [43] found *Populus* and *Castanea* in propolis samples from Portugal. *Castanea sativa* dominates in samples from northern Portugal, while *Populus* pollen is present in southern sites with Mediterranean climate.

Propolis chalcones and chromones from Jeju Island, Korea, contain species such as *Psoralea corylifolia*, *Musineon divaricatum* and *Angelica keiskei*. This island has a humid subtropical climate that makes it different from other sectors of that country [44]. Continental propolis is chemically similar to *Populus* [45]. *Hernandia nimphaefolia* has been suggested as a source of oriental propolis from Okinawa due to the presence of prenylflavonoids [46], but the source observed was *Macaranga tanarius*.

Lotti et al. [47] distinguished Mexican red propolis using a combination of markers: arizonicanol A and melitocarpan A and D present in *Dalbergia* species. Although isoflavones and pterocarpans are common in red propolis, their presence in Mexico propolis is recent [48].

Volpi and Bergonzini [34] analyzed several samples from Argentina, Europe, Azerbaijan, China, Ethiopia and Kenya, finding more similarities between propolis from Argentina and Europe, than from Asia. In the case of Italy and Spain, their samples are rich in polyphenols.

Chaillou and Nazareno [49] compared the propolis from Santiago del Estero (Argentina) and the one from southern Brazil, finding similarities. Salgado-Laurenti et al. [50] found in Argentina, in addition to pollen, the species *Schinus*, particularly in northeastern Argentina [51]. Similarly, Barth and da Luz [52] identified *Schinus terenthifolius* pollen in red propolis, instead of *Dalbergia* pollen. Unfortunately, *Schinus* species are present throughout America, grown in locations as far away as Hawaii.

Zunini et al. [53] selected the coelution of fisetin and myricetin as Uruguayan propolis representatives.

The method of electrospray ionization is suitable for low concentrations of balms, i.e. pharmaceutical hydroalcoholic solutions of low concentration. Similarly LC-MS, liquid chromatography method plus mass spectrometry, allows the separation of other compounds of the matrix. Several authors described that the most polar components are not drawn in such hydro-alcoholic mixtures, but derived from caffeic acid and the ESI negative mode, among others, as a variant of unusual sensibility.

Popova et al. [54] established that the quantitative evaluation of chemical groups is better than the assessment of specific markers, determining flavones and flavonols, total phenolics, total flavanones and total dihydroflavonol of typical *Populus* resin propolis.

The gas chromatographic method plus silylation has been set aside due to its complexity [55].

Kumazawa et al. [31, 46] identified prenylflavonoids in Taiwanese and Okinawa propolis of *Macaranga* (Salatino IV Type) and photographed bees visiting *M. tanarius* [46]. Popova et al. [56] used DPN for the quantification of prenylated flavanones in Taiwanese *Macaranga* propolis using C-D-F-G propolis as taxonomic markers.

Trusheva et al. [57], in East Java (Java Timur), isolated and identified 11 compounds: four alk (en) yl) resorcinols (as inseparable mixture), with four prenylflavanonas and three cicloartan-type triterpenes, and with *Mangifera indica* and *M. tanarius* as resin source. Trusheva et al. [57] indicated that there are similarities in the compounds of propolis from *Macaranga tanarius* and *Mangifera indica* plants from Indonesia.

Thus, the Brazilian approach is to search for a specific marker for green propolis from *Baccharis*. In Chile, it was suggested that Chilean propolis may contain *Baccharis* resins, based on the presence of viscidone [58, 42]. *Baccharis dracunculifolia* (common name: *Alecrim do campo*), although it is a recognized source of viscidone, it is not an antibiotic agent [40]. Brazilian green propolis is characterized by the presence of prenylated compounds [59]. Similarly, Trusheva et al. [60] described prenylated coumarins in Iranian products. Direct observation of foraging insects appears to be an easy way to standardize.

Sawaya et al. [8, 13] described Brazilian propolis, in contrast to European, American and African descriptions, they found seven types of propolis using the EASI-MS analysis (easy ambient sonic-spray ionization), which corresponds to the final analysis solution, and had been used in other matrices including biodiesel.

Sawaya et al. [61] described, through the m / z 247 molecular ions, samples from Portugal, Spain and Iran, which had been observed in Italy and corresponded to dihydroxyflavone, chrysin, pinocembrin, apigenin / galangin, CAPE, and acetate of pinobanksine found in propolis from *Populus*. A second group, analyzed by the same authors, is composed of samples from various countries with temperate climates (South Korea, Australia, India, USA, Canada, Chile and S Brazil), where the ions characteristic of this group similarly corresponded to *Populus* flavonoids. The main components of the Korean samples, located in this group (K39-Geochang, K41 and K38-Muju-Sangju), were also identified by Ahn et al. [62] using HPLC. These authors concluded that Korean propolis also comes from *Populus*.

Flavonoids described above are common in products from southern Brazil and central Chile [63] and their ions have been observed in samples from U.S. and Europe using EASI-MS [13].

## 2. Propolis as Standardized Methods

There are tests in Chile to determine the palynological profile, which together with chemical analysis, can be a quality assurance standard [63, 64, 65]. Montenegro et al. [36] studied a combination of pollen and vegetative plant element microscopy, foraged in the vicinity of the beehive, characterizing *Baccharis* by the presence of trichomes and pollen grains in the sediment.

Remarkably, despite how powerful modern analytical procedures may be, typical markers such as CAPE can be difficult to separate and characterize; something recently mentioned by Pellati et al. [66] in a study of HPLC-diode array. The only limitation in the analysis is the separation of caffeic acid phenylethyl ester and 3 pinobanksine acetate peaks 28 and 29.

Other authors have tried combinations of pharmacological studies and chemical analysis, but their purpose has not been an implementation towards standardization [17]. Seasonal variation can be an obstacle to standardize [67, 68].

The study of seasonal variability theorizes the knowledge of stable, non-taxonomic and ecological variable compounds that are available as markers. For example, Artepillin C increases during the growing season, while Baccharin and isosakuranetin are quite stable. The authors also found a correlation between the rainy period and phenolic contents [69]. Castro et al. [67] found seasonal variation in 6-type propolis in northeastern Brazil and in the 12 zone of southeastern Brazil, measured in terms of antibiotic activity.

Erdogan et al. [70] succeeded in separating polyphenols using pressure extraction, which subsequently analyzed via HPLC, including catechins and phenolic acids.

Martena et al. [71] determined levels of polycyclic in Dutch commercial products, finding levels above LOQ (limit of quantification). These authors recommended certain PAHs exposure levels.

Gonzalez et al. [72] stated that the Folin-Cicolteu method remains the most reproducible method for phenolic-high samples, 30%. The inclusion in β cyclodextrin could improve the solubility of certain bioactive compounds, and ensure the quality of the products [73]. Marker molecules are fundamental in standardization given that they decrease the solubility of aromatic phenolic acids such as vanillin and benzoic.

In the late 90's, it was already pursued to integrate spectral methods to neuronal networks. Watson et al. [74] proposed to analyze the 1 H NMR data by principal components. Custodio et al. [75] combined hierarchical clustering methods regarding main components, failing to identify propolis waxes vs. beeswax using either gas chromatography or infrared spectroscopy methods.

Many authors emphasized their belief in the difficulty of developing a suitable analytical procedure for propolis and have recommended an overall assessment, rather than determining a specific marker, that everything can be seen as the epistemology of taxonomy. Both American and European authorities recommend this type of method. Similarly, China recommends analytical methods for medicinal plant extracts that have been endorsed by the Guidelines for the assessment of herbal medicines [76, 77]. Recently, fuzzy clustering [5] was added, which corresponds to a fast and efficient method for discrimination and authentication of various samples of propolis on the basis of slight classification of data through CCF image analysis. The results are consistent with local and geographical origin of the Romanian propolis flora and illustrate the lack of clarity about the similarities and differences of propolis samples.

Liang et al. [78] proposed the fingerprint (chromatographic digital impression shape) as an element to consider, and that the relationship among the chromatographic fingerprints could be analyzed by comparing, in terms of affinities and specificities, the data presented as a correlation coefficient or a coefficient of congruence. Finally, it is suggested that the estimation of similarity is used, along with the original digital impression.

The normalization of Argentine propolis by spectrophotometric methods, gives a great variability of samples; the ones from Mendoza had higher concentration of bioactive compounds using *Populus* as plant [51]. Galan Martinez [79] found variability of Colombian propolis using TLC. Similarly, Campo Fernandez et al. [80], using the CCF method, identified three types of Cuban propolis, which correlate with color, and were determined by chromatographic profiles.

The spray drying may alter some chemical parameters [81]. Baccharin content in the spray-dried propolis was altered by the drying temperature in a 5% significance level, while coumaric acid content up to 15%.

Kalogeropoulos et al. [73] found a better antimicrobial activity in Greece and Cyprus propolis, compared to nisin protein, a GRAS-type additive. The microbes identified, which are inhibited by propolis balm and not by nisin, were *L. monocytogenes*, *B. cereus* and *S. aureus*. Kalogeropoulos *et al.* [74] found chemical affinities with samples from Turkey, although the latter contained anthraquinones [9].

Recently, Cutujar et al. [82] identified totarolone and considered it as a *Tetraclinis articulata* marker in Malta, along with other compounds of Cupresaceae and Pinaceae. Thus, Mediterranean propolis contains many diterpenes, including isocupressic, pimaric, communic acids, isoagathoial, agathadiol and totarol, as main compounds [83].

In general, compounds found in propolis flavonoids seem to have very low pharmacodynamic potential; other substances have been cited as having the highest bioactivity, such as benzophenones, hydroxamic acids, prenylated compounds or terpenoids and artepillin C phenol [28, 84, 85, 86, 87, 88, 89, 90].

The properties of propolis are mentioned in the Old Testament as tzori (balsam in Hebrew) [91].

Highly prevalent microbial diseases could benefit from standardized known-profile products, i.e. with anti-candid [9, 92], antiprotozoal [93], *Trypanosoma cruzi* or *Leishmannia* [94] and anti-caries applications [95]. Liberio et al. [96], mentioned that diseases could be reduced using geopropolis.

Some of microbial disease, described by several authors that used propolis are: gingivitis, plaque control in humans [97], as neuroprotector [98] and hypolipidemic [99]; in the latter, caffeoylquinic acid was responsible of the disease. Saavedra et al. [100] determined an anticariogenic effect on *Lactobacillus fermentum* and Ferreira et al. [86] described an intracanal effect, in combination with calcium hydroxide against a number of specialized microbes.

Banskova [101] mentioned that phenolic compounds are mentioned as the responsible of this bioactivity.

Also, an antimicrobial activity has been described [102, 103], where benzophenones are described as responsible for this bioactivity, an antioxidant activity [4] that is attributed to phenolics and flavonoids. The antioxidant effects include several models, like Herrera et al. [104] who found that a protective effect is attributed to the pattern of flavonoids on animal steatosis [4].According to Sforzin and Vankova [105], it is necessary to develop studies about propolis before entering the market, investigating not only the chemical composition, effectiveness, experiments either positive or negative, but also other pharmacological and clinical history in healthy humans to obtain a usage profile in therapy.According to Medić-Šarić [3], nutraceutical products should have a similar approach to registered drugs, including standardization of their physicochemical and biological properties. Chromatographic and spectrophotometric methods are probably sufficient for "natural" products as chemical-biological methods for drugs [106]. These authors called the type of propolis the determination of source, mostly known as the palynological profile.The matrix honey, contrary to propolis, is primarily sugar and residual polyphenols. An electrophoretic analysis looks promising [107], which includes pretreatment, SPE solid phase separation in C18 cartridges, applying HPLC and electrophoresis to its samples.

## 3. Honeys as Standardized Methods

As Bogdanov et al. [108] described for honey quality control, it is not possible to identify a monofloral honey, the same happens when using propolis, which happens to be a complex matrix, and it takes many botanical-palynological and physicochemical trials to obtain a standardized characterization. The organoleptic properties are a real analytical challenge; for example, Piasenzotto et al. [109] conclude that when analyzing six unifloral honeys of different origins via solid-phase extraction, the gas chromatographic profiles are very similar. Using the SPME method, all samples of honey with the same botanical origin have remarkably similar profiles.

The total ash content, total acidity and dynamic viscosity are sufficient for honey identification. The analysis is easy and no time consuming at all [110]. The results obtained were not the expected regarding the pigments (flavonoids) or about the color pattern in this study, the latter was measured using La * b * and XYZ systems.

Radovic et al. [111], using a method of disposal of volatile compounds that were analyzed using GC-MS, created a system to identify honeys; nine markers were detected in the 43 unifloral varieties: scent markers for acacia, chestnut (*Castanea*), eucalyptus, *Erica*, linden, lavender, rapeseed or canola, rosemary and sunflower. *Escallonia* was identified by its safranal content.

Other studies have described that cetophorone and isophorone are typical of Ulmo honey [112]. However, linalool detected for quillay is not a specific feature, as it has also been detected in *Robinia pseudoacacia* (false acacia).

Terrab et al. [113] considered that 20% of *Helianthus*, *Mentha* and *Teucrium scorodonia* pollen is enough for unifloral honey characterization, and 10% for Citrus honey [114], considering that these species are poor in pollen, as the rules usually describe 45% of pollen marker. Other cases, such as eucalyptus honey, are characterized by over 70% of pollen marker [115].

Montenegro et al. [116], by principal components, divided the Chilean Mediterranean climate into three geographic areas, their melisopalinological profiles of *Escallonia* made possible to describe three landscapes that are correlated with bioclimatic zones.

The European Commission, seeking to harmonize national legislation, now requires floral and geographical origins [111]. These authors suggest that the aroma fingerprint may be more effective than the melisopalinological analysis.

Pyrzynska and Biezaga [107] recommended as an alternative to HPLC, capillary electrophoresis as CZE (Capillary zone electrophoresis) and MKE (micellar electrokinetic chromatography), separating and identifying common phenolic compounds (present in unifloral honeys of *Citrus, Thymus, Rosmarinus* and *Lavandula*). According to Hurtado-Fernández et al. [22], the advantage of the capillary electrophoresis method is the lesser degree of manipulation of samples without pre-cleaning.

The propolis future research should be directed to its origin description, as it has been in the development of honey. The analytical methods available especially tandem methods, would make better industry standards possible [108].

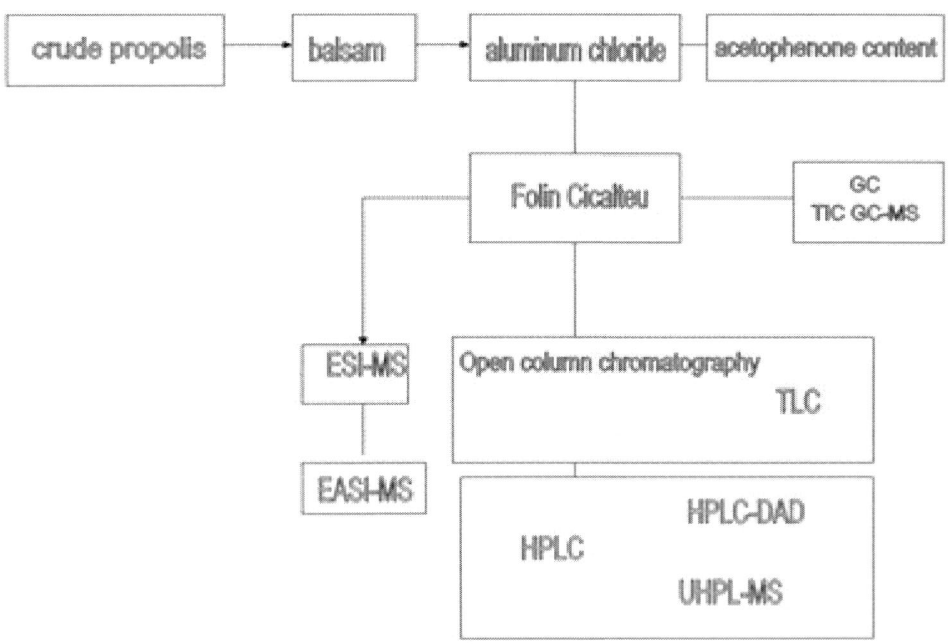


Figure 2. Sequence of analytical methods to identify propolis origin.

## CONCLUSION

One of the oldest applications of propolis is against diseases caused by microbial contamination. The synergy of propolis with standard antibiotics has neither been exploited nor explored, particularly in terms of pharmacoeconomics. Once standard products are designed, these can custom made.

Propolis has proven to be ideal for the screening of new biodynamic molecules.

Most honey analysis techniques can be applied to the characterization of propolis, including palynology, chromatographic methods and physico-chemical assessments. Like honey, the future will determine the amount of tests required, either for use in food or nutraceutical industry.

## ACKNOWLEDGMENTS

The authors also wish to thank the Fondo Nacional de Desarrollo Científico y Tecnológico (FONDECYT-REGULAR 2011), for funding within the scope of the project: "Bioindicators of botanical and geographical origin of Chilean endemic honeys", Project 1110808 to G. Montenegro.

## REFERENCES

[1] Ahn M.R., Kumazawa S., Hamasaka T., and Nakayama T. 2004. Antioxidant activity and constituents of propolis collected in various areas of Korea. *J. Agr. Food Chem.*, 52: 7286–7292.

[2] Ahn M.R., Kunimasa K., Ohta T., Kumazawa S., Kamihira M., Kaji K., Uto Y., Hori H., Nagasawa H., and Nakayama T. 2007. Suppression of tumor-induced angiogenesis by Brazilian propolis: Major component artepillin C inhibits in vitro tube formation and endothelial cell proliferation. *Cancer Letters,* 252: 235–243.

[3] Ahn, M.R., Kunimasa, K., Kumazawa, S., Kaji, K., Uto, Y., Hori, H., Nagasawa, H. Nakayama, T., and Ohta, T. 2009. Correlation between antiangiogenic activity and antioxidant activity of various components from propolis. *Mol. Nut. Food Res.*, 53(5): 643−651.

[4] Bankova V. 2005. Recent trends and important developments in propolis research. *Ecam,* 2: 29–32.

[5] Bankova V., and Marcucci M.C. 2000. Standardization of propolis: present status and perspectives. *Bee World,* 81(4): 182–188.

[6] Banskova V. 2005. Chemical diversity of propolis and the problem of standardization. *J. Ethnopharmacology,* 100:114–117.

[7] Barth O., and Pinto da Luz C.F.P. 2009. Palynological analysis of Brazilian red propolis samples. *J. Apicultural Res. and Bee World,* 48:181–188.

[8] Bogdanov S., Ruoff K., and Persano Oddo L. 2004. Physico-chemical methods for characterization of unifloral honeys: a review. *Apidologie,* S5-S17.

[9] Cabral I. S.R., Oldoni T.L.C., Prado A., Becerra R.M.N., Alencar S.M., Masaharu Ikegaki M., and Rosalen P.L. 2009. Composiçao fenólica, atividade antibacteriana e antioxidante, da propolis vermelha brasileira. *Quimica Nova,* 32: 1523–1527.

[10] Campo Fernández M., Cuesta Rubio O., Márquez Hernández I., Rosado Pérez A., and Porto R.M. de O. 2008. Análisis cualitativo de propóleos cubanos por cromatografía en capa delgada. *Latin American Journal of Pharmacy,* 27:380–386.

[11] Casaroto A.R., and Lara V.S. 2010. Phytomedicines for Candida-associated denture stomatitis. *Fitoterapia,* 81:323–328.

[12] Castro M. L., Cury J.A., Rosalen P.L., Alencar S.M, Masaharu I.; Simone I., Duarte S., and Koo, H. 2007. Própolis do sudeste e nordeste do Brasil: influência da sazonalidade na atividade antibacteriana e composição fenólica. *Quimica Nova,* 30: 1512–1516.

[13] Castro M.L., Vilela W.R., Zauli R.C., Ikegaki M., Rehder V.L.G.R., Foglio M.A., Alencar S.M., and Rosalen P.L. 2009. Bioassay guided purification of the antimicrobial fraction of a Brazilian propolis from Bahia state. *BMC Complementary and Alternative Medicine,* 9:25.

[14] Chaillou, L.L., and Nazareno, M.A. 2009. Chemical variability in propolis from Santiago del Estero, Argentina, related to the arboreal environment as the sources of resins. *J. Sci. Food Agric.*, 89: 978–983.

[15] Chang C., Yang M.H, Wen H.-M., and Chern J.-Ch. 2002 Estimation of total flavonoid content in propolis by two complementary colorimetric methods. *Food and drug Analysis,* 10: 178–182.

[16] Cottica S., Sawaya, A.C.F.H., Eberlin M.N., Franco S.L., Zeoula L.M. and Visentainer J.V. A. 2011. Antioxidant activity and composition of propolis obtained by different methods of extraction. *J. Braz. Chem. Soc.*, 22: 929-935.

[17] Cushnie T.P., and Lamb A.J. 2005. Antimicrobial activity of flavonoids. *Int. J. antimicrobial Agents,* 26: 343–356.

[18] Custudio A., Ferreira M.M.C., Giuseppina Negri G., and Salatino A. 2003. Clustering of comb and propolis waxes based on the distribution of aliphatic constituents. *J. Brz. Chem. Soc.*, 14: 354–357.

[19] Cutajar S., Farrugia C., Mifsud D., Popova M., Antonova D., and Bankova V. 2010. Chemical characterisation of maltese propolis in relation to botanical sources. Presented at the Seventh World Meeting on Pharmaceutics, Biopharmaceutics and Pharmaceutical Technology, Malta.

[20] da Silva Filho A., de Sousa J.P.B., Soares S., Niege A. J. C. Furtado, Márcio L. Andrade e Silva, Cunha W.R., Gregório L.E., N. P. Dhammika Nanayakkara, and Bastos J.K. 2008. Antimicrobial activity of the extract and isolated compounds from Baccharis dracunculifolia D. C. (Asteraceae). *Z. Naturforsch.*, 63c: 40–46.

[21] Daugsch A., Moraes C.S., Fort P., and Park Y. 2007. Brazilian red propolis composition and botanical origin. *Ecam,* 5:435–441.

[22] De Andrade Ferreira F.B., Torres S.A., da Silva Rosa O.P., Ferreira C.M., Garcia R.B., Marcucci M.C., and Gomes B.P.F.A. 2007. Antimicrobial effect of propolis and other substances against selected endodontic pathogens. Oral Surg. Oral Med. Oral Pathol. *Oral Radiol. Endod.*, 104:709–716.

[23] De Brito G., Ortigao-Farias J.R., Gaithier M., Liu F., and Giurfa M. 2007. Taste perception in honeybees:just a taste of honey? *Arthropod-Plant Interactions,* 1: 69–76.

[24] De Castro S.L., and Higashi K.O. 1995. Effect of different formulations of propolis on mice infected with *Trypanosoma cruzi*. *J. Ethnopharmacol.*, 46: 55–59.

[25] Duailibe S., Gonçalves A.G., and Ahid F.J.M. 2007. Effect of a propolis extract on Streptococcus mutans counts in vivo. *J. Appl. Oral Sci.,* 15: 420–423.

[26] El-Bassuony, A.A. 2009. New prenylated compound from Egyptian propolis with antimicrobial activity. *Rev. Latinoamer. Quím.* 37: 85–90.

[27] Erdogan S., Ates B., Durmaz G., Yilmaz I., and Seckin T. 2011. Pressurized liquid extraction of phenolic compounds of Anatolia Region. *Food and Chemical Toxicology,* 49: 1592–1597.

[28] Farooqui T., and Farooqui A.A. 2010. Molecular mechanism underlying the therapeutic activities of propolis: A critical review. *Current Nutrition and Food Science,* 6: 188–199.

[29] Fokt H., Pereira A., Ferreira A. M., Cunha A., and Aguiar C. 2010. How do bees prevent hive infections? The antimicrobial properties of propolis. Current Res. Technol. and Edu. In Méndez –Vilas (ed.).Topics in Applied Microbiology and Microbial Biotechnology. Badajoz, Spain, pp. 481-493.

[30] Fonseca Y.M., Marquele-Oliveira F., Vicentini F.T.M.C., Furtado, N.A.J.C., Sousa J.P.B., Lucisano-Valim Y.M., and Fonseca M.J. V. 2011. Evaluation of the potential of Brazilian propolis against UV-Induced oxidative stress. Evidence-Based Complementary and Alternative Medicine, pp. 8.

[31] Fujimoto T., Nakamura J., Matsuka M. 2001. Diversity of propolis Part 1., Propolis from the world. *Honeybee Sci.*, 22:9–16.

[32] González M., Guzmán B., and Rudyk R. 2003 Spectrophotometric determination of phenolic compounds in propolis. *Acta Farmaceutica Bonaerense,* 22: 243–248.

[33] Groh C., Brockmann A, Altwein M., and Tautz J. 2002. Selective blocking of contact chemosensilla in *Apis mellifera. Apidologie,* 33: 33–40.

[34] Hegazi A.G., Abd El Hady F.K., and Shalabi H.A. 2007. Inhibitory effect of Egyptian propolis on Fasciola gigantica eggs with reference to its effect on *Clostridium oedematiens* and correlation to chemical composition. *Pakistan J. Biol. Sci.*, 10:3295–3305.

[35] Herrera C.L., Fritz O., Montenegro G., Alvear M., del Sol M., and Salazar L.A. 2010. Propolis decrease diet-induced hepatic steatosis in mice. *Int. J. Morphol.,* 28:75–84.

[36] Hurtado-Fernández E., Gómez-Romero M., and Carrasco-Pancorbo A. 2010. Application and potential of capillary electroseparation methods to determine antioxidant phenolic compounds from plant food material. *J. Pharm. and Biomed. Analysis,* 53: 1130–1160.

[37] Isla M.I., Paredes-Guzman J.F., Nieva-Moreno M.I., H. Koo H, and Park Y.K. 2005. Some chemical composition and biological activity of Northern Argentine propolis. *J. Agric. Food Chem.,* 53: 1166–1172.

[38] Kalogeropoulos N.K., Konteles S., Mourtzinos I., Troullidou E., Chiou A., and Karathanos V.T. 2009. Encapsulation of complex extracts in β–cyclodextrin: An application to propolis ethanolic extract. *J. of Microencapsulation,* 26: 603–613.

[39] Koedam D., Jungnickel H., Tentschert J., Jones G.R., and Morgan, E.D. 2002. Production of wax by virgin queens of the stingless bee Melipona bicolor (Apidae: Meliponinae). *Insectes Sociaux.,* 49: 229–233.

[40] Koya-Miyata S., Arai N., Mizote A., Taniguchi Y., Ushio S., Iwaki K., and Fukuda, S. 2009. Propolis prevents diet-induced hyperlipidemia and mitigates weight gain in diet-induced obesity in mice. *Biological and Pharmaceutical Bulletin,* 32: 2022–2028.

[41] Kumazawa S., Nakamura J., Murase M., Miyagawa M., Ahn M., and Fukumoto S. 2008. Plant origin of Okinawan propolis: honeybee behaviour observation and phytochemical analysis. *Naturwissenschaften,* 95: 781–786.

[42] Kumazawa S., Suzuki S., Ahn M.R., Kamihira M., Udagawa Y., Bang K.-S., and Nakayama T. 2006. A new chalcone from propolis collected on Jejeu Island, Korea. *Food Sci. Technol. Res*., 12:67–69.

[43] Kumazawa S., Yoneda M., Shibata I., Kanaeda J., Masaka T., and Nakayama T. 2003. Direct evidence for plant origin of Brazilian propolis by the observation of honeybee behaviour and phytochemical analysis. *Chem. Pharm. Bull*., 51: 740–742.

[44] Li F., Awale S., Tezuka Y., and Kadota S. 2009. Cytotoxic constituents of propolis from Myanmar and their structure–activity relationship. *Bio. and Pharmaceutical Bull.,* 32: 2075–2078.

[45] Liang Y.-Z., Xie P., and Chan K. 2004. Quality control of herbal medicines. *J. of Chromatography B,* 812: 53–70.

[46] Liberio S.A., Pereira, A.L.A., Araújo, M.J.A.M. Dutra R.P., Nascimento F.R.F.,Monteiro-Neto V., Ribeiro M.N.S., Gonçalves A.G., and Guerra R.N.M. 2009. The potential use of propolis as a cariostatic agent and its actions on mutans group Streptococci. *J. Ethnopharmacol.,* 125: 1-9.

[47] Lotti C., Fernández M.C., Piccinelli A.L., Cuesta-Rubio O., Marquez Hernández I., and Rastrelli L. 2010. Chemical constituents of red Mexican propolis. *J. Agric. Food Chem.,* 58: 2209–2213.

[48] Lozina L.A., Peichoto M.E., Acosta O.C., and Granero, G.E. 2010. Estandarización y caracterización organoléptica y físico-química de 15 propóleos Argentinos. *Latin American Journal of Pharmacy,* 29: 102–110.

[49] Machado G., Leon L.L., and Castro S.L. 2007. Activity of Brazilian and Bulgarian propolis against different species of Leishmania. Mem. *Oswaldo Cruz.,* 102: 73–77.

[50] Marcucci M.C. 2008. HPLC and ESI-MS typification: New approaches for natural therapy with Brazilian propolis. In Nada Oršolić and Ivan Bašić (eds.). Scientific Evidence of the Use of Propolis in Ethnomedicine, pp. 33-54.

[51] Martena M., Grutters M.M.P., De Groot H.N., Konings E.J.M., and Rietjens I.M.C.M. 2011. Monitoring of polycyclic aromatic hydrocarbons (PAH) in food supplements containing botanicals and other ingredients on the Dutch market. Food additives and contaminants. Part A, Chemistry, analysis, control, exposure and risk assessment, First published, pp. 1-18.

[52] Martinez J.P. 2009. Caracterización físico-química y evaluación de la actividad antifúngica de propóleos recolectados en el suroeste antioqueño. Universidad Nacional de Colombia sede Medellín, Facultad de Ciencias Agropecuarias. Tesis de Maestría en Ciencia y Tecnología de Alimentos. Medellín, Colombia. 101 p.

[53] Medić-Šarić M., Rastija V., Bocic M., and Males Ž. 2009. From functional food to medicinal product: systematic approach in analysis of polyphenolics from propolis and wine. *Nutr. J.,* 8: 33.

[54] Michalska K., Stojakowska A., Malarz J., Doležalová I., Lebeda A., and Kisiel W. 2009. Systematic implications of sesquiterpene lactones in *Lactuca* species. *Biochem. Syst. and Ecol.*, 37: 174–179.

[55] Miorin P.L., Levy Junior N.C., Custodio A.R., Bretz W.A., and Marcucci M.C. 2003 Antibacterial activity of honey and propolis from Apis mellifera and Tetragonisca angustula against Staphylococcus aureus. *Journal of Applied Microbiology,* 95: 913–920.

[56] Mohammadzadeh S., Shariatpanahi M., Hamedi M., Admadkhaniha R., Samadi N., and Ostad S.N. 2007. Chemical composition oral toxicity and antimicrobial activity of Iranian propolis. *Food Chem.,* 103: 1097–1103.

[57] Molnár-Perl I., and Füzfai Zs. 2005. Chromatographic, capillary electrophoretic and capillary electrochromatographic techniques in the analysis of flavonoids. *J. Chromatography A1,* 073:201–227.

[58] Montenegro G., Gómez M., Casaubon G., Belancic A., Mujica A.M., and Peña R.C. 2009. Analysis of volatile compounds in three unifloral native Chilean honeys. *Phyton, (B. Aires)* 78: 61–65.

[59] Montenegro G., Mujica A.M., Peña R.C., Gómez M., Serey I., and Timmermann B.N. 2004. Similitude pattern and botanical origin of the Chilean propolis. *Phyton,* 73: 145–154.

[60] Montenegro G., Peña R.C., and Pizarro R. 2010. Multivariate analysis of pollen frequency of the native species *Escallonia pulverulenta* (Saxifragaceae) in Chilean honeys. *Revista Brasil. Bot.,* 33: 615–630.

[61] Montenegro G., Peña R.C., Avila G., and Timmermann B.N. 2001. Botanical origin and seasonal production of propolis in hives of central Chile. *Bol. Bot. Univ. Sao Paulo,* 19: 1–6.

[62] Montenegro G., Timmermann B.N., Peña R.C., Mujica A.M. and Avila G. 2000. Pollen grains and vegetative structures in propolis as indicators of potential drugs in Chilean plants. *Phyton,* 66: 15–23.

[63] Moreira L., Dias L.G., Pereira J.A., and Estevinho L. 2008 Antioxidant properties, total phenols and pollen analysis of propolis samples from Portugal. *Food and Chemisry Toxicology,* 46:3482–3485.

[64] Muñoz O., Peña R.C., Ureta E., and Montenegro G. 2000. Propolis from Chilean Matorral Hives. *Z. Naturforsch,* 56c: 273–277.

[65] Muñoz O., Peña R.C., Ureta E., and Montenegro G. 2001. Phenolic compounds of propolis from Central Chilean Matorral. *Z. Naturforsch,* 56c: 273–277.

[66] Murase M., Kato M., Sun A., Ono T., Nakamura J., Sato T., and Kumazawa S. 2008. Rhus javanica var. chinensis as new plant origin of propolis. Biosci. *Biotechnol. Biochem.,*72: 2782–2784.

[67] Park Y.K., Alencar S., and Aguiar C.L. 2002. Botanical origin and chemical composition of Brazilian propolis. *J. Agric. Food Chem.,* 50: 2502–2506.

[68] Patricio E.F.L.R.A., Cruz-López L., Maile R., Tentschert J., Jones G.R., and Morgan E.D. 2002. The propolis of stingless bees: terpenes from the tibia of three Frieseomelitta species. *J. Insect Physiology,* 48: 249–254.

[69] Pellati F., Orlandini G., Pinetti D., and Benvenuti S. 2011. HPLC-DAD and HPLC-ESI-MS/MS methods for metabolite profiling of propolis extracts. *Journal of Pharmaceutical and Biomedical Analysis,* 55: 934–948.

[70] Peña, R.C. 2008. Propolis standardization: a chemical and biological review. *Cien. Inv. Agr.*, 35: 11–20.

[71] Pereira E.M.R., da Silva J.L.D.C., Silva F.F., de Luca M.P., Ferreira E.F., Lorente T C M., and Santos V.R. 2011. Clinical evidence of the efficacy of a mouthwash containing propolis for the control of Plaque and Gingivitis: A Phase II Study. Evidence-Based Complementary and Alternative Medicine Volume 2011, Article ID 750249, 7 p.

[72] Piasenzotto L., Gracco L., and Conte L. 2003. Solid phase microextraction (SPME) applied to honey quality control. *J. Sci. Food Agric.*, 83:1037–1044.

[73] Popek, S. 2002. A procedure to identify a honey type. *Food Chemistry,* 79: 401–406.

[74] Popova M., Bankova V., Butovska D., Damyanova B. Sabatini A.G., Marcazzan G., and Bogdanov S. 2003. Poplar type propolis and analysis of its biological active components. *Honey Bee Science,* 24:61–66.

[75] Popova M., Bankova V., Butovska D., Petkov V., Damyanova B., Sabatini A.G., Marcazzan G.L., and Bogdanov S. 2004. Validated methods for the quantification of biologically active constituents of poplar-type propolis. *Phytochem. Anal.*, 15: 235–240.

[76] Popova M., Graikou K., Chinou I., and Bankova V. 2010. GC-MS Profiling of diterpene compounds in Mediterranean propolis from Greece. *J. Agric. Food Chem.*, 58: 3167–3176.

[77] Popova M., Silici S., Kaftanoglu O., and Bankova V. 2005. Antibacterial activity of Turkish propolis and its qualitative and quantitative chemical composition. *Phytomedicine,* 12: 221–228.

[78] Popova M.P., Bankova V., Bogdanov S., Tsvetkova I., Naydenski C., Marcazzan G.L., and Sabatini A.G. 2007. Chemical characteristics of poplar type propolis of different geographic origin. *Apidologie,* 38: 306–311.

[79] Popova, M., Chen C.N., Chen P.Y., Huang C.Y., and Bankova V. 2010. A Validated spectrophotometric method for quantifi cation of prenylated flavanones in Pacific propolis from Taiwan. *Phytochemical Analysis,* 21: 186–191.

[80] Pyrzynska K., and Biezaga M. 2009. Analysis of phenolic acids and flavonoids in honey. *Trends in Analytical Chemistry,* 28: 893–902.

[81] Radovic, B. S., Careri M., Mangia A., Musci M., Gerboles M., and Anklam E. 2001. Contribution of dynamic headspace GC±MS analysis of aroma compounds to authenticity testing of honey. *Food Chemistry,* 72: 511–520.

[82] Saavedra N., Barrientos L., Herrera C.L., Alvear M., Montenegro G., and Salazar L.A. 2011. Effect of Chilean propolis on cariogenic bacteria *Lactobacillus fermentum. Cien. Inv. Agr.*, 38:117–125.

[83] Salatino A., Fernandes-Silva C.C., Righi A.A. and Salatino M.L.F. 2011. Propolis research and the chemistry of plant products. *Nat. Prod. Reports,* 28:925–936.

[84] Salgado Laurenti C.R., Sosa López, A., and Pire, S. 2002. Análisis polínico de propóleos en apiarios del Nordeste Argentino. XIII Reunión de Comunicaciones científicas y técnicas Facultad de Ciencias Agrarias Universidad Nacional del Noreste. Argentina.

[85] Sârbu C., and Catalin Mot A. 2011. Ecosystem discrimination and fingerprinting of Romanian propolis by hierarchical fuzzy clustering and image analysis of TLC patterns. *Talanta,* 85: 1112–1117.

[86] Sawaya A. C. H. F., Tomazela D.M., Cunha I.B.S., Bankova V.S., Marcucci M.C., Custodio A.R. and Eberlin M.N. 2004. Electrospray ionization mass spectrometry fingerprinting of propolis. Analyst 129:739–744.

[87] Sawaya A.C.H.F., Cunha H., Marcucci M.C., Oliveira Rodrigues R.F. de, and Eberlin M.N. 2006. Brazilian propolis of *Tetragonisca angustula* and *Apis mellifera. Apidologie,* 37:398–407.

[88] Sawaya A.C.H.F., Cunha. I.B. da S., Marcucci M.C., Aidar D.S., Silva E.C.A., Carvahlo C.A.L., and Eberlin M.N. 2007. Electrospray ionization mass sspectrometry fingerprinting of propolis of native Brazilian stingless bees. *Apidologie,* 38: 93–103.

[89] Sawaya A.C.H.F., da Silva Cunha I.B., and Marcucci M.C. 2011. Analytical methods applied to diverse types of Brazilian propolis. *Chemistry Central Journal,* 5: 27.

[90] Sforcin J.M., and Bankova V. 2011. Propolis: Is there a potential for the development of new drugs? *J. Ethnopharmacol.,* 133:253–260.

[91] Shimazawa M., Chikamatsu S., Morimoto N., Mishima S., Nagai H., and Hara H. 2005. Neuroprotection by Brazilian green propolis against in vitro and in vivo Ischemic Neuronal Damage. *Ecam,* 2(2):201-207.

[92] Silici S., and Kutluca S. 2005. Chemical composition and antibacterial activity of propolis collected by three different races of honeybees in the same region. *J. Ethnopharmacol.,* 99: 69–73.

[93] Silva B.B., Rosalen P.L., Cury J.A., Ikegaki M, Souza V.C., Esteves A., and Alencar S.M. 2007. Chemical composition and botanical origin of red Propolis, a new type of Brazilian Propolis. *Ecam,* 5:313-316.

[94] Sousa J.P., Leite M.F., Jorge R.F., Resende D.O., da Silva Filho A.A., Furtado N.A., Soares A.E., Spadaro A.C., de Magalhães P.M., and Bastos J.K. 2009. Seasonality role on the phenolics from cultivated *Baccharis dracunculifolia. Ecam,* July 15.

[95] Sousa J.P.B., Tacon L.A., Correia C.C., Bastos J.K., and Freitas, L.A.P. 2007. Spray-dried extract, II: prenylated components of green propolis. *Pharmazie,* 62:488–492.

[96] Sulaiman, G.M., Sammarrae K. W. Al, Ad'hiah A.H., Zuccheti M., Frapolli R., Bello E., Erba E., D'Incalci, and Bagnati R. 2011. Chemical characterization of Iraqi propolis samples and assessing their antioxidant potentials. *Food Chem. Toxicol.,* 49: 2415–2421.

[97] Teixeira E.W., Message D., Meira, R.M. S. A., and Salatino A. 2003. Indicadores da origem botânica da própolis: importância e perspectivas. *B. Indus. Animal,* 60: 83–106.

[98] Teixeira É.W., Message D., Negri G., Salatino A., and Stringheta P.C. 2010. Seasonal variation, chemical composition and antioxidant activity of Brazilian propolis samples. *Evidence-Based Complementary and Alternative Medicine,* 7: 307–315.

[99] Teixeira É.W., Negri G., Meira R.M.S.A., Message D., and Salatino, A. 2005. Plant origin of green propolis: bee behavior, plant anatomy and chemistry. *Ecam,* 2:85–92.

[100] Terrab A., Díez M.J., and Heredia F.J. 2003a. Palynological, physico-chemical and colour characterization of Moroccan honeys: III. Other unifloral honey types. *Int. J. of Food Science,* 38: 395–402.

[101] Terrab A., Díez M.J., and Heredia F.J. 2003b. Palynological, physico-chemical and colour characterization of Moroccan honeys. II Orange (*Citrus* sp.) honey. *Int. J. of Food Science,* 38: 387–394.

[102] Terrab A., Díez M.J., and Heredia F.J. 2003c. Palynological, physico-chemical and colour characterization of Moroccan honeys: I River red gum (*Eucalyptus camaldulensis* Dehnh) honey. *Int. J. of Food Science,* 38: 379–386.
[103] Thomas Barberan F.A., García-Viguera C., Vit-Olivier P., Ferreres F., and Tomás-Lorente F. 1993. Phytochemical evidence for the botanical origin of tropical propolis from Venezuela. *Phytochemistry*, 34: 191–196.
[104] Trusheva B., Popova M., Bankova V., Simov A. S., Marcucci M.C., Laguna M. P., Rocha P. F., and Tsveskova I. 2006. Bioactive constituents of Brazilian red propolis. *Evidence-Based Complementary and Alternative Medicine,* 3: 249–254.
[105] Trusheva B., Popova M., Koendhori E.B., Tsvctkova I., Naydenski C., and Bankova V. 2011. Indonesian propolis: chemical composition, biological activity and botanical origin. *Natural Product Research,* 25(6): 606 – 613.
[106] Trusheva B., Todorv I., Ninova M., NAjdenski H., Daneshmand A., and Bankova V. 2010. Antibacterial mono- and sesquiterpene esters of benzoic acids from Iranian propolis. *Chemistry Central Journal,* 4:8.
[107] Valcic S., Montenegro G., Mujica A.M., Avila G., Franzblau S., Singh M.P., Maiese W., and Timmermann B. 1999. Phytochemical, morphological, and biological investigations of propolis from Central Chile. *Z. Naturforsch,* 54: 406–416.
[108] Velikova M., Bankova V., Marcucci M.C., Tsvetkova I., and Kujumgiev A. 2000. Chemical composition and biological activity of propolis from Brazilian Meliponinae. *Z. Naturforsch.,* 55: 785–789.
[109] Volpi N. 2004. Separation of flavonoids and phenolic acids from propolis by capillary zone electrophoresis. *Electrophoresis,* 25: 1872–1878.
[110] Volpi N., and Bergonzini G. 2006. Analysis of flavonoids from propolis by HPLC electrospray mass spectrometry. *J. Pharm. Biomed. Analysis,* 42: 354–361.
[111] Watson D.G., Peyfoon E., Zheng L., Lu D., Seidel V., Johnston B., Parkinson J.A., and Fearnley J. 2006 Application of principal components analysis to 1H-NMR Data obtained from propolis samples of different geographical origin. *Phytochemical Anal.,* 17: 323–331.
[112] WHO - World Health Organization. 1991. Guidelines for the Assessment of Herbal Medicines. WHO, Munich, Geneva.
[113] Woisky R.G., and Salatino A. 1998. Analysis of propolis: some parameters and procedures for chemical quality control. *J. Apicultural Res.*, 37: 99–105.
[114] Yao H., Shi P., Shao Q., and Fan X. 2011. Chemical fingerprinting and quantitative analysis of a *Panax notoginseng* preparation using HPLC-UV and HPLC-MS. *Chin. Med.*, 6: 9.
[115] Zhang S., Bock F., Si A., Tautz J., and Srinivasan M.V. 2005. Visual working memory in decision making of honey bees. *PNAS,* 102: 5250–5255.
[116] Zunini M.P., Rojas C., De Paula S., Elingold I., Migliaro E.A., Casanova M.B., Iribarne Restuccia F.I., Aguilera Morales S., and Dubin. M. 2010. Phenolic contents and antioxidant activity in central-southern Uruguayan propolis extracts. *J. Chil. Chem. Soc.*, 55:141–146.

# INDEX

## B



## C

## D



## E

## F



## G

## H

## L



## M

## N



## O

## P

## Q



## R



## S

## T